X-Ray Computed Tomography in Biomedical Engineering

Robert Cierniak

X-Ray Computed Tomography in Biomedical Engineering

Springer

Dr. Robert Cierniak
Department of Computer Engineering
Technical University of Częstochowa
Al. Armii Krajowej 36
42 200 Częstochowa
Poland
e mail: cierniak@kik.pcz.czest.pl

ISBN 978 0 85729 026 7 e ISBN 978 0 85729 027 4

DOI 10.1007/978 0 85729 027 4

Springer London Dordrecht Heidelberg New York

British Library Cataloguing in Publication Data
A catalogue record for this book is available from the British Library

Library of Congress Control Number: 2010936694

Translation: Mike Butynski

Cover design: eStudio Calamar S.L.

Printed on acid free paper

Springer is part of Springer Science+Business Media (www.springer.com)

To my Parents

Preface

This book is an attempt at a comprehensive treatment of those medical imaging techniques commonly referred to as Computed Tomography (CT) and sometimes known as Computerised Tomography, which rely on X-rays for their action. As this is a place to explain my reasons for writing the book, I would like to begin by assuring the reader of my passion for the medical technology discussed here. My main motivation in publishing this work was a desire to share with the widest possible readership my fascination with the topic. I would expect the target audience for this account to be primarily academics, students and technicians involved with biomedical engineering, as well as doctors and medical technicians concerned with medical imaging. The structure and content of the book place particular emphasis on issues related to the reconstruction of images from projections, a key problem in tomography. This reflects my area of interest in the field. Other problems will be treated as technical and physical background to the reconstruction algorithms, in so far as is necessary for an understanding of how they work (and perhaps a little more). The reconstruction algorithms covered relate to all the basic designs of tomographic equipment, from the first Hounsfield scanner to the most recent spiral CT devices for reconstructing images in three dimensions. I hope that the summaries of various practical implementations of the algorithms will help people to test the individual reconstruction methods for themselves. The final chapter contains an account of a virtual test environment so that those without access to physical measurement data from a real scanner can carry out these tests. Perhaps it is a good point here to wish you the best of luck.

There is another reason for engaging the reader at this point, in addition to spreading enthusiasm for the subject. It is to thank those particularly who have made significant contributions to the conception of "the work". I would like to start with my lecturer Professor Ryszard Tadeusiewicz. It was at his lecture that I first heard about the reconstruction problem. It was then, perhaps thanks to his eloquence, that I was quite simply struck by the "beauty" of the problem. The second person who, in my academic life, had a decisive influence on the direction of my research was Professor Leszek Rutkowski. He, as my academic supervisor, always gave me enough freedom to choose the direction of my own interests.

However, I also cannot forget those individuals and institutions that, during the writing of this monograph, enabled me to bring the project to fruition. Amongst these I would like to stress the contribution of Dr. Marek Waligóra from the Private Health Care Group "Unimed" in Czestochowa, who provided me with the tomographic images contained in the book, and offered advice on all contentious medical issues. I would like to thank Mr Marcin Gabryel for his assistance in preparing the program listings included in the book. These should prove very useful to those wishing to test the reconstruction algorithms described here. I would also like to offer my special thanks to Japan Industries Association of Radiological Systems (JIRA) and Sumio Makino for allowing the publication of historical photographs related to the development of computed tomography techniques. A significant role was also played by Ms. Claire Protherough, on behalf of Springer Publishing. She showed great patience with such an ill-disciplined author as myself and took such care during the editorial work on the publication. This book would probably not have arisen at all without Mike Butynski, who not only translated the text from the Polish language but also, thanks to his physics background, helped me with many of the basic problems that arose during the writing of this monograph. Thank you, Mike, for the heart that you put into the book. To others not mentioned here by name, but who helped with this work, I apologise and ask for understanding.

In conclusion, I would like to hope, dear reader, that you are willing to spare the book a moment of your attention and not regard it as time ill spent.

Częstochowa, March 2010 Robert Cierniak

Contents

Chapter 1
Introduction

Only a few devices in the rich arsenal of medical equipment can match the popularity of the computed tomography scanner (or CT scanner). Its invention undoubtedly initiated a revolution in diagnostic technology by allowing us to look inside a person and obtain a very clear anatomical image without violating the outer surface of his body, in other words, non-invasively. Throughout the industrialised world, it would be difficult to find anyone who was not familiar with CT scanning either personally or indirectly, perhaps via an acquaintance or a popular science television programme.

Anyone who encounters CT is amazed by its research possibilities and its diagnostic precision. However, the CT scanner is more than just a collection of technical solutions or an example of a successful implementation of long-term biomedical engineering research. This wonderful instrument unquestionably represents the embodiment of the power of human thought and the proud spirit of man, who throughout the ages has worked on the problem of how to look inside his earthly form without the use of a scalpel and without causing haemorrhaging. When we stand before such a complex machine, we find ourselves asking: where does this seemingly inconceivable idea come from, this bloodless “cutting” of a person slice by slice, then to reassemble the slices to describe in detail the result of this incredible journey deep into the human body? It is worth therefore looking a little closer at this piece of medical history, to have a more complete understanding of the field of tomography.

The examination of a person’s anatomy, as a preliminary to performing various diagnostic procedures, is a technique that has been used for centuries. However, people have not always been convinced that it was necessary to know about the structure of the human body, let alone about the physical diagnosis of internal illnesses. The belief in a link between the body and the suffering of sick people probably arose by the way of observation of the changes that occurred in the appearance of people afflicted with various kinds of illness. This also probably aroused a curiosity about the structure of the human body, the operation of its individual parts, and the links between symptoms and the pattern of pathology. A number of historical sources indicate that people first investigated the internal

R. Cierniak, *X Ray Computed Tomography in Biomedical Engineering*,
DOI: 10.1007/978 0 85729 027 4 1, © Springer Verlag London Limited 2011

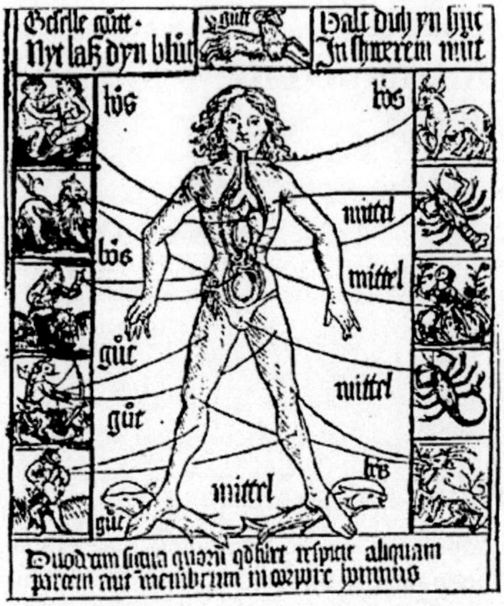

Fig. 1.1 The transcendental human

structure of the body through human dissection, a process that aroused ambivalent emotions.[1] Dissections were probably already being performed in ancient times by scholars such as Alcmeon, Erasistratus, Galen and Herophilos of Alexandria.

In the middle ages, there was a reluctance to continue this earlier work and so there was a reduction in the number of such procedures performed. At that time, people perceived the human body to be the seat of the soul and thus the property of the Creator. They endowed it with a kind of inviolability clause and surrounded it with a special taboo. It was forbidden to carry out any kind of human dissection, thereby removing the only possible source of knowledge about the human anatomy at that time. Until the sixteenth century, therefore, the only available description of the inside of a person was the ancient work of Galen *De usu patrium*, based on which people created a variety of ideas about the human body, its nature and structure (see Fig. 1.1).

A fundamental shift in the perception of the body and knowledge of anatomy came with the renaissance. The new ideological and philosophical trends of this period very much favoured anthropological research. It is significant, for those interested in human affairs, that it was at this time that geographical exploration was being carried out on a large scale. In the course of their distant journeys, travellers discovered new lands, previously unknown animal and plant species, and, in the eyes of people from the Old World, strange peoples with strange customs and different attitudes to the body. These journeys had a great effect on European imagination and consciousness. Differences between peoples not only

[1] The word tomography comes from the Greek words *tomos*, meaning slice, and *graphia*, meaning writing or description.

aroused curiosity but also induced a deeper reflection on their own organism and its structure.

At the turn of the fifteenth and sixteenth centuries, people began to perform dissections openly. Yet secret dissections had already taken place earlier, in fifteenth century Florence. Leonardo da Vinci carried out 30 such procedures in 1470, producing descriptions and drawings. However, it was Andreas Vesalius, professor of medicine at the University of Padua, who profoundly transformed our way of thinking about the nature of man. In 1543, he published his work *De humani corporis fabrica*. It signalled a revolution in the understanding of man and his body. Anthropologists started to think of homo sapiens exclusively as an arrangement of bones and muscles, disregarding those elements of human nature, important to medieval scholars, which were supposed to emphasize the relationship of the human being with the Transcendent. The renaissance conception of man as a carnal being was dominant for many centuries. The development of empirical investigation of the body and the observation of variations in the structure of tissues permitted the drawing of conclusions about the normal and abnormal functioning of the human organism. This, in turn, led to the evolution of the field of medicine known today as pathophysiology.

Of course, pathophysiology owes a great deal to a certain accidental discovery by Wilhelm Conrad Röntgen at the end of the nineteenth century, that is, to the discovery of X-rays. Thanks to pictures taken using röntgen radiation, it was now possible to look at the internal organism of a person without violating the outer surface of his body (see Fig. 1.2). The use of X-ray apparatus to diagnose many serious illnesses and complex post-traumatic complications quickly became standard clinical practice. This type of apparatus still forms the basic equipment of departments of imaging diagnostics in hospitals, and devices making use of X-rays in varying degrees find their application in operating theatres, dental practices or even mobile mammographic screening units. Moreover, although it soon transpired that X-radiation is harmful to the human organism, this did not alter the fact that its impact on our understanding of the human interior was nothing less than

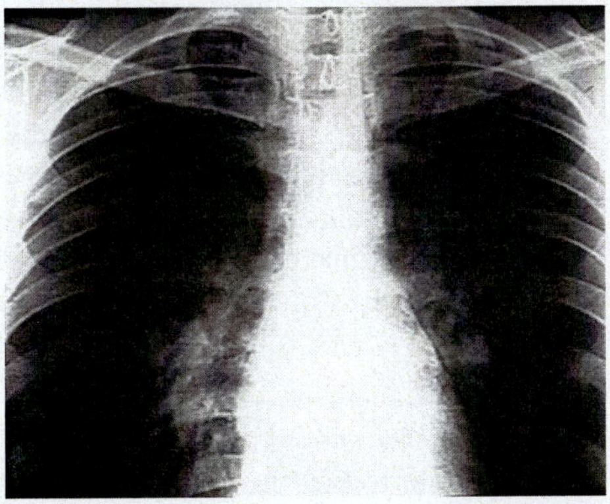

Fig. 1.2 X ray picture of a chest

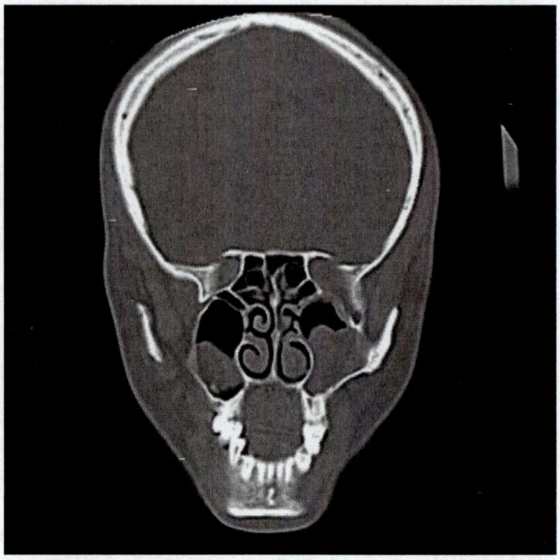

Fig. 1.3 Tomographic image of the sinuses in the frontal plane

astonishing. With time, one of the more important applications of this radiation turned out to be CT.

If we compare the use of X-ray techniques in medicine to the revolution that brought about the industrial age, then we can certainly argue that the formulation of the principles of computed tomography and the design of the CT scanner is evidence of the arrival of a new period in the history of knowledge and technology: the third phase, the information age.[2] The arrival of a new era inevitably involves the enrichment of familiar earlier technologies with new ideas and their practical application. In the case of CT, this has meant the application of not only X-rays but also of the mathematical algorithms that allow the reconstruction of an image of any given cross-section of a person's body. By suitably arranging a set of these cross-sections, it is possible to visualise, in three dimensions, the anatomical structure of any part of a human body. A spatial image such as this is of enormous help in medical diagnosis. An example of a tomographic cross-section is shown in Fig. 1.3.[3]

Tomographic examination is currently one of the basic techniques of medical diagnosis. Indeed, the significance of tomographic techniques in contemporary medicine is clearly demonstrated by the fact that when this type of apparatus in a hospital breaks down, doctors will avoid making a definitive diagnosis until an examination can be carried out in another centre.

This book is an attempt at a comprehensive and detailed portrayal of the subject of X-ray CT, beginning with its history, followed by its physical and technical concepts, its parameters and principles of operation, and concluding with methods of solving the image reconstruction problem. Much space is devoted to this last issue because it is of fundamental significance for the operation of the equipment,

[2] Toffler A.: *The third wave*. Bantam Books, New York, 1980

[3] Image made available by the Private Health Care Group "Unimed", Czestochowa, Poland.

whereas a more modest amount of space is devoted to the section discussing the physical and technical concepts. The aim of the chapters on the technical aspects of CT scanners is to raise awareness of the nature of the image reconstruction problem. Chapters 3 and 4 therefore are concerned with topics relating to the construction of CT scanners and the physics of their operation. This then allows us to formulate the reconstruction problem for every type of projection system.

Chapter 9 completes the remaining two parts of the work, discussing the technical parameters describing practical CT scanners, together with methods and procedures for determining values that indicate the quality of the reconstructed image.

The fundamental issue of image reconstruction methods has been organised by taking into consideration the two most important approaches: transformation (analytical) reconstruction methods and algebraic reconstruction techniques (ART). The first of these methods is covered in Chaps. 5, 6 and 7, while the second is covered in Chap. 8.

The prevalence of certain transformation reconstruction methods in practical scanners has meant that Chaps. 5, 6 and 7 are dominated by discussion of algorithms. Chapter 5 also considers issues that are fundamental for other approaches to solve the reconstruction problem. ART algorithms are considered in Chap. 8. Chapter 10 contains descriptions of standard methods of obtaining projection values using mathematical modelling. These are extremely useful for carrying out computer simulations of various types of projection systems.

Finally, I hope that you will share, at least to some degree, my passion for the subject of this book and that you will kindly forgive any possible mistakes that you may find. As the medieval scribes used to say, "God did not create this, but the hand of a sinner". Following their example and after wishing you a fruitful read, there only remains for me to say:

> I beg you dear reader if you find any mistake or shortcoming [...] don't despise me because of my human frailty, but forgive me all and that shortcoming or error correct.[4]

---

[4] *The Liturgikon*, pp. 1727 1738, Supraśl, Poland

Chapter 2
Some Words About the History of Computed Tomography

We could limit the story of the beginnings of computed tomography to mentioning Allan MacLeod Cormack and Godfrey Newbold Hounsfield, the authors of this groundbreaking invention, and to placing their achievements on a timeline, from Cormack's theoretical idea in the late 1950s to Hounsfield's development of a practical device in the late 1960s. However, perhaps we should broaden our horizons and look back through the centuries to obtain a more complete view of the development of human thought and aspirations, which led to the invention of a device without which it would be difficult to imagine contemporary medicine.

This story begins in ancient times about 400 BC, when the Greek philosopher Democritus first described matter as a cluster of invisible and at the same time indivisible particles. He called these particles atoms, from the Greek, atomos, meaning indivisible. He also studied the invisible forces which caused attraction and repulsion. Their action was observed for example, when, after being rubbed with fur, amber attracted various small objects. Today we know that the cause of this mysterious attraction is the electric force. We can see the evidence of Democritus' research in the use of the word "electron", which in Greek means amber, to name one of the elementary particles. Now, over two thousand years later, this physical phenomenon, first observed by ancient scholars, is exploited in the modern X-ray tube.

X-radiation, used in X-ray computed tomography, is an electromagnetic wave. The English physicist Michael Faraday (1791 1867) observed the phenomenon of electromagnetism and in 1831, he formulated his famous laws of electromagnetic induction. Twenty-nine years later, in 1860, this discovery by the "father of electromagnetism" allowed another pioneer, the Scot, James Clark Maxwell, to formulate the laws, which are included in the equations that bear his name. Maxwell's equations comprehensively expressed the ideas of electricity and magnetism in their dynamic form and provided a revolutionary stimulus, which led to the development of the later technologies of radio and television and of course, radiology.

R. Cierniak, *X Ray Computed Tomography in Biomedical Engineering*,
DOI: 10.1007/978 0 85729 027 4 2, © Springer Verlag London Limited 2011

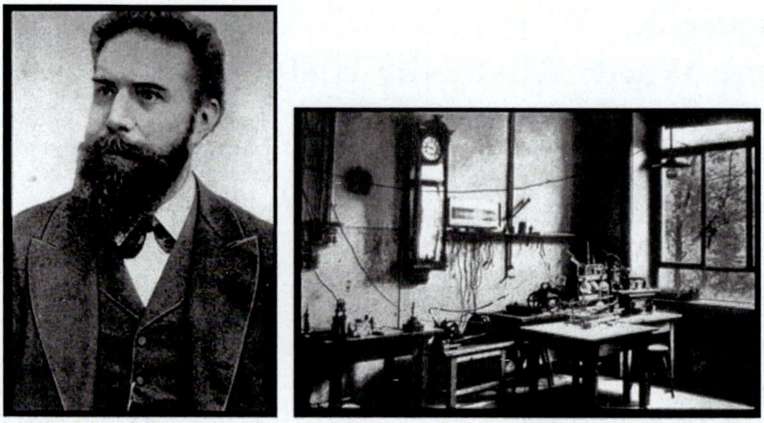

(a) (b)

Fig. 2.1 Wilhelm C. Röntgen (**a**) and the room where he discovered X rays (**b**)

The accidental discovery of the radiation, known today as X-radiation,[1] triggered a revolution in our knowledge of the inside of the human body. The discovery was made on 8th November 1895 by the German scientist Wilhelm Conrad Röntgen (1845 1923) (see Fig. 2.1a) and it marked the beginning of his glittering career and fame. Röntgen, at that time professor of physics at the University of Würzburg, was in his blacked out laboratory (see Fig. 2.1b) investigating the glow that occurred during electric discharges inside an evacuated glass tube, a Crookes tube. An example of a Crookes tube and ancillary equipment, similar to that used in his famous experiment, is shown in Fig. 2.2a.

Röntgen was working on the properties of cathode rays, and in particular on the determination of their range outside the tube (his description of the experiment is shown in Fig. 2.2b). During the experiment, completely unexpectedly, he observed something unusual; a screen coated with crystals of barium platinocyanide started to glow. The screen was made of fluorescent paper, which at that time was used routinely to detect ultraviolet radiation. While he was carrying out the experiment, the screen happened, by chance, to be in the laboratory within range of the radiation coming from the tube. Röntgen noticed that the screen was too far away from the source for the cathode rays to have been the cause of the glow. He was also surprised that tightly covering the tube with cardboard did not eliminate the effect; this contradicted his assumption that the glow, occurring during the electrical discharge inside the tube, was the cause of this phenomenon.

If anyone today wanted to reproduce Röntgen's experiment of the evening of 8th November 1895, he would need to the follow these instructions:

[1] X radiation (or X rays) seemed to Röntgen to be so inexplicable and mysterious that he took inspiration from mathematicians and named it after the symbol X: the symbol of the unknown in mathematics.

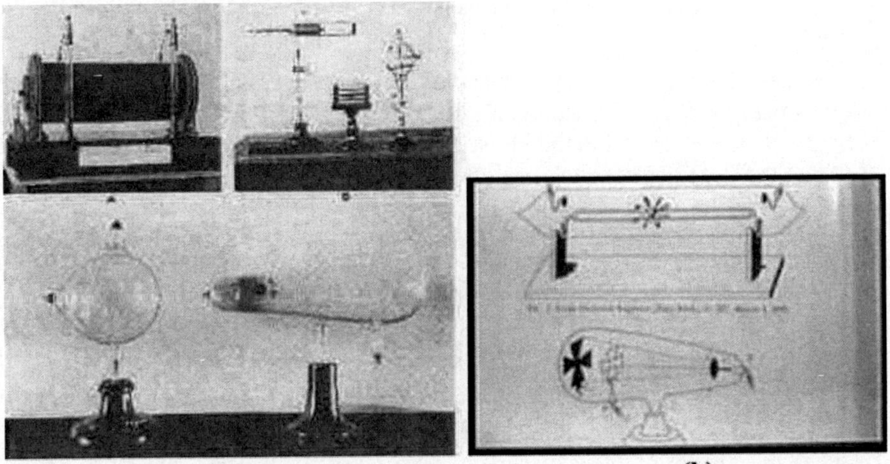

(a) (b)

Fig. 2.2 Crookes tube from the time of Röntgen (**a**) and circuitry similar to that used in his famous experiment (**b**)

Recipe for X rays á la Röntgen. Take an induction coil consisting of a primary coil with a few hundred turns of thick wire (the current in this coil is about 20A), a secondary coil with 200 thousand turns of thin wire, and a contact breaker (invented by Deprez) with platinum contacts (this breaks the current in the primary coil 15 20 times a second). Transform the constant primary voltage from a 32V battery to an alternating secondary voltage of 40 60 kV. Apply this voltage to a Crookes vacuum tube which has previously been evacuated to a pressure of 0.01 Torr (mmHg) using a mercury pump. Cover the tube with blackened cardboard. Put aside a little time for pumping out the tube. This can take a number of hours, but may well extend to several days. Place a screen coated with crystals of barium platinocyanide near the cathode end of the tube. While the electric discharge is taking place inside the tube, place various objects between the tube and the screen and observe the image appearing on it. Try to resist experimenting on your own hands.

During the few days following the 8th November, Röntgen carried out a series of tests in which he placed various objects between the tube and the screen. It was then that he also noticed, clearly outlined on the screen, the skeleton of his own hand.

He was not sure however, to what extent his observations were scientifically valid, as he mentioned in letters to friends. Röntgen confided to them: "I have discovered something interesting but I don't know if my observations are correct". Nevertheless, he conducted further experiments. When, on 28 December 1895, he was finally certain that the mysterious rays really existed, he sent a report of his research to the Würzburg Physical Medical Society, in which he wrote:

If the discharge of a fairly large induction coil is put through a Hittorf vacuum tube or through a Lenard tube, Crookes tube or other similar apparatus, which has been evacuated, the tube covered with thin, quite tightly fitting, black cardboard, and if the whole apparatus is placed in a completely dark room, then with every discharge a bright flickering is observed on a paper screen coated with barium platinocyanide, placed near the induction coil [4].

Attached to the 11-page report was the famous X-ray picture of a hand, which most probably belonged to Röntgen's wife, Bertha (see Fig. 2.3).

The report contained a detailed list of the properties of X-rays. From the point of view of the medical applications of the radiation, the most significant of these were:

- the ability of various materials of the same thickness to transmit X-rays depends to a great extent on their densities,
- the ability of samples of the same material to transmit X-rays depends on their thickness; an increase in thickness of the material decreases the transmission of the rays,
- photographic plates are sensitive to X-rays.

After the results of the experiment were reported in The New York Times, Röntgen's career, and that of X-rays, took off. By January 1896, the whole world knew about the wonderful discovery, and people, not just those connected with science, were overwhelmed by a peculiar "X-ray mania". Röntgen's success culminated in 1901 with the Nobel Prize, the first in history to be awarded for physics.

The technique of making X-ray photographs, to enable the observation of the internal features of a person without any surgical intervention, quickly found

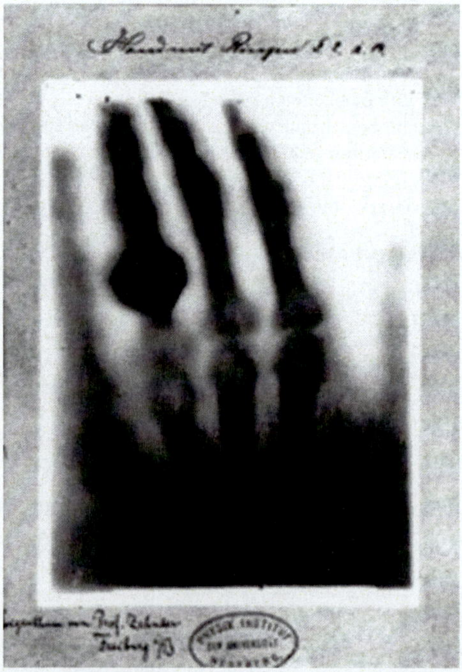

Fig. 2.3 Röntgen's report on his research into X rays the enclosed X ray picture of the hand of his wife, Bertha

justified recognition among doctors and spread around the whole world. People began to build devices for taking X-ray pictures for medical purposes, and X-ray research developed so quickly that by 1897, William Morton had taken the first picture of a whole skeleton using X-rays. Figure 2.4 shows a picture of one of the pioneering devices in an X-ray room of the time.

We should not forget however, that Röntgen's epoch-making discovery was made possible by the inventions of several earlier innovators. Among those, we should mention the Italian Evangelista Torricelli, inventor of the mercury barometer (1643) and the German Otto von Guericke, creator of the vacuum pump. Their work contributed to William Crookes' (1832 1919) construction of the vacuum tube. This was widely known in Röntgen's time and, of course, was used by him in his first experiments. Other elements of the equipment used by Röntgen came directly from the ideas of Gaston Plant, the designer of the electric battery that Röntgen used as his source of electrical energy.

Over the years, the design of X-ray equipment was refined to obtain better and better two-dimensional images of the inside of the human body. The American Thomas Alva Edison (1847 1931), for example, made a significant contribution to the development of medical imaging techniques. He was, among other things, the author of many improvements to the design of X-ray tubes. The German Hermann von Helmholtz (1821 1894), on the other hand, investigated the nature of X-rays; he was interested in the mathematical equations describing their properties and in measuring their penetration through different materials.

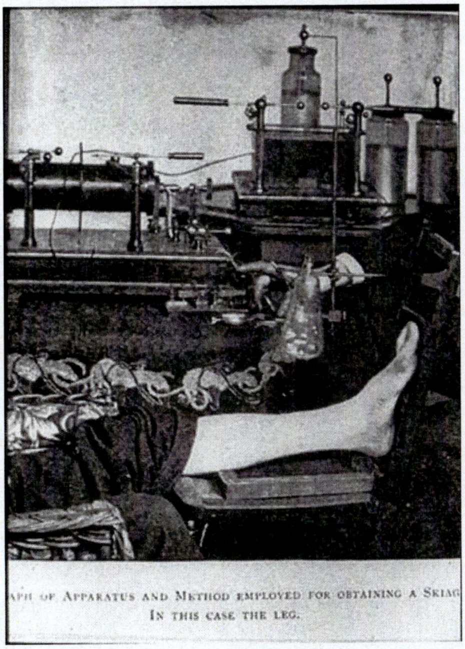

Fig. 2.4 X ray room from the early years of radiography

The initial euphoria surrounding the diagnostic possibilities of X-ray pictures gradually gave way to a realisation of the limitations of body imaging methods in only two dimensions. In the year after the discovery of X-rays, E. Thompson was already attempting to obtain a three-dimensional X-ray image using stereoscopic techniques. The solution he proposed involved taking two X-ray pictures, displaced with respect to each other, of a patient who remained motionless. The diagnostician could then use a stereoscope to view the images with depth perspective.

At this point, it is worth mentioning that Poles also made their contribution to the improvement of X-ray imaging techniques. In particular, the experiments of Doctor Karol Mayer from the Krakow Clinic of Internal Medicine are acknowledged as a prelude to tomography. In 1916, he obtained stratigraphic images using a moving X-ray tube and a stationary film cassette, a method which resembles the process of scanning by computed tomography. Carlo Baese patented a similar imaging method in 1915 and described it in his paper *Methods and equipment for the location of foreign bodies in the human body by use of X-rays*. The technique devised by Baese depended on the simultaneous movement of tube and film cassette.

In 1922, the CT scanner came still closer to fruition; A.E.M. Bocage obtained a patent entitled *Methods and equipment for obtaining radiological images of cross-sections of the body not obscured by tissue structures in front of or behind the cross-section*. During the same period, B.G. Ziedses des Plantes conducted research into his concept of planigraphy, which was put into practice by Massiot in 1935.

A further step along the road towards contemporary scanners was the use, by the German doctor Willy Kuhn, of gamma radiation to obtain a layered image of tissues, in 1963.

The discovery of X-rays was a necessary but insufficient condition for the rise of computed tomography. Its design also depended on the development of computational techniques, which enabled the building of the computer, a device having fundamental significance for modern imaging techniques.

Perhaps we could think of the "computer" story as having started with the human hand, undoubtedly the first calculating device. By means of an ingenious system of counting, using the fingers, the early peoples of Europe and the Near East could calculate up to 9999. The Chinese even pushed the upper limit of calculation to ten billion. The results of calculations were recorded in various ways such as by making cuts in animal bones and in wooden tablets. The Incas used a so-called *kipu*, that is, a system of strings with knots on them. However, people were soon dissatisfied with such an approach to calculations; they needed instruments that were capable of carrying out complicated arithmetic and even of interpreting the data obtained.

One of the first "calculating machines", consisting of a tablet and stones, was the abak; this would be familiar to the ancient Greeks and Romans. Its operation was very straightforward. A series of columns of stones[2] were arranged on the

---

[2] It is not by accident that the word calculation has its roots in the Latin word for *pebble* calculus.

tablet and the stones moved to perform the arithmetical operations. It is interesting that in China they still use an abacus which they call the *suan-pan*, based on similar principles.

In the 17th century, a mathematician from Scotland, John Napier, well-known today as the creator of logarithm tables, built a system for the multiplication of numbers, a set of rods of square cross-section known as *Napier's bones*. To use them to multiply, it was necessary to sort through the rods to find the appropriate digits, place the rods next to each other in the appropriate order and then read off the result. In about 1630, the German Wilhelm Schickard, amongst others, mechanised this idea using systems of cogs and dials.

Further innovations were introduced by some of the most outstanding figures in the world of science. Among these was Blaise Pascal (1623 1662), who designed a machine to perform addition and subtraction. Contemporary computer scientists have shown their appreciation of his services to computational technology by naming one of the most popular high-level computer languages after him. At this point, it is impossible not to mention Gottfried W. Leibniz (1646 1716), who significantly reduced the degree of complexity of his predecessors' calculating machines by introducing a drum with teeth of unequal length. The next step in the evolution of calculating machines was the arithmometer, examples of which were built independently by F.S. Baldwin and W.T. Odhner; the mechanics of calculating machines reached their zenith with these devices.

Today's computers owe their computational power to progress in the fields of electricity and electronics. Scientists designed prototypes of new components which were soon manufactured and applied practically. Particularly noteworthy here are the inventions of the electronic valve (produced by the Philips company in 1917), the transistor (developed by the Americans John Bardeen and Walter H. Brattain in 1948) as well as the integrated circuit (developed by a group of researchers at Intel under the direction of Ted Hoff in 1969). These innovations might well have contributed only to the improvement of the calculating function of existing instruments, if it were not for the appearance of the English mathematician, physicist and philosopher Alan Turing.

Turing (1912 1954) transformed the ordinary calculating machine into a device that could be regarded as a prototype computer. In his paper *On Computable Numbers with an Application to the Entscheidungsproblem* [5], he discussed the possibility of building a programmable calculating machine. He considered three factors: logical instructions, the equivalent of today's microprocessor instructions; a thought process, in effect an algorithm; and a "machine". Turing argued that it was possible to write down an analytical thought process as a finite series of simple instructions, and then to execute these using the machine. He reasoned therefore that every process, which could be expressed logically, could be implemented by means of tables described in his work, these constituting the essence of the Turing machine.

The universal Turing machine contained the idea of creating a device, which knew a "code" that it could use to record each computational procedure. It was now only a step away from the creation of a computer programming language. It is not by accident that the word code has been used at this point. During World War II, Turing became an expert in cryptography while engaged in decoding German Enigma cipher machines. This kind of experience was undoubtedly to be of great help in his work on computing languages.

It is worth commenting on the significant contribution to the process of decoding the famous Enigma cipher system made by the Polish mathematicians: M. Rejewski, J. Różycki, and H. Zygalski. It was they who broke the code of the early versions of Enigma.

The first computer in the world to be officially recognised as such is the ENIAC machine (*Electronic Numerical Integrator and Calculator*) from 1946. In fact, the first computer was three years older and was built during the war at the Bletchley Park centre, by a group under the direction of Max Newman. The existence of the computer, called Colossus I, was kept secret until 1976. It is worth remembering that the first computers were far from perfect. They contained about 18 thousand very unreliable valves; this meant that the time that the computers were out of commission considerably exceeded the time that they worked. Over the years, engineering advances and progress towards the miniaturisation of components in computers led to the development of microcomputers.

It is at this point that the two separate strands of discovery and invention come together; the path leading to the discovery and exploitation of X-rays meets that leading to the refinement of computational techniques. Without this convergence, there would probably not have been computed tomography today.

The two people generally credited with inventing computed tomography were awarded the Nobel Prize for Physiology or Medicine in 1979: Allan MacLeod Cormack (1924 1998) and Godfrey Newbold Hounsfield (1919 2004). Although the Norwegian Abel conceived the idea of tomography significantly earlier (in 1826), and then the Austrian Radon developed it further,[3] it was only the solution proposed by Cormack and Hounsfield that fully deserves the name computed tomography.

Born in South Africa, Allan MacLeod Cormack first encountered issues associated with tomography during his work at the Department of Physics at the University of Cape Town; he was working on the measurement of the X-ray absorption of various body tissues. He later moved to Harvard University and, in 1956, began work on the problem of image reconstruction of X-ray projections. First, he solved the problem theoretically and then confirmed the results of his research experimentally using cutlets of horsemeat and pork, and apparatus that he had built himself. Figure 2.5[4] shows the apparatus which Cormack used for his first experiments in 1963.

[3] The Radon transform forms the basis of methods of image reconstruction from projections, the fundamental mathematical problem in computed tomography.

[4] The Homepage of the Japan Industries Association of Radiological Systems (JIRA) and Sumio Makino: *Key words for success or failure of enterprises From case study of X ray CT business*, Japan Planning Center.

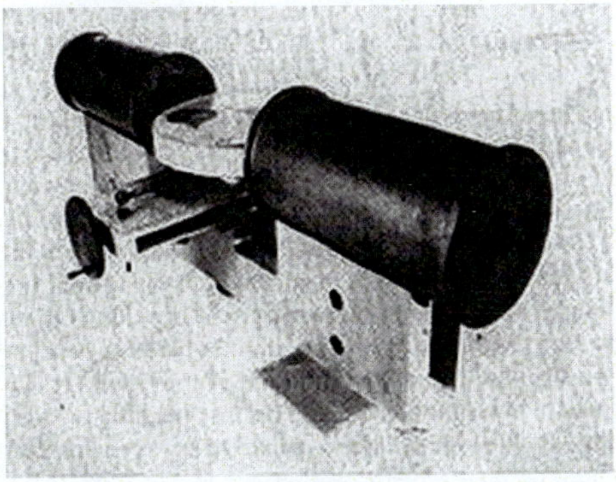

Fig. 2.5 Tomographic device built by Cormack in 1963

Cormack published the results of his research in an article entitled *Representation of a Function by its Line Integrals*, in *The Journal of Applied Physics* and later in *Physics of Medical Biology* [2].

As a theoretical physicist, Cormack was not concerned about the practical application of his research. It was the work of the Englishman Godfrey Newbold Hounsfield, employed at the Central Research Laboratories of EMI Ltd., which led to the construction of the first CT scanner; Hounsfield and his creation are shown in Fig. 2.7a.[5] During World War II, Hounsfield had worked on the technical development of radar air defence systems; this undoubtedly influenced his later achievements in the field of tomography. In 1967, independently of Cormack, he began his research on tomography, initially using gamma radiation, which has similar properties to X-radiation. Hounsfield developed a different approach to the problem of image reconstruction from that of his predecessor and he used the power of the computers available at that time to carry out the complicated calculations needed. In this way, the concept of computed tomography found its practical expression. A photograph of the CT scanner, which Hounsfield used in the laboratory, is shown in Fig. 2.6a.

The first laboratory tests revealed the great complexity of the technical problems facing the builders of the scanner; because of the low output of the gamma ray source (Americium, Am) individual exposures took a long time, so scans took as long as nine days. The first experiments were carried out on a human brain prepared in formalin, the brain of a living calf and the kidneys of a pig and it was difficult to differentiate the healthy tissues from the unhealthy. Nevertheless, after about 28 thousand measurements and a process of reconstruction taking about 2.5 hours, an image was obtained with enough contrast to enable the observation of the differences between the tissues of the brain. The resolution of the image was 80×80 pixels (see Fig. 2.6b). Hounsfield finally patented his device in 1968.

In order to confirm the results of his initial research, further experimental work was necessary, this time using living tissues. Hounsfield also took the opportunity

[5] In 1958, Hounsfield was, among other things, leader of the group, which built the EMIDEC 1100, the first computer in Great Britain to be made entirely of OC72 transistors.

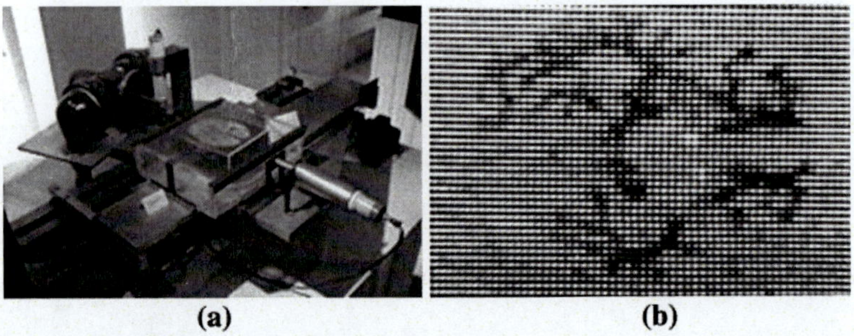

Fig. 2.6 Laboratory scanner used by G.N. Hounsfield (**a**) and an image of a preserved brain, obtained using this equipment in 1968 (**b**)

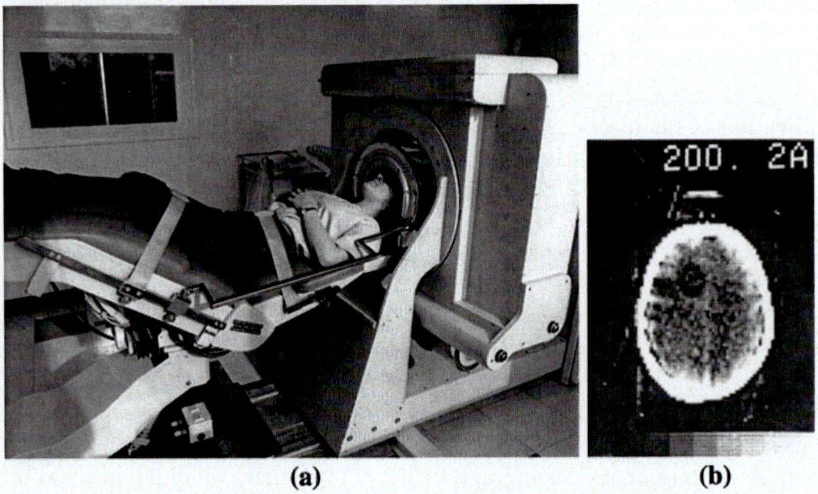

Fig. 2.7 The EMI Mark I scanner (**a**) and a transverse image of the brain (**b**)

to refine the design of the scanner. As a result, he was in a position to begin the clinical test phase, during which an X-ray tube replaced the source of gamma radiation. This shortened the time spent taking the measurements to nine hours. The actual process of image reconstruction was reduced to 20 minutes.

In September 1971, with the participation of the neurologists James Ambrose and Louis Kreel, an improved prototype scanner, the EMI Mark I, was installed at the Atkinson Morley's Hospital in Wimbledon (CT scanners at that time were known as EMI-scanners; see Fig. 2.7a). Because of the small size of the opening in which the scan was carried out, this apparatus could only be used to produce images of the head. In order to reduce the range of radiation intensities registered by the detectors, the head was placed in a rubber membrane filled with water.

The first tomographic examination of a patient took place on 1 October 1971. It was of a woman with a suspected brain tumour. On the image obtained, it was

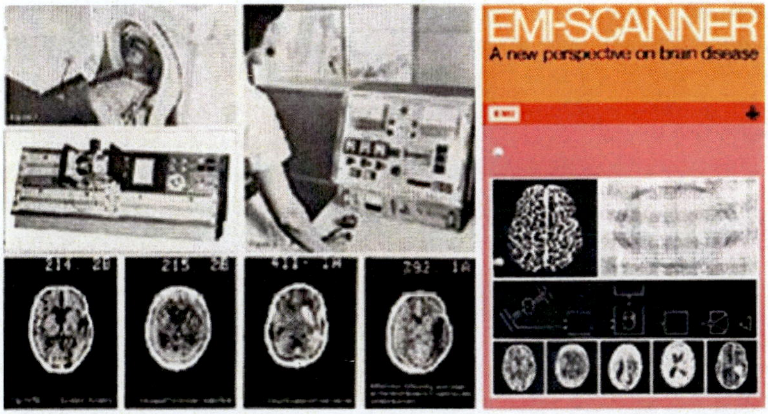

(a) (b)

Fig. 2.8 The EMI scanner with instrumentation and images obtained with it (**a**), and the front cover of a company brochure describing the new technology

possible to differentiate clearly between the physiological areas of the brain and the round, darker pathological area where a cyst was developing (see Fig. 2.7b).

The basic parameters of the scanner used at that time were as follows:

- scan time: about 4.5 min,
- reconstruction time: 20 s,
- cross-section thickness: 13 mm,
- image matrix: 80 × 80 pixels, where each pixel represented an area 3 × 3 mm.

In his first scanner, Hounsfield used a reconstruction algorithm, which is known today as the algebraic reconstruction technique (ART).

In April 1972, at a seminar at the British Institute of Radiology, Hounsfield formally presented the results he had obtained using the EMI scanner, and descriptions of the device appeared in many publications, including for example in the *British Journal of Radiology* [1, 3].

After these first successes, Hounsfield's group continued its research at the Atkinson Morley's Hospital and at The National Hospital, Queen Square in London. At this point, the fascinating story of the development of computed tomography began to gather momentum; numerous neurologists, radiologists, physicists, engineers and data processing specialists all started working on methods of obtaining and interpreting tomographic images.

By the end of 1973, the first commercial CT scanner was on the market; this was the EMI CT 1000, a development of the Mark I computer (see Fig. 2.8).[6] Due to the increased pace of development, in the course of 1973, the time to acquire an

---

[6] The Homepage of the Japan Industries Association of Radiological Systems (JIRA) and Sumio Makino: *Key words for success or failure of enterprises From case study of X ray CT business*, Japan Planning Center.

image was reduced to 20 s. Next, the number of detectors was increased to 30; this allowed the acquisition of a reconstructed image with a resolution of 320 × 320 pixels.

From the very beginning, computed tomography was commercially significant. Six EMI CT 1000 models were sold in 1973, two of them to the United States, and

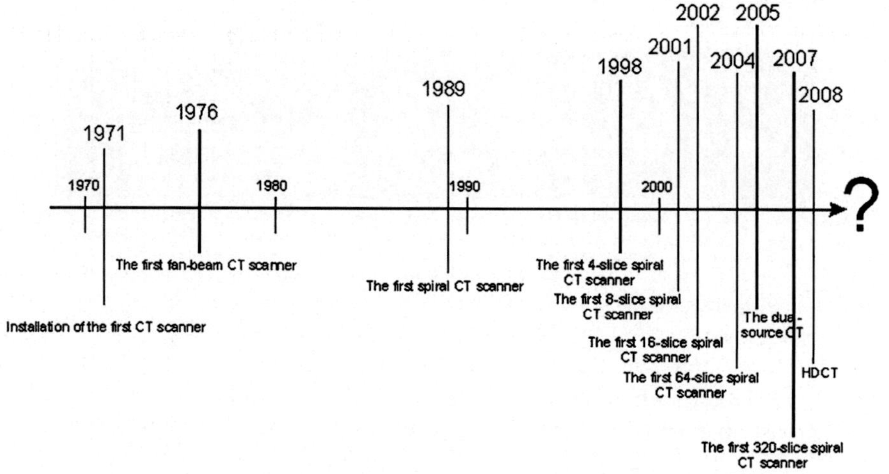

Fig. 2.9 Turning points in the history of computed tomography

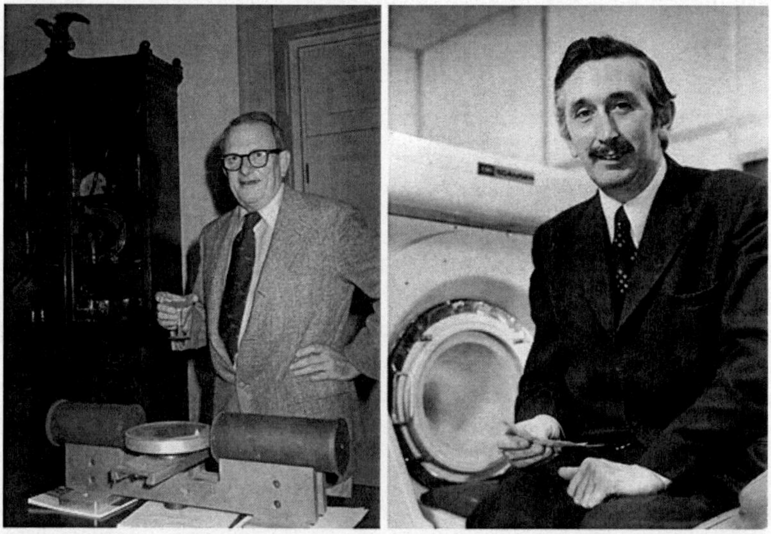

(a) **(b)**

Fig. 2.10 Co creators of computed tomography: Allan MacLead Cormack (**a**), Godfrey Newbold Hounsfield (**b**) each for the not inconsiderable sum of approximately £100,000. In the course of the following two years, the market for CT scanners reached a value of about £40,000,000.

In 1974, competition for the EMI scanner appeared in the form of designs by such firms as Neurscan (head scanner) and Disco (whole body scanner). The year 1975 brought an avalanche of different models. Unfortunately, the production capacity of EMI did not allow it to hold on to its leading position, which was soon taken by such giants as Technicare and General Electric, who quickly took a major share of the scanner market. Manufacturers from continental Europe, such as Siemens and Philips (in 1974 and 1975, respectively) soon followed in the footsteps of the Americans. They all joined in the race to capture as much of this very important medical technology market as possible.

If we compare the first scanners with today's successors, it is striking how much progress has been made in their design and manufacture in such an extremely short time. Contemporary CT scanners can scan in a few hundred milliseconds and reconstruct an image of 2048 × 2048 pixels. The most important events in the history of the development of computed tomography are shown on a timeline in Fig. 2.9.

Finally, it is also interesting to note that the two people, who are recognised by historians of science as the fathers of computed tomography (see Fig. 2.10a and 2.10b), only met each other for the first time in 1979 at the presentation ceremony, where they jointly received the Nobel Prize in Psychology or Medicine.

References

1. Ambrose J (1973) Computerized transverse axical scanning (tomography) part 2. Clinical applications. Br J Radiol 46:1023 1047
2. Cormack AM (1973) Reconstruction of densities from their projections, with applications in radiological physics. Phys Med Biol 18(2):195 207
3. Hounsfield GN (1973) Computerized transverse axial scanning (tomography) part 1. Description of the system. Br J Radiol 46:1016 1022
4. Röntgen CW (1895) Uber eine neue Art von Strahlen. Vorläufige Mitteilung
5. Turing A (1936 1937) On Computable numbers with an application to the entscheidungs problem. In: Proceedings of the London Mathematical Society, series 2, vol 42, pp 230 265

Chapter 3
Technical Concepts of X-ray Computed Tomography Scanners

Medical examinations using computed tomography are currently standard hospital practice. Back in the 1980s, its use was relatively rare, and was available only in a limited number of specialised medical centres. Today it is hard to imagine medical diagnosis without it.

Nowadays, hospitals in most major cities are equipped with CT devices. They are deployed, taking into account the prevailing demographic situation, so that optimal use is made of the equipment and the time needed for a patient to reach a centre is minimised. Computed tomography is used in the diagnosis of many conditions, both chronic and acute.

The installation of a CT scanner requires complex preparatory work. For a medical centre to be able to carry out on-site tomographic examinations, it must first adapt a suite of rooms for the purpose. The CT room must meet several requirements

- it must have floors with adequate load-carrying capacity,
- its walls must be constructed of X-ray absorbing material (this is usually a barium (Ba) plaster),
- the floor should be lined with material that is both anti-slip and antistatic.

Separate rooms should be provided for the CT scanner and for the radiographers; the rooms must be separated from each other by special window-glass (containing lead, Pb), to protect against X-rays. In addition, a suite of CT rooms must comply with all the health and welfare regulations, which are typically required for units carrying out medical X-ray examinations. A typical CT suite showing the location of the various elements of the scanner is illustrated in Fig. 3.1.

We can consider the CT scanner as being composed of two layers: the computer layer and the physical layer. The computer layer consists of the operating system[1] responsible for running the tomography application, file management and communication with external devices; and the tomography application itself. The latter

[1] As a rule, the UNIX operating system.

R. Cierniak, *X Ray Computed Tomography in Biomedical Engineering*,
DOI: 10.1007/978 0 85729 027 4 3, © Springer Verlag London Limited 2011

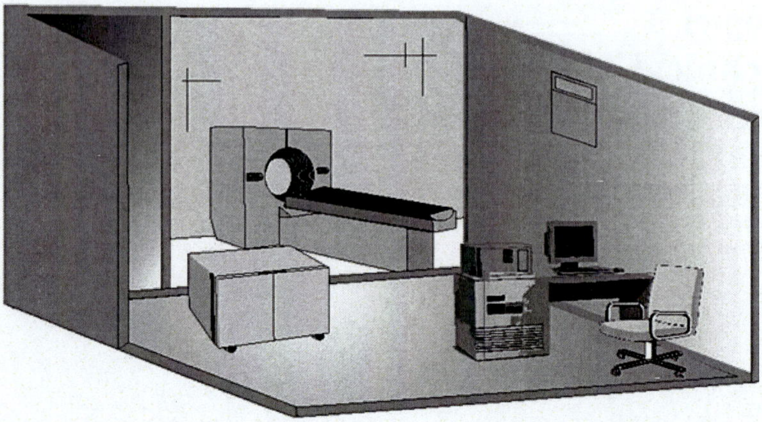

Fig. 3.1 A general view of a CT scanner installation

has two basic functions: user and utility. The user function carries out the tasks associated with the preparation of the scanner for operation, the management of the scanning process itself, the acquisition of the projection data, image reconstruction, support functions aiding diagnosis from the reconstructed images and archiving of the tomographic images. The utility function deals with the technical parameters of the scanner, the diagnosis of errors and other service tasks.

A CT scanner consists of the following main elements

- a data acquisition system that carries out the X-ray projections,
- a computer to reconstruct the images from the projections and to assist in the analysis of the reconstructed images,
- a variable power supply,
- a monitor to display the routine operation of the computer system and to act as an interactive interface in the diagnosis of the reconstructed images,
- a documentation camera to produce an image on film similar to traditional X-ray images,
- other data archiving systems, such as tape or disk, collectively referred to as storage devices,
- other elements.

As can be seen from Fig. 3.1, the scanner itself is situated behind a screen to protect the operators from the harmful effects of the X-rays emitted by the tube. The other components of the CT system are located in the same room as the technicians and doctors.

3.1 Data Acquisition Systems

Whatever the differences in design of the different generations of scanners, the main elements remain the same. Figure 3.2 presents three orthogonal views of a

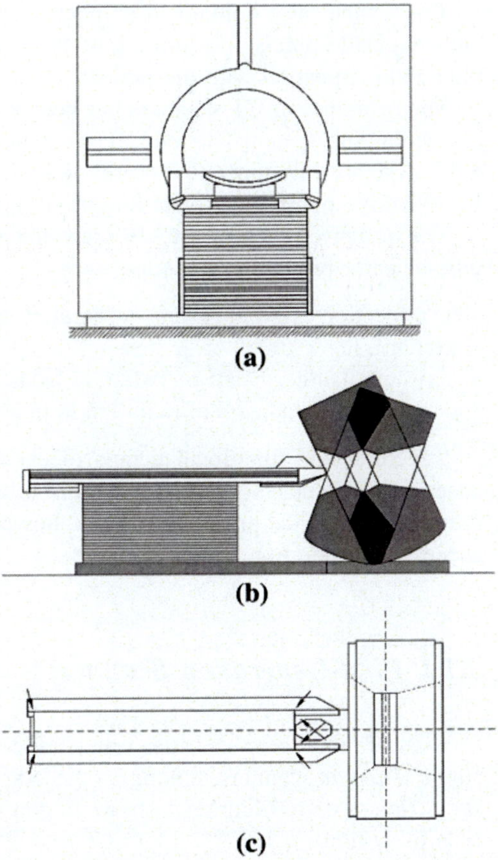

Fig. 3.2 Views of a CT scanner; **a** from the front, **b** from the side, **c** from the top

standard design of data acquisition system. Some elements of the apparatus shown in Fig. 3.2 are immediately recognisable, while others are part of the larger units and are not visible. The main components of the scanner design are:

- *The gantry* with a central opening, into which the patient is moved during the examination. This is the most recognisable element of the CT scanner;
- *The X-ray tube,* the source of the X-rays that pass through the body situated in the gantry and carry the information about the structure of the body to the detectors. The information is in the form of a series of projections;
- *The detector array* converts the projection values, in the form of radiation intensities, into electrical quantities. Usually, the whole detector array rotates synchronously with the X-ray tube around the test object;
- *The table* allows the patient to be manoeuvred easily into position. The table can be controlled manually before the actual scan begins, but it moves automatically during the scan. The table can be moved into or out of the gantry along the axis of the patient's body, as well as up and down. This allows the patient to be appropriately positioned depending on which part of the body is being examined.

The scanner also contains a number of sub-systems that drive and control the device, enable precise positioning of the patient during the scan as well as facilitate communication with the patient.

The evolution of CT scanners has been marked by changes to the design of the projection sub-systems of the data acquisition system [2, 3, 18]. In comparing these designs, only those that represent commonly used classes of CT devices are listed below; non-typical or prototype designs have been omitted.

The design of each of the CT scanner generations contains one of three basic tube-detector projection systems

- a projection system using a parallel beam of radiation (a parallel-beam system),
- a system using a beam of radiation in the shape of a fan (a fan-beam system),
- a system using a beam of radiation in the shape of a cone (a cone-beam system).

Structural and functional details of each of these projection systems will be described in Chaps. 5, 6 and 7 when discussing the algorithms used to reconstruct the images from the projections. Here, however, we will focus on the evolution of successive generations of scanners.

3.1.1 First-Generation Scanners

First-generation scanners, sometimes called *pencil beam* or *translation/rotation single detector* scanners, belong to the class of device that uses a parallel-beam projection system. Figure 3.3 shows how a single projection is carried out in this type of system [3, 18].

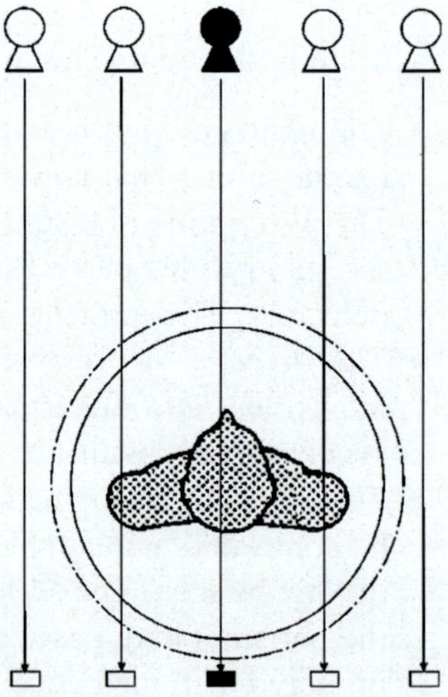

Fig. 3.3 A parallel beam projection system

In this type of scanner, there are two components to the movement of the rigidly coupled tube-detector system: a lateral movement to make a single projection and a circular movement about the central opening in the gantry to gather all the projections necessary to reconstruct the image.

The acquisition of the individual projections can be either continuous or discrete, but each of these projections is obtained only at a discrete angle of rotation of the projection system. It is easy to see how this method of scanning is not fast enough (it takes approximately 5 min); both the single detector and the X-ray tube must travel a distance equal to the diameter of the gantry opening, twice during each projection. A sequence of two projections for this type of scanner is shown in more detail in Fig. 3.4.

First-generation scanners are prime examples of devices having a parallel-beam projection system. The procedure for obtaining images of successive cross-sections with this type of scanner is explained in Fig. 3.5.

The short arrows in the diagram show the positioning of the patient lying on the table while successive cross-sections are obtained. They represent the small sliding movements of the table that take place after all the projections needed to reconstruct the image of a single slice have been performed. After each movement, the procedure for the collection of the projections for the next image is repeated.

3.1.2 Second-Generation Scanners

Great progress was made (compared to the design of first-generation scanners) when scanners with a larger number of detectors in the array were introduced around 1972. These second-generation scanners, sometimes called *partial fan-beam* or *translation/rotation multiple detector* scanners, had between 3 and 52 detectors in the array. The use of the fan-shaped radiation beam [3, 18] enabled the projections to cover a larger area of the patient's body at any one time and resulted in the reduction of the number of projections needed to reconstruct an image of satisfactory quality. Figure 3.6 illustrates the scanning sequence for this generation of scanner.

In this approach, the time to obtain the projections necessary for the reconstruction of one image was reduced to about 300 s, even though the movement of the tube-detector array was still a combination of lateral and rotational motion. This system can be considered as a transitional stage between the parallel-beam projection system and the fan-beam system.

3.1.3 Third-Generation Scanners

Further steps to improve the CT scanner were next directed towards the elimination of the lateral movement of the tube-detector system. In 1976, scanner

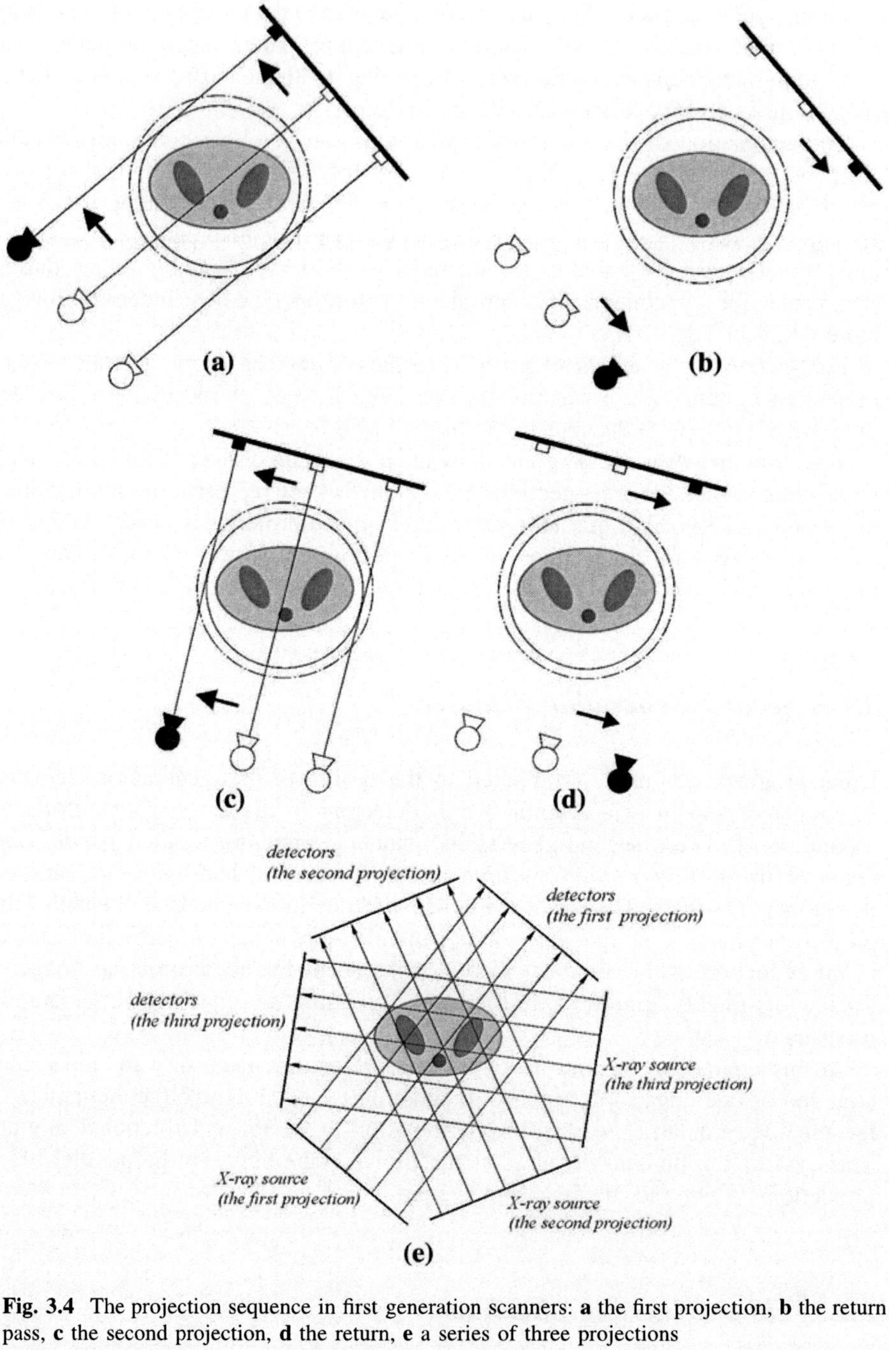

Fig. 3.4 The projection sequence in first generation scanners: **a** the first projection, **b** the return pass, **c** the second projection, **d** the return, **e** a series of three projections

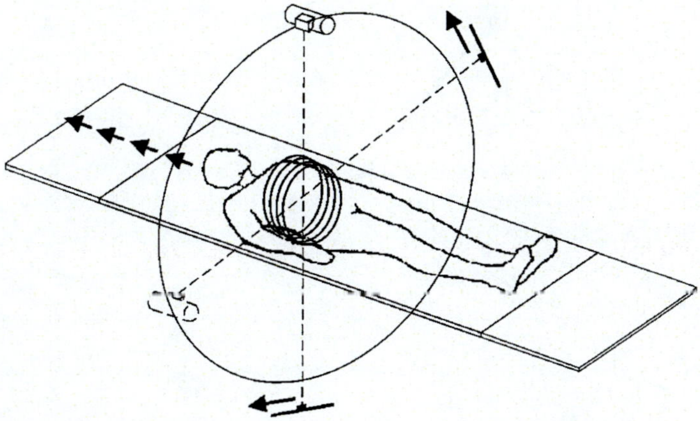

Fig. 3.5 Obtaining a sequence of image slices in a parallel beam scanner

designers managed to limit the movement in the projection system exclusively to rotational movement [3, 18, 22, 25]. This was the so-called *fan-beam* or *continuous rotation scanner*. By fan-beam, we mean here a projection system with a beam of radiation in the shape of a fan with an angular spread of between 40 and 55 degrees, enough to encompass the whole of the test object, as shown in Fig. 3.7.

The sequence of individual projections for this type of scanner is shown in Fig. 3.8. An obvious consequence of this modification was the need to increase the number of detectors in the array moving synchronously with the rotating X-ray tube (up to 1,000 detector elements). As a result of these design changes, the time to acquire a reconstructed image was reduced to about 5 s. Scanners of this generation are examples of the implementation of the fan-beam projection system in its purest form.

In this scanner, after all the projections have been made for the first image, the table moves and the whole procedure is repeated for the next cross-section of the body. The sequence of projections for reconstructing the images of successive slices of the patient's body is shown in Fig. 3.9, where the short arrows once again indicate the positioning of the patient lying on a table.

3.1.4 Fourth-Generation Scanners

The next, fourth generation of scanners, introduced in 1978, differed only slightly from the third generation. In the earlier designs, the detector array moved around the test object together with the X-ray tube. Now the rotation of the array was eliminated by arranging it on a stationary ring with a radius larger than the radius of the circle described by the tube [3, 18]. The result was a scanner known as the *rotate-fixed* scanner; the word rotate in the name refers to the movement of the tube and the word fixed to the array of detectors. In order to maintain an adequate

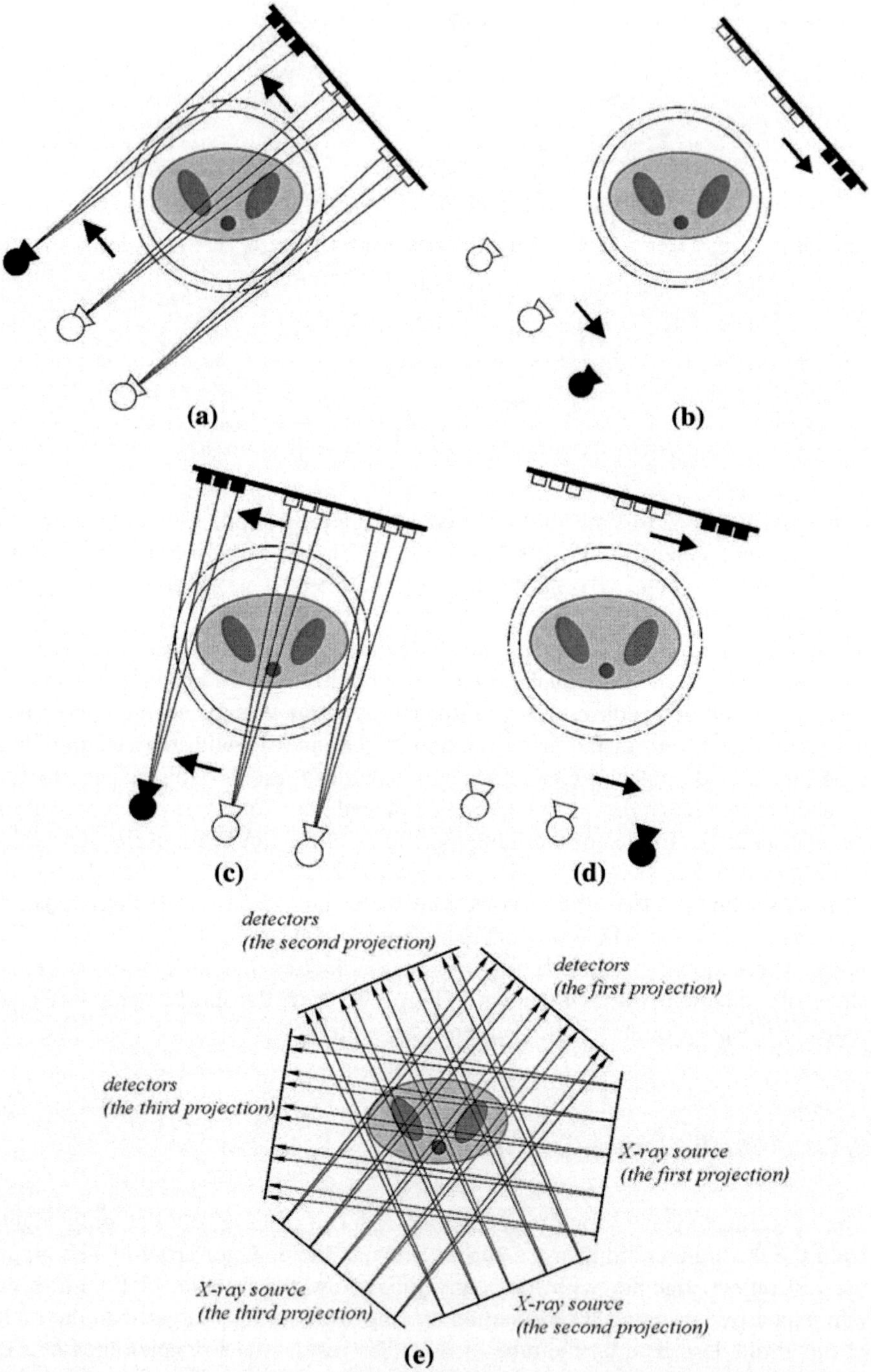

Fig. 3.6 The projection sequence in second generation scanners: **a** the first projection, **b** the return pass, **c** the second projection, **d** the return, **e** a series of three projections

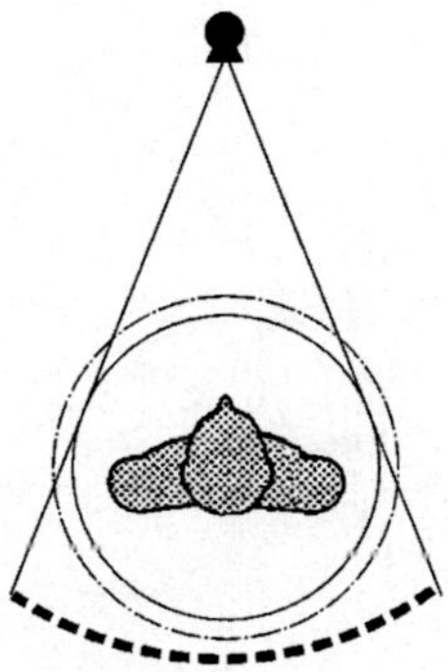

Fig. 3.7 A fan beam system

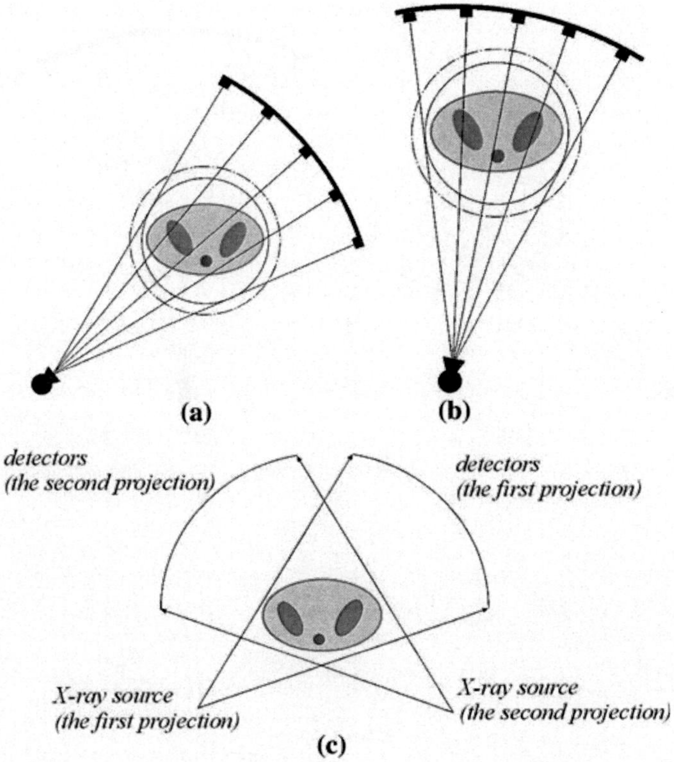

Fig. 3.8 The projection sequence in third generation scanners: **a** the first projection, **b** the second projection, **c** a set of two projections

resolution of the radiation intensity measurements, the number of detectors in the array was increased and now ranged from 600 to 5,000 detector elements. The time taken to obtain one image using this design however was still about 5 s. The group

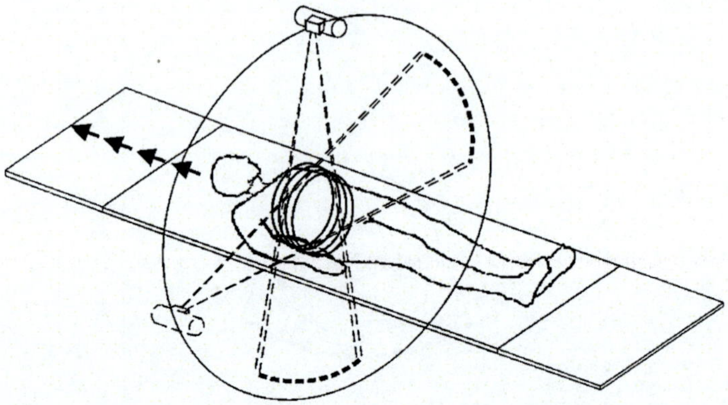

Fig. 3.9 Obtaining a sequence of image slices in a fan beam scanner

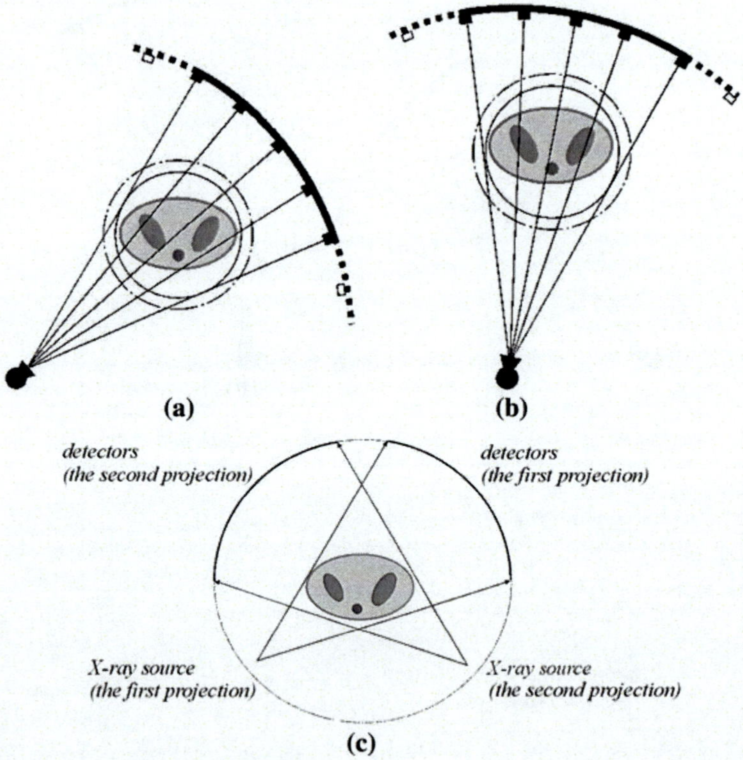

Fig. 3.10 The projection sequence in fourth generation scanners: **a** the first projection, **b** the second projection, **c** a set of two projections

to which this scanner belonged remained the same; it was still classified as a fan-beam scanner. The projection sequence for this type of scanner is shown in Fig. 3.10.

3.1.5 Spiral Scanners

We saw earlier that successive generations of scanners used either parallel beams of radiation or fan beams. On closer analysis, a problem becomes apparent with the projection systems used in these generations: there is no movement along the axis of the patient during each of the projections. In 1989, to remedy this situation, the first designs of scanners appeared which combined the movement of the tube around the patient with a simultaneous smooth displacement of the patient into the opening of the gantry [3, 18, 26]. The projection system moved in a spiral around the patient.

In the initial phases of the development of spiral tomography, the scanners used a detector array in shape of an arc of a circle, similar to the design of third-generation scanners.[2] The device was called a *single-slice spiral computed tomography* scanner or SSCT. Figure 3.11 shows the spiral motion of the tube and detectors around the patient.

In 1998, an improved design of scanner emerged: the *multi-slice spiral computed tomography* scanner (MSCT) [1, 14]. The projection system still moved in a spiral but the detector array was made up of between 8 and 34 rows of detectors, making it possible for this design of scanner to obtain four adjacent slices simultaneously.

The beam now took the shape of a cone (see Fig. 3.12); this cone-beam was the most natural shape for a beam of X-rays. Previous designs of spiral scanner had used a radiation beam in which the individual rays were almost parallel to each other. The new design permitted three-dimensional projection techniques to be mastered and so paved the way for the development of reconstruction techniques operating in three dimensions.

The first *cone-beam spiral CT* scanners (CBCT) were put into operation in the years 2001 2002 [21, 33]. The cone-shaped radiation beam made it possible to increase the width of the detector array to 16 or even 320 elements, thereby allowing the simultaneous acquisition of up to 256 adjacent image slices with these scanners. The main advantages of this design were the increased scanning speed and the reduction of the impact of collimation inaccuracies on the quality of the reconstructed image. The reduction in collimation losses had the additional advantage of allowing a reduction in the power of the X-ray tube. The combination of the cone-beam and the spiral motion of the projection system resulted in a significant reduction in the time taken to complete the scan (down to 2 min, or even less) and during this time, the images of many adjacent slices could be reconstructed. The spiral movement of the projection system also enabled the slice resolution to be increased so that a slice could be obtained with resolution 0.23 mm. The principle of the spiral path cone-beam scanner is illustrated in Fig. 3.13.

[2] In practice, using an array consisting of two rows of detectors.

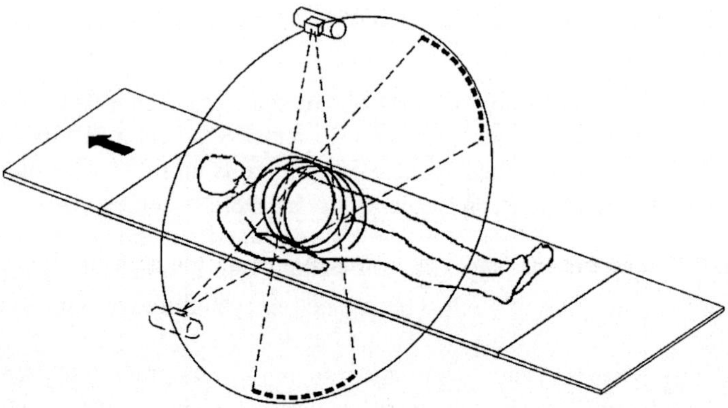

Fig. 3.11 Rotation of the tube around the patient combined with a smooth displacement of the patient through the gantry

Fig. 3.12 A cone beam projection system

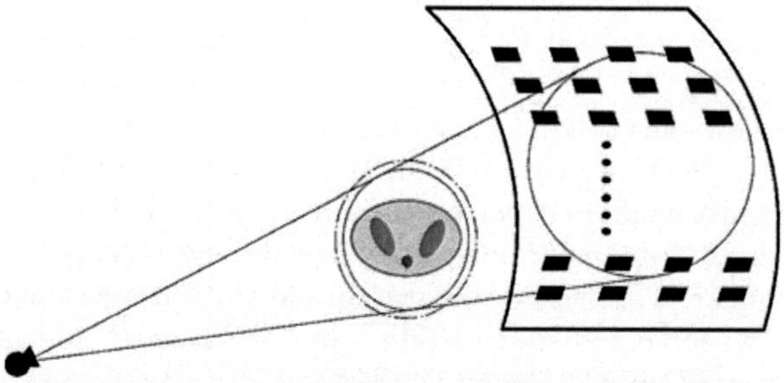

Spiral scanners are currently the standard tomographic equipment used in clinical practice. Because of the reduced time needed to complete a scan, they can be used to study organs, such as the heart or lungs, which are physiologically in motion. In addition, by synchronising the working phases of the heart with the acquisition of the projections, it is even possible to obtain a dynamic tomographic image. Spiral tomography with its short exposure time also makes it possible to examine people, who for various reasons, cannot remain motionless for long, such as children or emotionally disturbed patients.

3.2 X-ray Sources

The X-ray tube is the fundamental element in the projection system of every CT scanner. Its operation is based on the complex physical principles involved in the generation of X-rays. Knowledge of these principles helps us to design improved X-ray equipment and apply them in a variety of different medical devices.

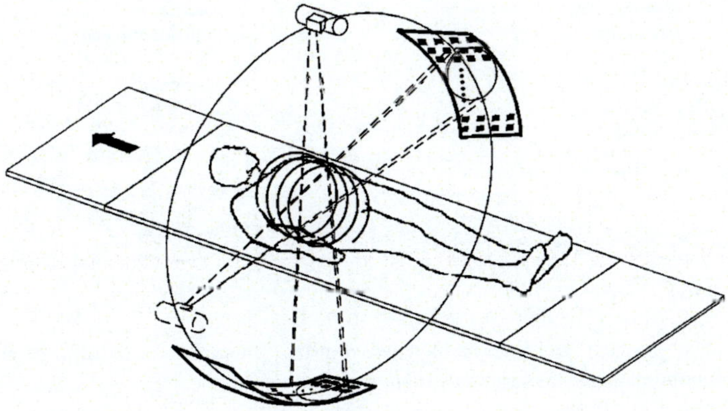

Fig. 3.13 The movement of the projection system relative to the patient in a spiral scanner

3.2.1 The Physics of X-ray Sources

X-rays are generated by physical processes that take place within matter at the atomic level. Quanta of electromagnetic radiation with wavelengths in the range 10^{-12} to 10^{-8} m (0.01 100 Å) (in medical applications, in the range 6×10^{-12} to 1.2×10^{-10}m (0.06 1.2 Å)) are produced as a consequence of two processes: the transition of electrons between the inner shells of an atom and the deceleration of charged particles caused by electromagnetic fields within matter. Both of these phenomena occur during the generation of X-radiation in X-ray tubes.

Each transition of an electron from a shell with a higher energy level to a shell with a lower level is accompanied by the emission of a quantum of radiation with energy equal to the energy difference between the shells [29]. Physicists call this characteristic X-ray radiation and it has typical quantum energies in the range 0.052 129.544 keV. As only shells with specific energy levels are allowed in atoms, the quantum energies of characteristic radiation can only have discrete values within this range. The generation of this type of X-rays is illustrated in Fig. 3.14a.

When electromagnetic fields within matter cause charged particles such as electrons, protons, α-particles or heavy ions to decelerate [29], the energy lost is emitted as X-ray quanta. This energy can take any value in a range reaching up to 20 MeV. This type of X-ray radiation is often called *bremsstrahlung*, which is German for *braking* or *deceleration radiation*. A diagram of the generation of bremsstrahlung or continuous X-rays is given in Fig. 3.14b.

Characteristic X-rays are emitted when matter is bombarded by charged particles with sufficiently large kinetic energies to be able to knock electrons out of their orbits in the atoms.

If we assume that an electron is knocked out of a shell that has an energy level E_1, then after a time interval of the order of 10^{-15} s, another electron from a shell

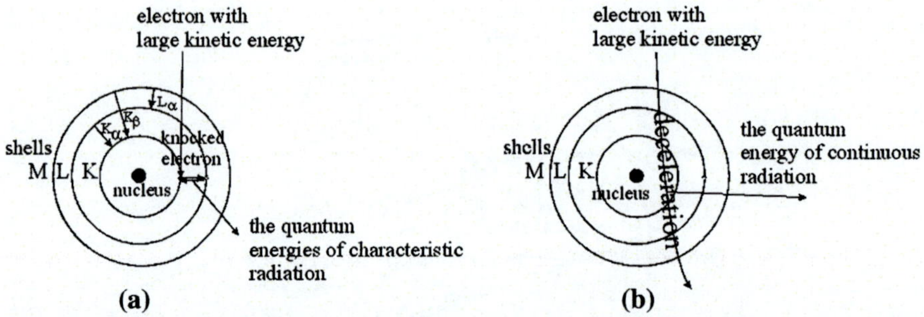

Fig. 3.14 The physical processes responsible for the generation of X rays: **a** characteristic radiation, **b** continuous X rays (*bremsstrahlung*)

of higher energy E_2 fills the resulting vacancy and simultaneously a quantum of radiation is emitted with energy

$$h\upsilon = E_1 - E_2, \tag{3.1}$$

where h is Planck's constant; υ is the frequency of the quantum of radiation emitted.

The energy levels in the atom can be defined by the following equation [29]

$$E(n,l,j) = c_1 \frac{m}{m+m_e}\left(\frac{(Z-\sigma_1)^2}{n^2} + c_2 \frac{(Z-\sigma_2)^2}{n^4}\left(\frac{n}{j-0.5} - 0.75\right)\right), \tag{3.2}$$

where c_1, c_2 are constants; m is the mass of the nucleus with charge Z; m_e is the mass of an electron; σ_1 is the total screening constant, which specifies the screening of the nuclear charge by all the electrons; σ_2 is the internal screening constant, which specifies the screening by the inner electrons; n, l, j are, respectively, the principal quantum number, the orbital momentum quantum number, the total angular momentum quantum number.

Since electrons can be found only at specific energy levels, the quantum energies emitted by the electrons when they fill the vacancies can only have discrete values. Every time an electron from a higher energy level fills a vacancy, a characteristic X-ray line is produced. The term "characteristic line" comes from the fact that atoms of different elements are characterised by different sets of lines, whereas the term "characteristic series" refers to a collection of all these characteristic X-ray lines. The so-called K, L, and M series are associated with the filling of vacancies in the K, L, and M shells of the atom, in order of increasing energy levels of the shells. The number of possible electron transition lines is also limited by the so-called selection rules. These establish conditions as to which transitions can occur between the quantum numbers n, l, j. The equations below describe the requirements imposed by these rules [29]

$$\Delta n \neq 0; \; |\Delta l| = 1; \; |\Delta j| = 0 \text{ or } 1, \tag{3.3}$$

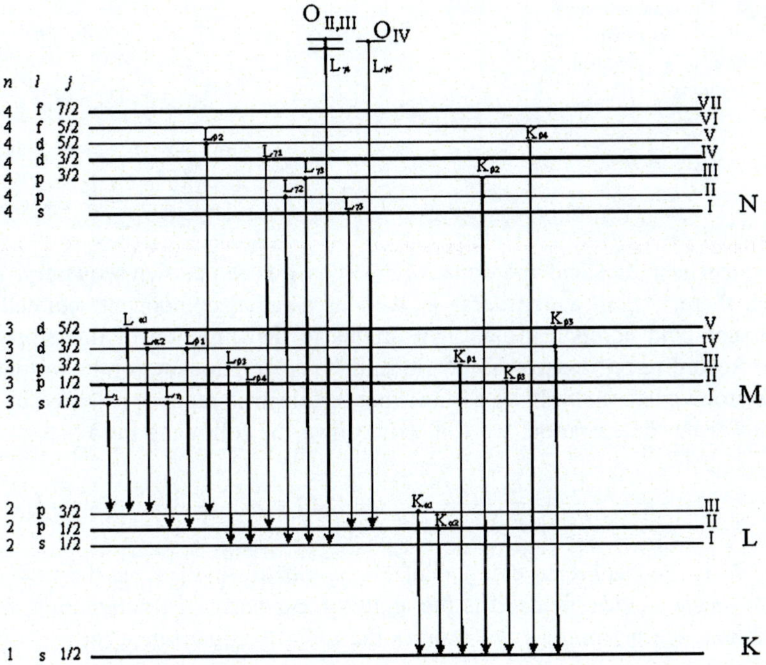

Fig. 3.15 The K and L series of characteristic X ray lines

where Δn, Δl, Δj are the changes in the quantum numbers during the transition of electrons between different energy levels.

The conventional symbols used to represent the characteristic X-ray lines of the K and L series are shown in Fig. 3.15.

When it comes to the practical use of individual characteristic X-ray lines, the relative probability of transition (i.e. the probability of filling a vacancy) is particularly important. It is this, which manifests itself through the emission of a specific characteristic X-ray line.

At this point, let us examine one of the explanations adopted by physicists to explain the generation of continuous X-rays. It is generally known that the electric field of a charge at rest has only a radial component E_r. The production of continuous X-rays however depends on the formation of a transverse electric field component E_t of the electron. This happens when an electron decelerates as it strikes a target material. The process is illustrated in Fig. 3.16.

In the diagram below, the electron moves along the x-axis at a speed $V \ll c$ (c, the speed of light) and is suddenly decelerated and brought to a complete halt in a time Δt. Within a radius $r = ct$ of the halted charge, the electric field is radial. However, at a distance greater than $r_\Delta = c(t + \Delta t)$, the electric field has only a transverse component, i.e. the field is the field of a moving charge. The zone of radius r expands at the speed of light. In the region $r_\Delta - r$ of width ct, the electric field pattern exhibits a smooth transition between the zone where the field

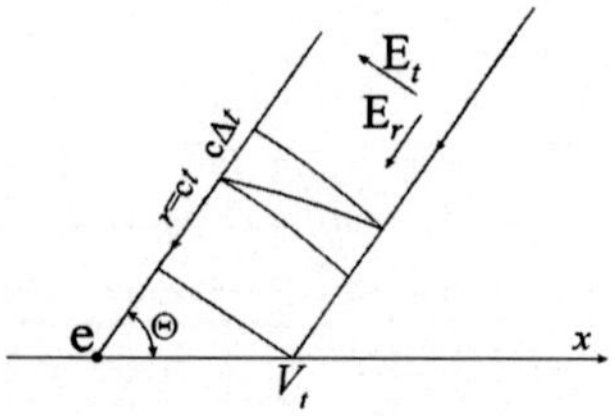

Fig. 3.16 The generation of continuous X rays during the deceleration of an electron (*bremsstrahlung*)

component is radial and the zone where it is transverse. Consequently, in that region, there is both a transverse as well as a radial component: mutually perpendicular field components at right angles to the direction of the propagating wave. According to Maxwell's equations, this is a prerequisite for the formation of an electromagnetic field. If we assume that the electron reduces its speed by ΔV as a result of the deceleration, we can write down the following ratio

$$\frac{|E_t|}{|E_r|} = \frac{E_t}{E_r} = \frac{t \cdot V \cdot \sin \Theta}{c} \cdot \Delta t = \frac{a \cdot t}{c} \sin \Theta, \tag{3.4}$$

where E_t is the transverse component of the electric field; E_r is the radial component of the electric field; Θ is the angle of incidence of the radiation; a is the retardation. Furthermore, if we express the radial component of the electric field by

$$E_r = \frac{e}{r^2}, \tag{3.5}$$

where e is the charge on the electron, we obtain the following equation

$$E_t = \frac{e \cdot a}{c^2 \cdot r} \sin \Theta. \tag{3.6}$$

This approximate relationship for the transverse component of the electric field can then be substituted into an equation expressing the intensity of the electromagnetic radiation as a function of E_t

$$I = \frac{c}{4\pi} E_t^2 = \frac{e^2}{4c^3 \cdot \pi} \cdot \frac{a^2}{r^2} \sin \Theta. \tag{3.7}$$

A prerequisite for the generation of bremsstrahlung is a non-zero value of the retardation a. This happens in the X-ray tube by the action of a force on the moving charge in the opposite direction to its movement. Because of the non-zero scattering cross-sections of the charged particles (whatever their angle of incidence) and the different amounts by which the retarded particles change their speed, the frequency spectrum of the radiation produced is continuous throughout its entire frequency range.

The X-ray spectrum produced by the tube is the sum of the energies of both of the above processes, in other words, a combination of discrete characteristic X-rays and continuous X-rays. An example of the combined X-ray spectrum

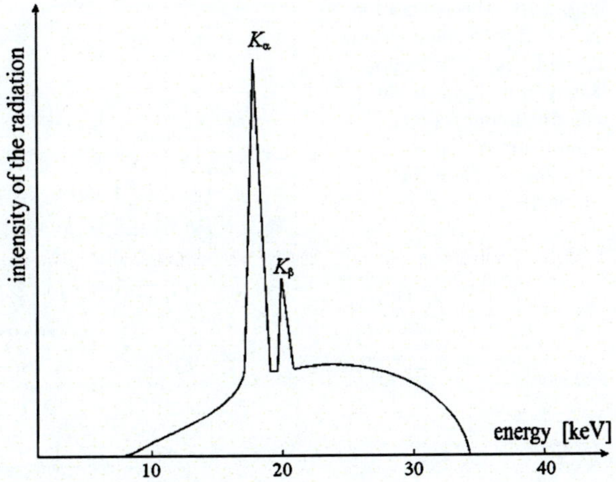

Fig. 3.17 The energy spectrum of X rays obtained by bombarding a sample of molybdenum

obtained by bombarding a sample of molybdenum (Mb) with electrons is shown in Fig. 3.17.

The description of the production of X-rays given above is by way of an introduction to the topic of X-ray tube design, in particular, to the design of the tubes used in computed tomography.

3.2.2 X-ray Tubes

Wilhelm Röntgen, while using a Crookes tube to examine the behaviour and properties of cathode rays and without realising it at the time, discovered X-rays and the mechanism that produces them (see Chap. 2). An insight into how the Crookes tube operates as an X-ray tube can be gained from the description of the physics of X-ray generation given in the previous section. A diagram of the experiment performed in 1895 is shown in Fig. 3.18.

Röntgen used two voltage sources: one to supply current to heat the cathode; the second, a high voltage source, to produce the cathode rays. By doing so, he produced a beam of electrons, which collided with the positively charged anode (the anticathode) with great energy and directly resulted in the production of X-rays.

The design of tubes used to produce X-rays has changed substantially compared to the early days. A diagram of an X-ray tube with a stationary anode is shown in Fig. 3.19.

The most important parts of the X-ray tube are situated inside an envelope made of Pyrex glass or metal where the pressure is in the range 10^{-3} 10^{-5} Pa. Two metal electrodes supply a low voltage (of the order of several volts) to the tube. This causes a current to flow through the coil, which heats the cathode. Two other electrodes, the cathode and anode (sometimes called the anticathode), supply a

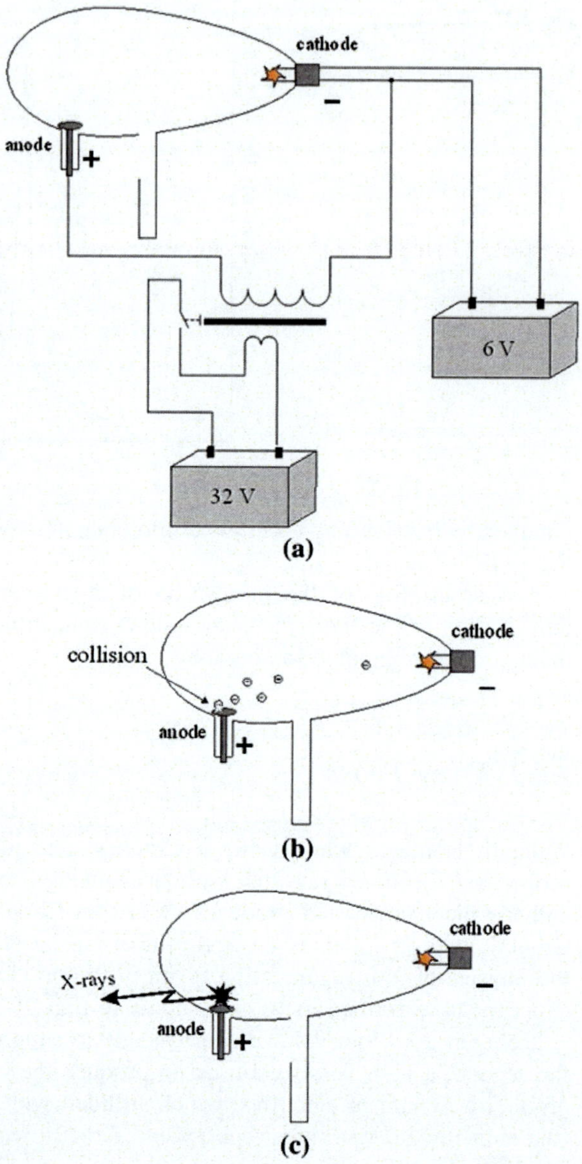

Fig. 3.18 The generation of X rays during the experiment carried out by Wilhelm Röntgen in 1895: **a** the electrical connections, **b** collision of the electrons with the anode, **c** the production of X rays

high voltage (between 5 kV and approximately 100 kV; in computed tomography between 80 and 140 kV). In order to reduce the number of electrical connections, a single electrode often combines the cathode with one of the heater coil connections.

An important element in the design of the cathode is the focus, the part of the cathode that emits the electrons. The more the focus resembles a point source, the sharper the images that are obtained during a projection [32]. The oldest method of

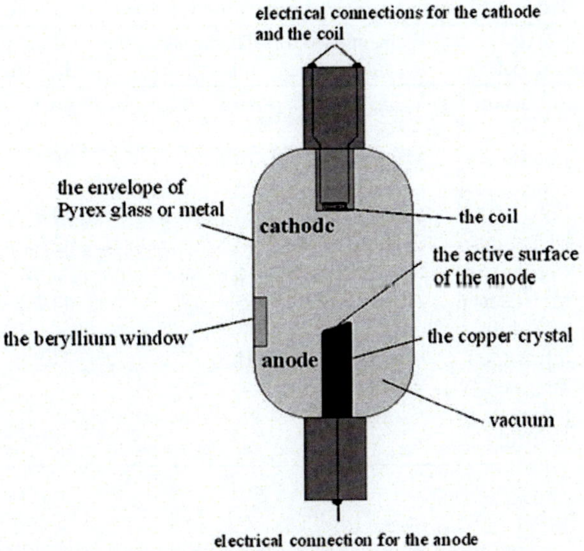

Fig. 3.19 A stationary anode X ray tube

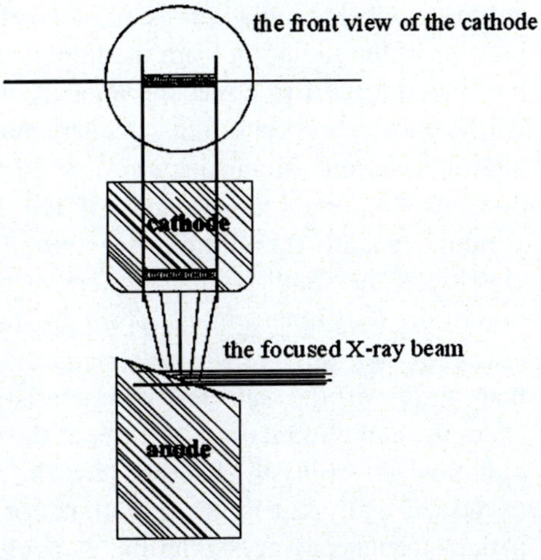

Fig. 3.20 Focusing the X rays in a tube with a linear focus

focusing the electron beam involved the use of metal shields and electrostatic lenses. Another design solution is a cathode in the form of an elongated coil emitting electrons through an elongated opening, whose longitudinal axis is parallel to the axis of the anode, as shown in Fig. 3.20 [29].

In this design, if we imagine a mirror placed on the anode, inclined at a slight angle to the cathode surface, the focus, as viewed from the screen, appears foreshortened. In this way, we artificially reduce the size of the focus of the tube.

The electrons emitted by the cathode are accelerated to high energies, up to 10^3 eV (sometimes even 10^6 eV), but only a fraction of them hit the anode, located opposite, with great speed.

Table 3.1 Comparison of elements used in anodes and filters

Anode material	Element used for the filter	Thickness of the filter [μ m]	Absorption of the K_α series [%]	Absorption of the K_β series [%]
Zirconium (Zr)	Vanadium (V)	15.3	46.7	99.6
Iron (Fe)	Manganese (Mn)	15.1	36.1	99.5
Cobalt (Co)	Iron (Fe)	14.7	44.7	99.4
Nickel (Ni)	Cobalt (Co)	14.3	42.9	99.2
Copper (Cu)	Nickel (Ni)	15.8	42.5	98.9
Molybdenum (Mo)	Zirconium (Zr)	63.0	44.2	98.4
Silver (Ag)	Lead (Pb)	41.3	44.8	74.3
Tungsten (W)	Various			
Rhodium (Rh)	Various			

The anode (anticathode) is a much more complex element of the X-ray tube. Its end face is cut at a slight angle of 10° 20° and has a layer of material with a large atomic number, such as tungsten, deposited on it. For radiological applications, it is better if the radiation from the tube is as monochromatic as possible. Therefore, the material used to cover the anode contains elements (such as Cu, Al or Mg), which emit appropriate lines of characteristic radiation, such as the $K_{\alpha_{1,2}}$ lines. In addition, various impurities are used to concentrate the radiation of the selected line. An important component of the X-ray monochromatising system is the window (usually beryllium, Be) through which the radiation leaves the glass envelope. The small atomic number of beryllium ($Z = 4$) minimises the absorption of the $K_{\alpha_{1,2}}$ lines while suppressing the remaining components of the radiation spectrum. Various types of filter can also be used to filter out frequencies other than those of the selected characteristic lines, suppressing the K_β lines, for example, and eliminating the parts of the spectrum in the soft radiation range. Soft radiation is strongly absorbed by the surface structure of the tissues being examined and, as it is not important for obtaining the projection, it exposes the patient to unnecessary radiation. A comparison of the elements most commonly used in this way is shown in Table 3.1. Figure 3.21 illustrates the process of shaping the X-ray spectrum.

An appropriate filter is matched by selecting the absorption threshold so that it lies between the K_α and K_β series of the X-ray spectrum. Materials with atomic numbers 1 or 2 less than the anode material have this property.

X-ray tubes are estimated to be only 1% efficient; the energy not used to produce radiation is converted into heat. Previously, in order to conduct the heat away more effectively, a tubular or cylindrical anode was often made from a single crystal of copper. Currently, in the newer types of X-ray tube, the anode is usually cooled using water or oil. It is also possible to cool the envelope of the tube in this way, as it is completely encased in a lead shield. The shield also has an opening

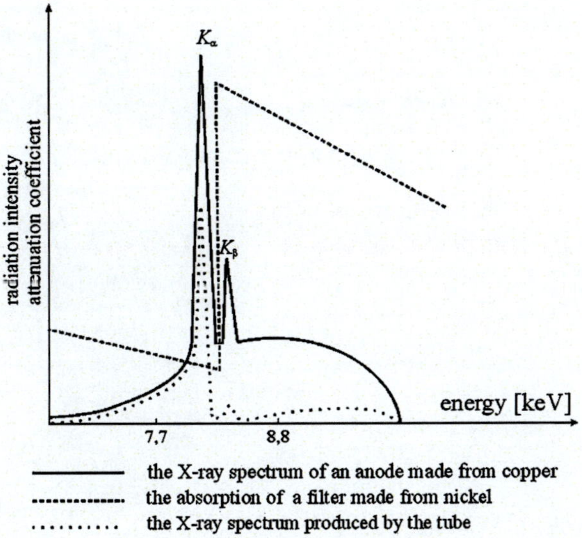

Fig. 3.21 Shaping the radiation spectrum of the X ray tube

that forms part of the collimator. Only a small part of the radiation produced by the tube passes through the collimator to the outside; the material of the shield absorbs the rest.

In order to build X-ray tubes for use in computed tomography, a design was needed that prevented the anode from overheating in conditions where the power could be as high as 50 kW. The solution proved to be a tube designed with a rotating cathode, as shown in Fig. 3.22.

Figure 3.22 shows a flat cylinder made of a material with a high melting point (e.g. graphite). The edge facing the cathode is bevelled and covered with a material that emits X-rays when bombarded by the high-energy electrons emitted by the cathode.

During the production of the beam of electrons, the cylindrical anode is rotated at a speed of about 3,000 rpm. This is made possible because the anode is attached to the rotor of a motor whose stator windings are located outside the envelope of the tube. When the tube is in operation, electrons hit the anode at different places, thus artificially increasing its active surface. In addition, the inclination of the active plane with respect to the longitudinal surface of the cathode increases the concentration of the radiation beam, as was explained for the case of the standard X-ray tube [29].

In 64-slice spiral scanners, a design of X-ray tube with two focuses was used [3], as illustrated in Fig. 3.23. In this tube, the deflection system switches the beam of electrons emitted by the cathode at a rate of 4,640 times per second. This produces two beams of electrons, which then hit the anode, generating two separate beams of X-rays. The use of this dual focus design of X-ray source allows us to obtain a reconstructed slice thickness of 0.4 mm. It also eliminates artefacts from the image, caused by the spiral motion of the projection system.

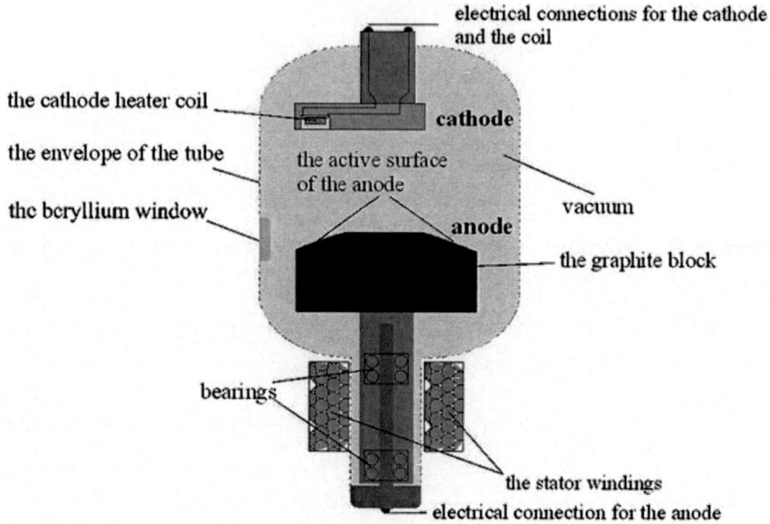

Fig. 3.22 An X ray tube with a rotating anode

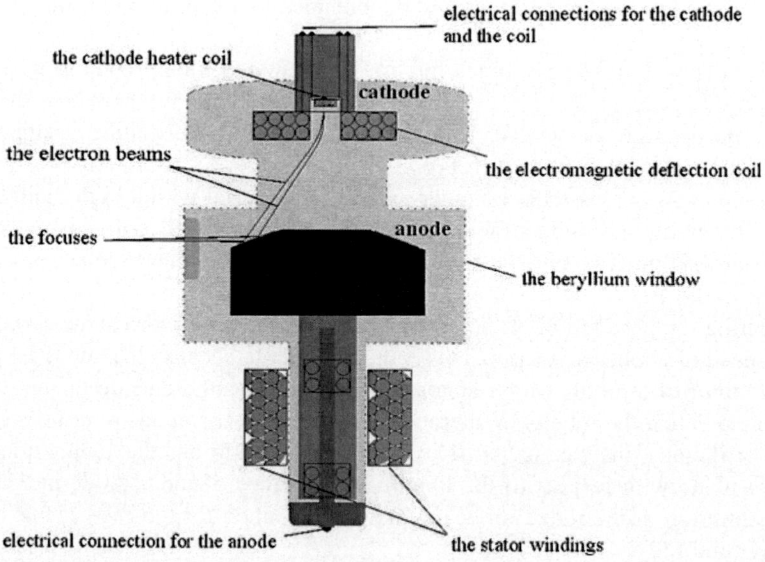

Fig. 3.23 A dual focus X ray tube

At this point, we will give a qualitative and quantitative description of the production of bremsstrahlung (i.e. continuous radiation). Most of the energy emitted by an X-ray tube is in the form of this type of radiation. We can say approximately that

$$\text{Power\_of\_tube} = k \cdot \mathcal{U}_R^2 \cdot I_R \cdot Z, \tag{3.8}$$

where $k \cong 10^{\;9}$ is a coefficient of proportionality; U_R is the voltage between the anode and cathode; I_R is the current flowing through the tube; Z is the atomic number of the element of the anode.

Note that the easiest way to alter the cathode current I_R in the tube is by changing the current flowing through the heater. The minimum wavelength obtained from the X-ray tube is determined however using the relationship

$$\lambda_{\min} = \frac{hc}{e\mathcal{U}_R}. \tag{3.9}$$

As we can see from the above, by adjusting the voltage between the anode and the cathode we can alter both the power of the tube and the wavelength of the radiation and so influence the high-energy components of the radiation spectrum. This voltage however does not affect the power of the characteristic radiation. All that is required to produce this component of the spectrum is a certain minimum level of voltage.

In medicine, the term "hard" is used to describe high frequency X-rays with their high penetrating power; the word "soft" is used for lower frequency radiation with lower penetrating power.

3.2.3 Electrical Aspects of X-ray Tubes

When considering the design and the operating principles of X-ray tubes, it should be pointed out that their electrical properties are not essentially different from those of other vacuum tubes, such as diodes. Let us start by considering a simple system (see Fig. 3.24), where a voltage is applied between the anode and cathode of the tube and a current flows.

We can use this system to examine the shape of the electrical characteristic of the X-ray tube, that is, the relationship between voltage U_R applied across the anode and cathode and the current I_R that flows through the tube, for a given heater current I_h. A plot of the characteristic curves is shown in Fig. 3.25.

It can be proved analytically that the shapes of the characteristics in Fig. 3.25 correspond to the Child Langmuir equation [4, 23]

$$I_R(\mathcal{U}_R) = 2.34 \cdot 10^{\;6}\frac{\mathrm{S_{anode}}}{\mathrm{d_{ak}^2}} \cdot U_R^{3/2}; \tag{3.10}$$

where $\mathrm{S_{anode}}$ is the active area of the electron beam, i.e. the area of the anode; $\mathrm{d_{ak}}$ is the distance between the anode and cathode.

The individual characteristic curves of the tube relate to different values of heater current I_h. The non-saturated, working region of the X-ray tube is called the Langmuir region. This is the active part of the characteristic curve. The saturated

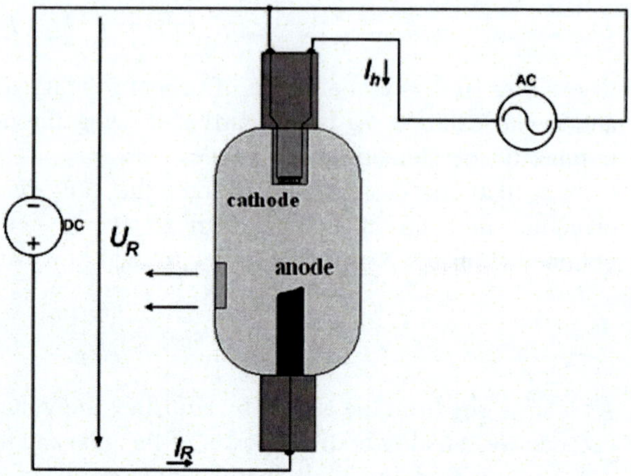

Fig. 3.24 A simple power supply for an X ray tube

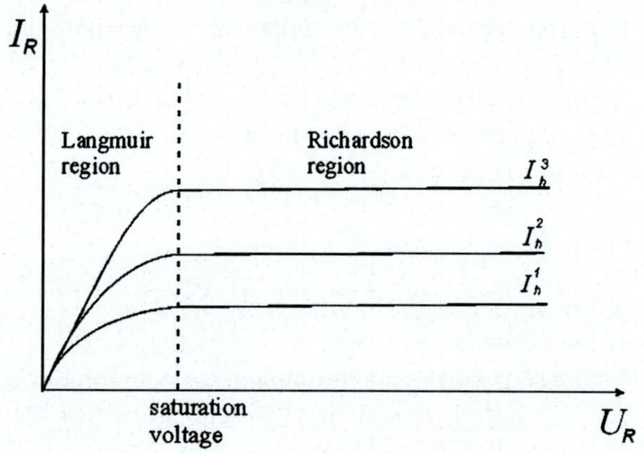

Fig. 3.25 The electrical characteristics of an X ray tube

area is called the Richardson region. This saturation of the tube's characteristic is due to the limited number of electrons that can be emitted from the cathode at any given temperature or heater current I_h.

From Eq. 3.10, we can conclude that the resistance of the tube while conducting a current is

$$R = \frac{U_R}{I_R} = c\frac{1}{U_R^{\frac{3}{2}}}, \tag{3.11}$$

where c is a coefficient of proportionality.

As mentioned earlier, an X-ray tube behaves like a diode; it conducts current in only one direction, the direction of the voltage applied between the anode and cathode. The equivalent circuit of an X-ray tube is shown in Fig. 3.26.

In order for it to generate X-rays, the tube should be connected to an electronic circuit such as that illustrated in Fig. 3.27, which is used to produce X-rays for medical applications.

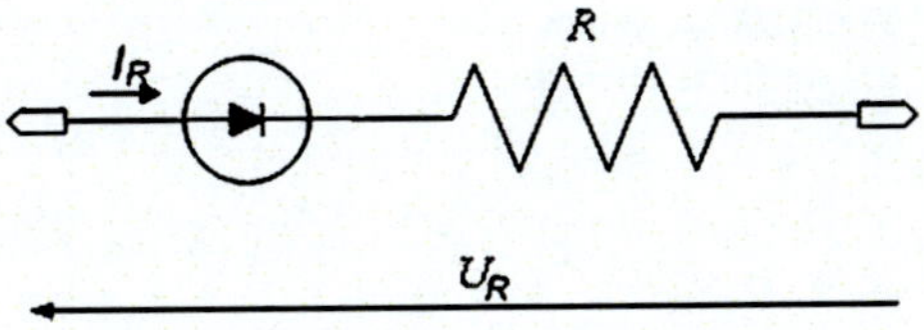

Fig. 3.26 The equivalent circuit of an X ray tube

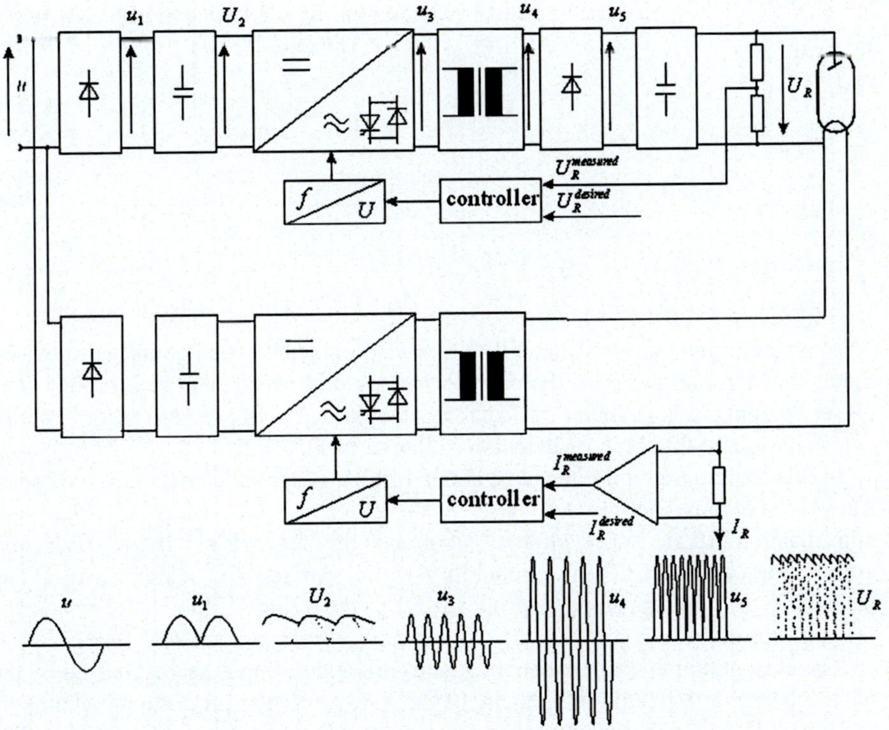

Fig. 3.27 A circuit diagram for an X ray tube used for medical purposes

3.3 X-ray Detectors

X-ray detectors have a similar function in computed tomography to photographic film in conventional X-ray radiography, that of creating the image from a projection of X-rays [1]. The following types of X-ray detector are currently used in computed tomography

- xenon proportional chambers, in which the electrical output signal is proportional to the intensity of the radiation that ionises the gas atoms inside *microgap gas chambers* (MGC) [27, 28];
- scintillation detectors [7, 8, 10, 12, 15].

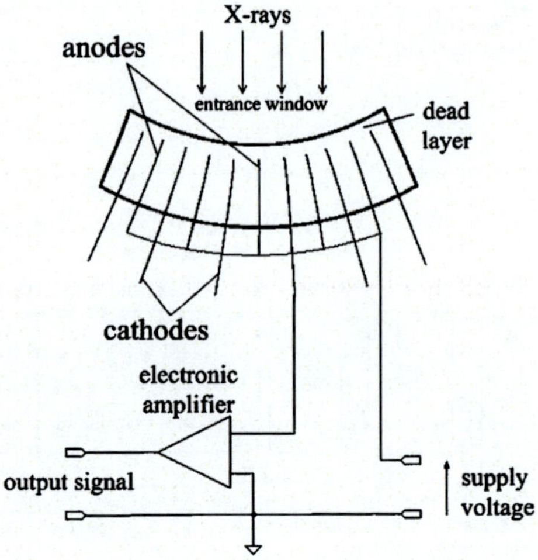

Fig. 3.28 A xenon proportional chamber

Most third-generation scanner use xenon proportional chambers, as they are much cheaper than the scintillation detectors used in subsequent generations. The gas in the ionization chamber of a xenon detector is at high pressure (about 10atm) [8]. A design of this type of detector is shown in Fig. 3.28.

In this detector, a high voltage of about 140 kV is applied across the electrodes. The voltage must not be too large however or it could cause so-called gas amplification. If an X-ray photon penetrates the detector's window (typically aluminium), there is a high probability of it ionizing the xenon inside. The probability of this happening is proportional to the length of the chamber and the pressure inside.

The current that flows between the electrodes and through the gas ionised by the X-rays is proportional to the intensity of the X-rays. Xenon proportional chambers work in such a way that almost no heating occurs after the ionization event, and so it only takes a short time for them to return to a state of readiness. This is highly significant when applying the technique to spiral projection systems. The high-voltage electrodes are often made of tantalum and the ion-collecting electrodes of copper. To get some idea of the dimensions of these detectors, the length of a xenon chamber is often quoted as 6 cm and the width of a single cell as about 1 mm (1.5 mm) [13]. Because of the difficulty of obtaining suitably convergent electrodes while maintaining the standard 8 cm length of chamber, chambers are currently produced with a length of 3 6 cm. In general, the efficiency of these detectors is about 60%, and their main advantages are low cost and small size.

In later generations of CT scanner, from the fourth generation onwards, ceramic (scintillation) detectors are used to measure X-ray intensity. The design of these detectors is described by Fig. 3.29 [13].

When X-rays strike a scintillator crystal a range of physical phenomena are produced, namely

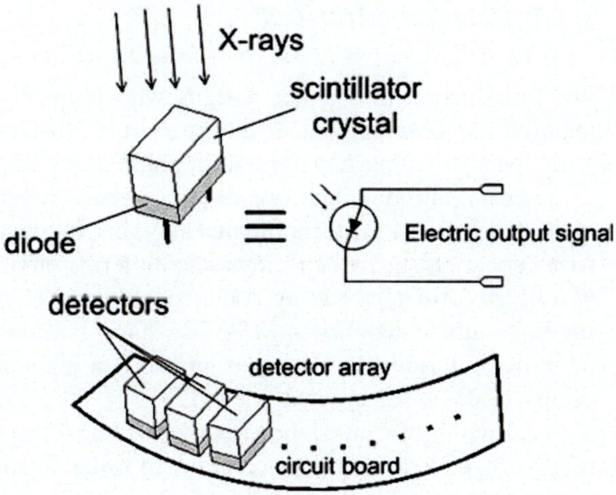

Fig. 3.29 Scintillation detectors

- the photoelectric effect,
- the Compton effect,
- pair production.

Scintillation detectors make use of the photoelectric effect. Photons of X-rays knock electrons out of their orbit and these, in the presence of a phosphor, produce a flash of light (luminescent radiation) in the ultraviolet or visible range of wavelengths [11, 30]. Detector arrays in the newer scanners are constructed with scintillation detectors made from materials such as sodium iodide (NaI) doped with thallium (Tl), caesium iodide (CsI), cadmium tungstate ($CdWO_4$), zinc sulphide (ZnS), naphthalene, anthracene and other compounds based on rare earth elements, or gadolinium oxysulfide (GD_2O_2S) [8] and finally from rare earth based garnet material (98% garnet, 2% rare earth cerium). The scintillator crystals have a thickness of 1 2 mm and are shaped so that the majority of the photons created as described above pass through the rear wall of the crystal. Here, a photomultiplier amplifies the light signal and photo-detectors convert the light into an electrical signal.

Scintillation detectors have a high time resolution [8]. This is because the duration of the flash in a scintillator is extremely short; for example for NaI, it lasts 0.25 ns. In addition, because the materials from which scintillators are made have a large atomic number, these sensors absorb radiation strongly and this affects their detection efficiency. Because there are two processes involved in this type of measurement, we have to take care that the light contact between the scintillator and the photo-detectors is good enough to maintain an adequate level of detection efficiency. An individual semiconductor detector has greater measurement sensitivity than an individual ionization chamber in a xenon detector, but ionization chambers can be packed much more densely, so that the overall sensitivities of the xenon and the semiconductor detectors are very similar.

3.3.1 Detector Matrices

The introduction of scanner designs with projection systems moving in a spiral required the development of detector arrays that could measure the intensity of X-ray beams having non-zero solid angle along the axis of the patient [20].

Since the introduction of multi-slice spiral tomography (MSCT), there has been rapid development of technologies allowing the manufacture of detector matrices with very sophisticated specifications in terms of size and efficiency. An example of a design of detector array, which enables the subsequent reconstruction of four slices simultaneously in an MSCT scanner, is shown in Fig. 3.30.

In the outermost detectors of an array, a phenomenon called image smearing occurs in the reconstructed slices [20, 31]. This happens because, for a slice of nominal width of 1 mm, the effective width of the outer slice is 6.6 mm (see the right half of Fig. 3.30b). In practice, in order to solve this problem, we sum the electrical signals from outer detectors to obtain a single slice (see the left half of Fig. 3.30b). This reduces the effective width of the slice in question (in this case, reduced to 4.7 mm).

The existence of certain design factors in detector arrays, such as gaps between the individual detectors, has led manufacturers of these components to carry out further research. In order to compensate for the increased angle of incidence of the X-rays on the screen, *adaptive array detectors* (AAD) have been used in some design solutions [18, 26]. In these, instead of separate electrical connections to each detector, some of the detectors in the array have been physically integrated. An example of this type of detector array is shown in Fig. 3.31.

Spiral cone-beam scanners that reconstruct 128 slices simultaneously use a technique called *z-Sharp* by one manufacturer and *z-Wobble* by another. These projection systems use a dual focus X-ray tube and a specially adapted detector array. The arrangement is shown in Fig. 3.32. By doubling the number of photodetectors in relation to the number of scintillator crystals and by changing the focus of the X-ray tube at high frequency, it has been possible to obtain images with very high contrast. At the same time, the width of the image slices has been reduced to less than 0.4 mm.

3.3.2 Detector Parameters

The literature lists the following parameters that describe the quality of measurements achieved by various X-ray detectors

- quantum efficiency,
- energy resolution,
- afterglow,
- stability over time,
- inertia,

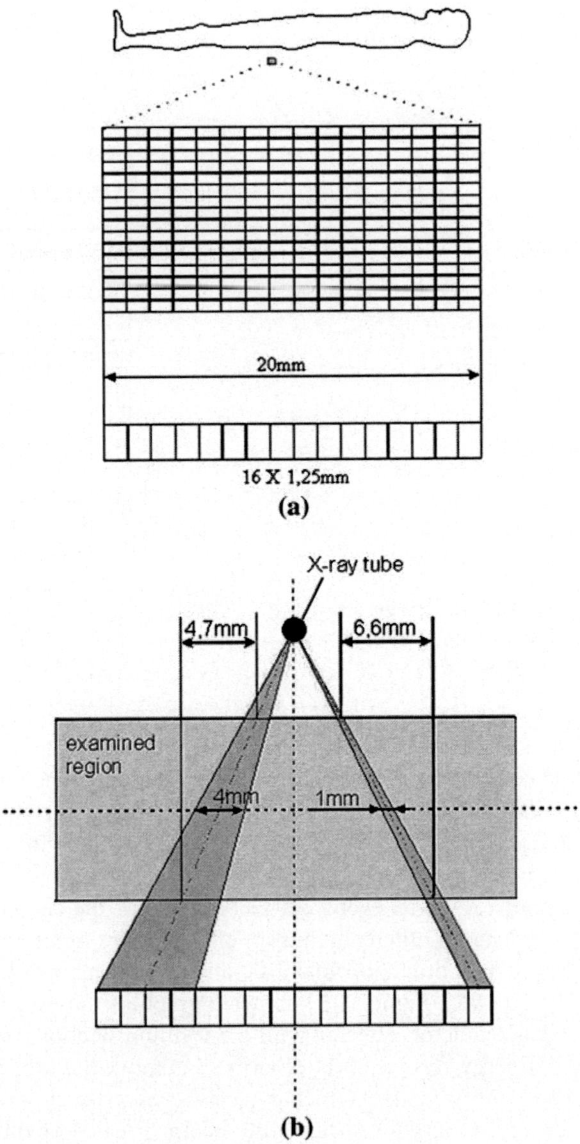

Fig. 3.30 A detector array used in spiral tomography: **a** front and side views of the array, **b** image smearing in the outer layers

- spatial resolution,
- resistance to irradiation damage,
- internal detector noise.

The quantum efficiency is defined as the ratio between the number of quanta registered by the detector and the total number of quanta striking the detector. The limited extent to which gas detectors absorb X-rays reduces their efficiency to between 30 and 60%. Because the atomic numbers of materials used to construct

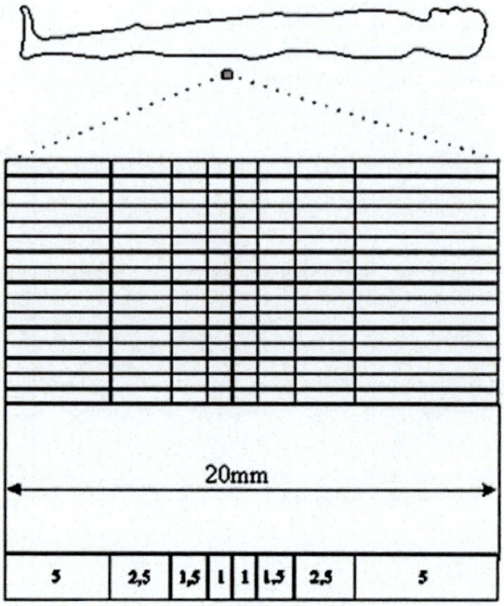

Fig. 3.31 A modified detector used in spiral tomography: front view of the array, and side view

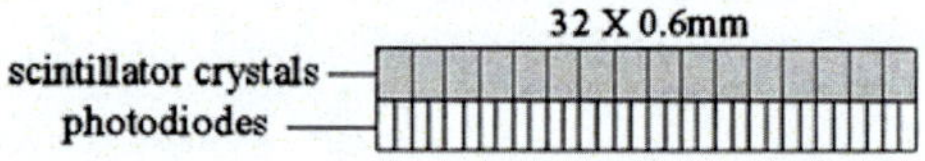

Fig. 3.32 A detector array using *z Sharp* or *z Wobble* technology (*side view*)

scintillators are much larger than the atomic numbers of gases, semiconductor detectors have significantly better quantum efficiencies than xenon proportional chambers (from 98 to 99.5%) [15]. On the other hand, the two-stage conversion process of X-ray quanta into an electrical signal in semiconductor detectors results in additional losses due to the conversion of the light photons into electrical impulses, which evens out the benefits of the two detection techniques.

Quantum efficiency has an effect on the minimum radiation dose that must be applied in order to obtain an image with a specific contrast and signal-to-noise ratio (*SNR*). Figure 3.33 shows a graph of the transfer characteristic of an Si (Li) semiconductor detector with a beryllium window of thickness 8 μm.

Energy resolution is described as the *full width at half maximum* (*FWHM*) of the detector's transfer characteristic as a function of the incident X-ray photon energy. Figure 3.34 shows the characteristics of three types of detector and how the *FWHM* is determined.

As shown in Fig. 3.34, we first find the X-ray frequency at which maximum detection occurs and then determine the maximum value and divide it by two to get the reference level. This is the level at which we estimate the width of the transfer function, which in turn determines the energy resolution of the detector. The smaller the width, the higher the energy resolution of the detector and the less image distortion caused by a polychromatic X-ray beam.

The stability over time of measurements obtained using different types of X-ray detectors is determined above all by the radiation intensity. Xenon proportional

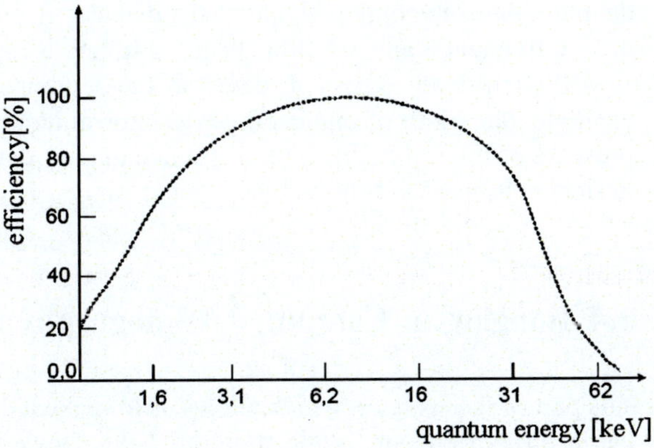

Fig. 3.33 The transfer characteristic of an Si (Li) semiconductor detector

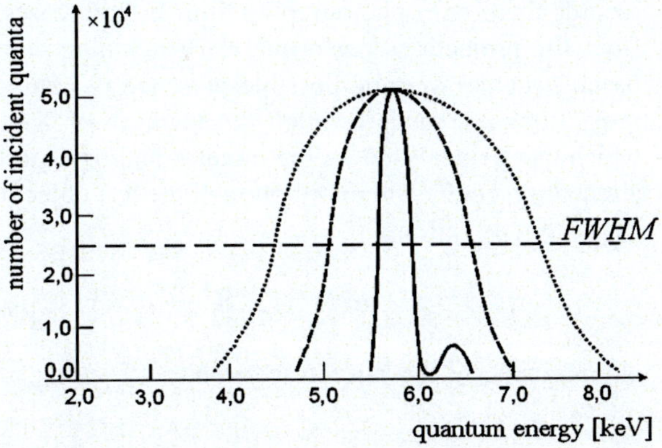

Fig. 3.34 Determination of the energy resolution

chambers meet the highest specifications in terms of their insensitivity to radiation overload. Semiconductor detectors have a tendency to change their properties during irradiation, resulting in a change in transfer characteristics. All semiconductor crystals however are able to return to their initial properties after a certain period after the irradiation has stopped. This time may be hours or minutes, depending on the type of material. At present, the aim is to obtain semiconductor detectors with a return time of the order of seconds [15].

After the X-rays have interacted with the sensors in the matrix, degradation of the output signal occurs. This can also happen when there are sudden large changes of attenuation coefficient along the path of the rays reaching the detector. Two parameters are used to quantify this degradation: *primary speed* and *afterglow*. The primary speed can be understood as one of the impulse response parameters of the detector, which is obtained after the input of a brief pulse of X-rays. Afterglow occurs following a sudden change in X-ray intensity, caused in turn by defects in the crystal structure in the detectors. The existence of electron traps where the crystal defects are situated causes optical recombination of the electrons. This shows up as thermal motion. Image distortions arising from the degradation of the output signal of the detectors (especially ceramic detectors) are of low frequency and are difficult to eliminate using algorithms [15, 19].

Although both types of detector have comparable spatial resolution (for example, the width of one ceramic detector in an array may be 0.95 mm [8]), the prospect of the miniaturisation of semiconductor detectors is encouraging scanner designers to use them in an ever greater range of components.

3.4 Imaging in Computed Tomography Devices

The part of the scanner, which allows us to make a diagnosis after the examination has been carried out, is the monitor. Note, however, that diagnostically useful images can also then be sent to a device (i.e. the documentation camera) that records them onto photographic film. In both cases, it is the image reconstructed from the projections performed earlier, which carries the information about the tissue structure and the possible presence of abnormalities. In a CT scanner, the projections are made through the medium of X-rays. The reconstructed image, which can be analysed on the monitor and/or exposed on film is simply the X-ray attenuation coefficient distribution of the test object (the patient's body), which can be written as follows

$$\mu : (x, y) \in \mathbb{R}^2 \xrightarrow{\mu} \mu(x, y) \in [\mu_{min}, \mu_{max}], \tag{3.12}$$

alternatively, in the discrete version

$$\hat{\mu} : \{1, 2, \ldots, I\} \times \{1, 2, \ldots, J\} \xrightarrow{\hat{\mu}} \hat{\mu}(i, j) \in [\mu_{min}, \mu_{max}]. \tag{3.13}$$

Both for technical as well as practical reasons, it is more convenient to use a digital image. Before tackling the issue of digital visualisation, we should first clarify the concept of luminance, which is a key term used to describe images.

3.4.1 Luminance of the Image

Luminance is defined by the following equation [16]

$$lum(x, y) \triangleq \int_0^\infty \Lambda(\lambda) I_{light}(x, y, \lambda) \mathrm{d}\lambda, \tag{3.14}$$

where λ is the wavelength of the light; $I_{light}(x, y, \lambda)$ is the distribution of the light emitted by the object; $\Lambda(\lambda)$ is a function relating the efficiency of the visual system to the wavelength of the light.

This function assigns a value for the luminous intensity to each point on an image and will be referred to as the luminance of the analogue image. The assignment can be described by the following transformation

$$lum : \Xi \xrightarrow{lum} [lum_{\min}, lum_{\max}] \subset \mathbb{R}, \tag{3.15}$$

where $\Xi = \{(x, y) : 0 \le x \le x_{\max}, 0 \le y \le y_{\max}\} \subset \mathbb{R} \times \mathbb{R}$; $lum_{\min}$ is the minimum luminance in the image; $lum_{\max}$ is the maximum luminance in the image, $x_{\max}$ is the horizontal size of the image; $y_{\max}$ is the vertical size of the image.

The analogue luminance of the image as defined above forms the basis of operations that change the appearance of the image on the computer monitor into a form that is useful for the radiologist. It is also important to look at the following two processes: discretisation of the analogue image and quantisation of the image.

3.4.2 Discretisation and Quantisation of the Image

In order to digitise an image, the analogue image as represented by its luminance must be subjected to sampling (discretisation) and quantisation [9, 16], in the order given in Fig. 3.35.

As shown in Fig. 3.35, the analogue luminance of the image is first subjected to sampling, using the following transformation

$$\hat{lum}(i, j) = lum(x, y) \cdot comb(x, y; \Delta_x, \Delta_y), \tag{3.16}$$

where $\Delta_x = \frac{1}{2f_{x0}}$ is the horizontal raster discretisation; $\Delta_y = \frac{1}{2f_{y0}}$ is the vertical raster discretisation; f_{x0}, f_{y0} are the horizontal and vertical cut-off frequencies of the image, and where

$$comb(x, y; \Delta_x, \Delta_y) \triangleq \sum_{i=1}^{I} \sum_{j=1}^{J} \delta(x - i\Delta_x, y - j\Delta_y), \tag{3.17}$$

where *I*, *J* are the number of image points sampled vertically and horizontally, respectively.

By combining Eqs. (3.16) and (3.17), we obtain the formula

$$\hat{lum}(i, j) = \sum_{i=1}^{I} \sum_{j=1}^{J} lum(x, y) \cdot \delta(x - i\Delta_x, y - j\Delta_y). \tag{3.18}$$

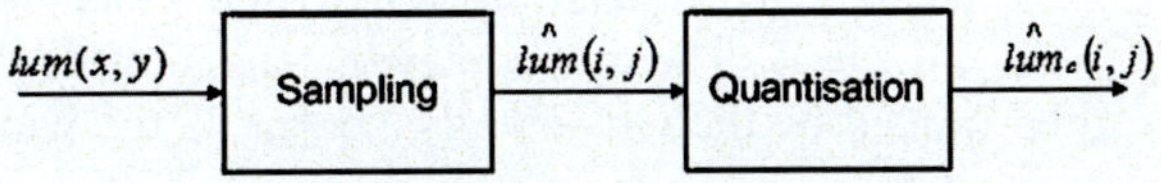

Fig. 3.35 Sampling and quantisation of an analogue image

In the image to be digitised, the units of area, to which uniform luminance values are assigned, are called pixels and are indexed using $i = 1, 2,\ldots, I; j = 1, 2,\ldots, J$. In practice, the display resolutions most often used for tomographic images are: 256 × 256, 320 × 320, 512 × 512, 1,024 × 1,024 and 2,048 × 2,048.

In the frequency domain, the following relationship corresponds to the transformation defined by Eq. (3.18)

$$\hat{LUM}(f_x,f_y) = LUM(f_x,f_y) * COMB(f_x,f_y). \tag{3.19}$$

The next step in converting the analogue image into a digital image is quantisation

$$\hat{lum}_c : \Xi_c \overset{lum_c}{\rightarrow} \Omega, \tag{3.20}$$

where $\Xi_c = \{(i\Delta_x, j\Delta_y) : 0 \le i \le x_{\max}, 0 \le j \le y_{\max}\} \subset \mathbb{I} \times \mathbb{I}$; $\Omega = \{0, 1, \cdot, 2^q - 1\}$; q is the number of bits used to encode the luminance value of the image point, in natural binary code.

The luminance as defined by (3.20) is called the digital luminance of the image, and each point on the image is defined by the digital luminance function $\hat{lum}_c(i,j)$. There are obvious similarities between the transformations (3.15) and (3.20) but the former describes the luminance distribution of the analogue image and the latter of the digital image. The range of values of $\hat{lum}_c(i,j)$ depends on the number of quantisation levels, which in turn depends on the number of bits assigned to encode the luminance of the pixels. This is usually 8 bits, representing 256 quantisation levels or 9 bits and 512 quantisation levels.

In order for the projections performed by the scanner to be subjected to the reconstruction process, we need to obtain the attenuation coefficient distribution in the cross-section of the test object. To display the reconstructed image of the attenuation coefficient distribution $\mu(x,y)(\hat{\mu}(i,j))$ on the computer screen in a way that will be diagnostically useful however, we need to apply the following non-linear transformation

$$imaging : \mu(x,y) \in \mathbb{HU} \overset{imaging(C,W)}{\longrightarrow} \hat{lum}_c \in \Omega \tag{3.21}$$

or in the discrete version

$$imaging : \hat{\mu}(i,j) \in \mathbb{HU} \overset{imaging(C,W)}{\longrightarrow} \hat{lum}_c(i,j) \in \Omega. \tag{3.22}$$

It is common practice in medical applications to use units on the Hounsfield scale: Hounsfield units (HU) [3, 17]. Their value usually varies in the range −1,000 to 3,000, making it necessary to apply a so-called *window*. This term defines a section of the scale, which is determined by two parameters: the *window centre C* and the *window width W*. The first parameter specifies the centre of the range of the scale to be framed by the window; the second is the width of this range.

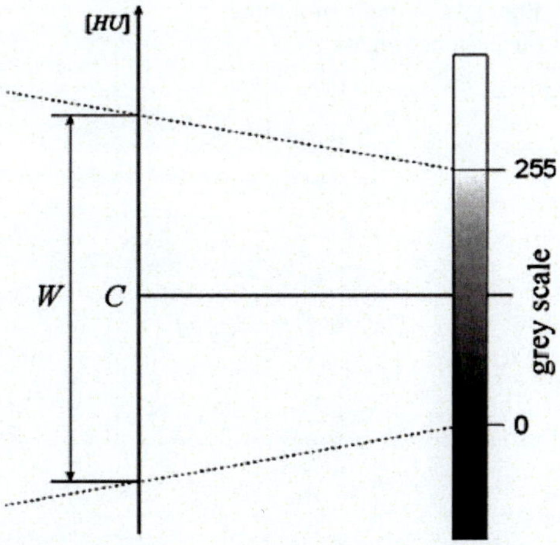

Fig. 3.36 Applying an imaging window to values on the Hounsfield scale

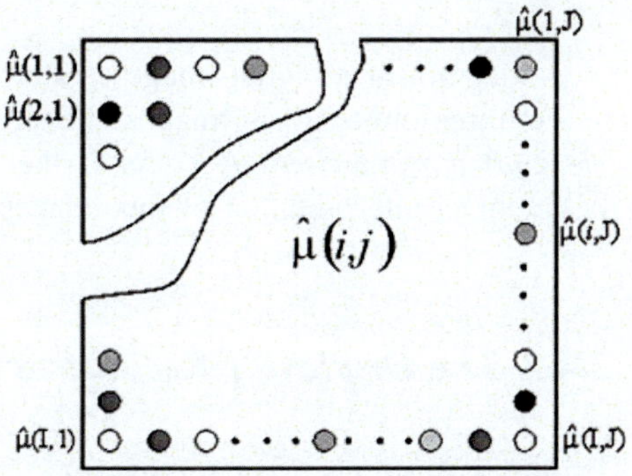

Fig. 3.37 Arrangement of pixels in a digital image

In practice, the assignment (3.22) is performed according to the following rules

1. the points at which the function $\hat{\mu}(i,j)$ is to be determined, are assigned to corresponding points on the screen;
2. the luminance values at these points are determined as follows

$$\hat{lum}_c(i,j) = \begin{cases} 0 & \text{for} \quad \hat{\mu}(i,j) \le C - \frac{W}{2} \\ 2^q - 1 & \text{for} \quad \hat{\mu}(i,j) \ge C + \frac{W}{2} \\ \left(\frac{\left(\hat{\mu}(i,j) - C + \frac{W}{2}\right) \cdot (2^q - 1)}{W} \right) \, div \, 1 & \text{for} \quad C - \frac{W}{2} < \hat{\mu}(i,j) < C + \frac{W}{2} \end{cases}, \quad (3.23)$$

A pictorial representation of this assignment, for $q = 8$ is given in Fig. 3.36.

In practice, a variety of different values of C and W are used, for example, $C = 1,000$ HU and $W = 2,500$ HU for bone imaging, $C = -50$ HU and $W = 400$ HU for the mediastinum, $C = -600$ HU and $W = 1,700$ HU for the lungs.

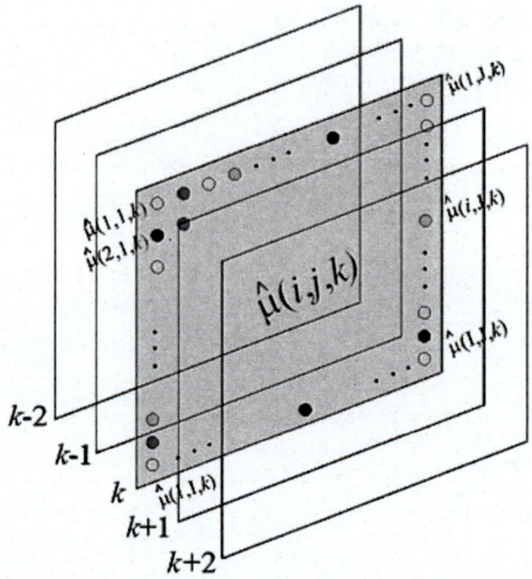

Fig. 3.38 Voxels in a three dimensional image

A diagram of a digital image created in this way is given in Fig. 3.37 [9].

For three-dimensional images, the term voxel (a contraction of the term *volume element*) is often used. A voxel is the three-dimensional equivalent of a pixel. A graphical interpretation of this concept is shown in Fig. 3.38.

3.4.3 The Display of Reconstructed Images

During a comprehensive tomographic examination, a series of actions are performed, the result of which is a set of images of successive slices of the patient's body. During the preliminary phase of the procedure, the table with the patient on it is positioned inside the opening of the gantry. The distance that the patient is inserted into the gantry, the height of the table, and the angle of inclination of the gantry are all factors that can be adjusted. All of these options are shown in Fig. 3.39.

The position of the patient at this stage depends on the part of the body that is to be scanned. In order to position the appropriate region of the patient's body accurately, a preliminary scan is performed to produce a reference image similar to a standard X-ray image (see the illustration in Fig. 3.40). Some scanner manufacturers call this a *topogram* or *toposcan*.

The main difference between this image and an ordinary X-ray image is that it is in electronic form. The scanner's application software uses this image to determine the positions at which subsequent projections will be performed. The places where image slices are planned are indicated using a feature of the application called *field of view* (FOV) markers, as shown in Fig. 3.40. Scans are then carried out on the motionless patient according to the parameters determined by the radiology staff.

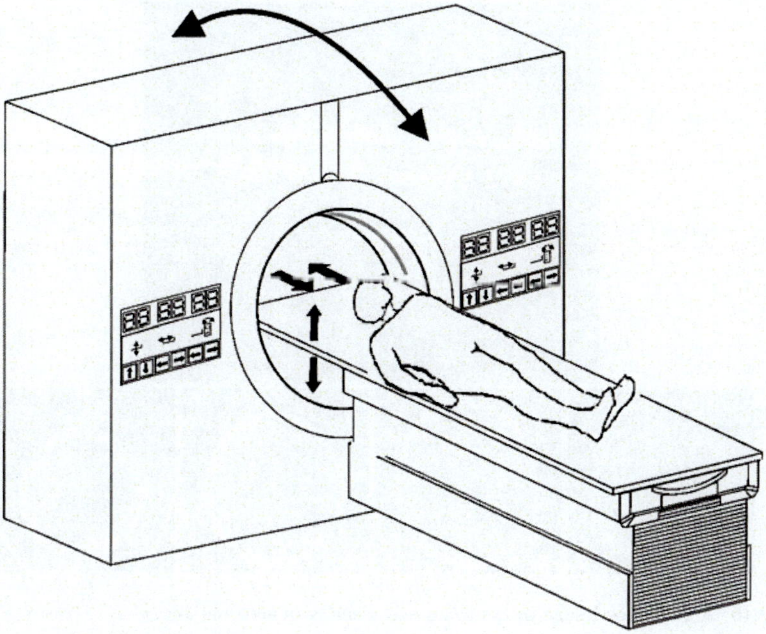

Fig. 3.39 Positioning the patient in the gantry

It is worth mentioning that, in order to enhance the view of certain organs, the scan is often preceded by the intravenous injection of a contrast agent into the patient.

The digital images obtained after reconstructing all the images of the individual slices of the patient's body are known as tomograms. Each of the tomograms may be visualised on demand as described below. An example of a set of tomograms is shown in Fig. 3.40.[3]

This set of tomographic images forms the basis of the next phase of the process: diagnosis. During diagnosis, the radiologist may use additional features of the tomography software to identify a *region of interest* (ROI) (and possibly enlarge it), to measure distances on the tomogram, calculate the radiation attenuation coefficients of selected areas and to display the attenuation coefficients of any of the slices, etc. In addition, the use of windows with different values of C and W presents the radiologist with a great opportunity to evaluate different diagnostic aspects of the image (see the displays of the same reconstructed image using windows with different parameters in Fig. 3.41 (see footnote 3).

[3] Image made available by the Private Health Care Group "Unimed", Czestochowa, Poland.

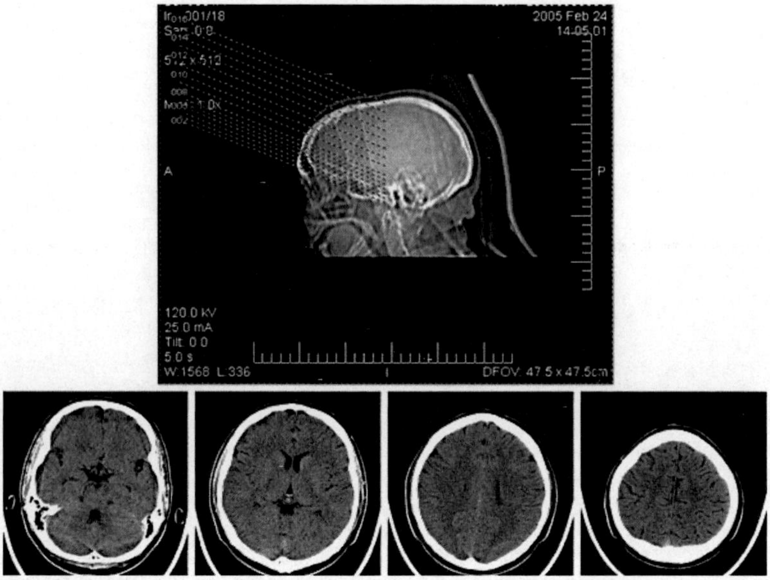

Fig. 3.40 A reference image of the brain and a series of selected slices

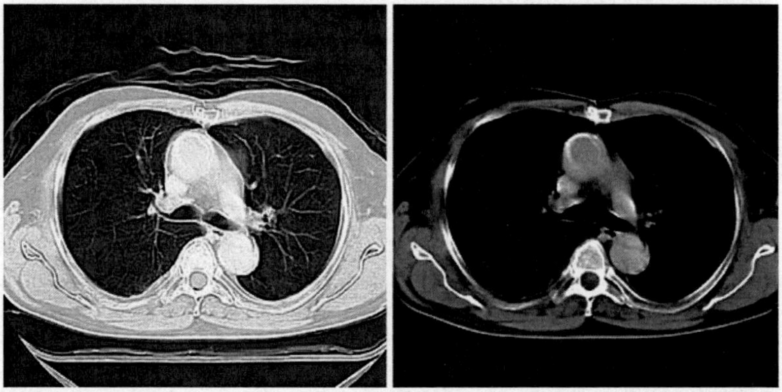

Fig. 3.41 The same slice viewed with different values of window parameters: the left image with the pulmonary window (C 600, W 1, 600), the right image with the mediastinal window (C 50, W 350)

After obtaining a complete set of tomographic images of neighbouring slices, it is possible to use special techniques to visualise the results of the scan in three dimensions.

One of these techniques is *multi-planar reconstruction* (MPR) also known as *multi-planar reformatting*. Using this technique, we can obtain images of any plane in the body (unlike standard X-ray images, these images represent the

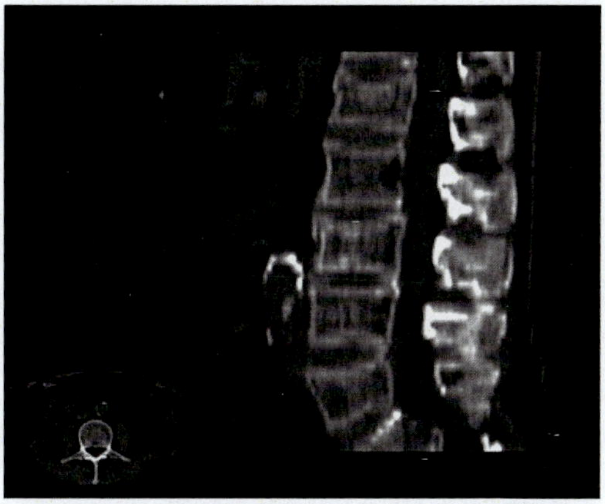

Fig. 3.42 An image of lumbar vertebrae obtained using the MPR technique

properties of the tissues in the selected layer only). An example of an image obtained in this way is shown in Fig. 3.42 (see footnote 3).

With a three-dimensional image of the human body at our disposal, we can construct a three-dimensional model of any organ, using a technique called *volume rendering* [34]. Because some organs have a relatively uniform structure, it is possible to obtain 3D images of such structures as blood vessels, soft tissue or bone.

One use of this imaging method is in the visualisation of internal voids in the body, so-called *virtual endoscopy*. This technique allows us to carry out a virtual examination of organs such as the bronchi, the gastrointestinal tract or blood vessels; it lets us "wander" around inside these organs and study their internal surfaces.

A variant of the image rendering technique mentioned above is an approach called *three-dimensional surface shaded display* (3D SSD) [6, 24]. In this method, the shading of the three-dimensional surface of the object is obtained by using simple thresholding. A virtual light source is placed near the test object, and the attenuation of the light intensity as it encounters elements of the object is simulated. It is easy to obtain images of objects such as bone, which have high values of HU, using this technique. An example of this visual effect is shown in Fig. 3.43 (see footnote 3).

Another approach, called *maximum intensity projection* (MIP) [5], enables us to visualise the structure of a test object by selecting the highest value of HU coefficient occurring along the path of the rays passing through the object at a given angle of observation. It allows us in particular to examine blood vessels, after the injection of a contrast agent. An example image obtained using this technique is shown in Fig. 3.44 (see footnote 3).

The scanner's user software also provides a number of additional visual effects to aid the correct interpretation of reconstructed images. These include various kinds of spatial rotation, shading, highlighting, etc. The radiologist can also choose to archive images that he thinks are diagnostically important. The number of

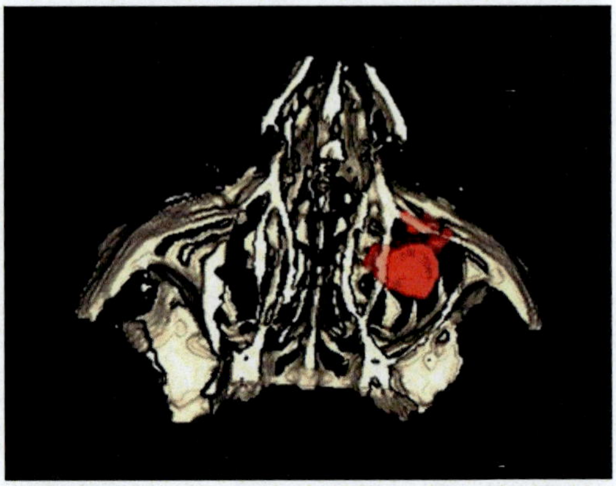

Fig. 3.43 An image of a polyp in the lower maxillary sinus obtained using the 3D SSD technique

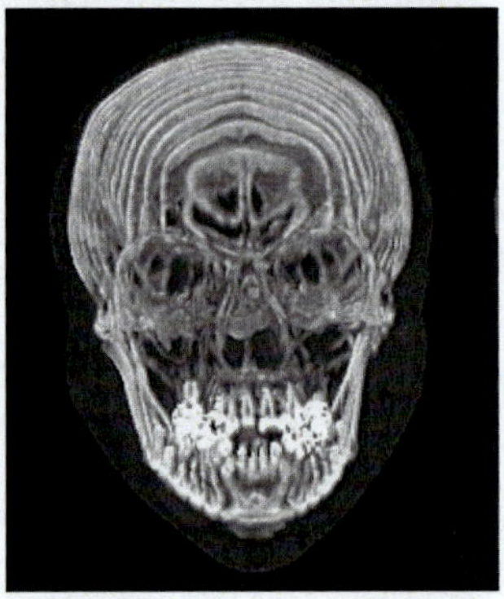

Fig. 3.44 An image of a skull obtained using the MIP technique

archived images is limited however by the large size of the image files and the limited capacity of the computer's permanent storage.

As a rule, after all the examinations and imaging have been completed, a collection of diagnostically useful images is selected and earmarked for physical archiving using the documentation camera. In this way, we obtain a film similar in appearance to a standard X-ray film, but with the images arranged on it in an appropriate order.

References

1. Arenson JS, Levinson R, Fruendlich D (1993) Dual slice scanner. U.S. Patent No. 5,228,069
2. Arenson JS (1995) Data collection strategies: gantries and detectors. In: Goldman LW, Fowlkes JB (eds) Medical CT and Ultrasound. Advanced Medical Publishing
3. Buzug TM (2008) From photon statistics to modern cone beam CT. Springer, Belin
4. Child CD (1911) Phys Rev (Series I) 32:492

5. Cline HE, Dumoulin CL, Hart HR et al (1987) 3D reconstruction of the brain from magnetic resonanse images using a connectivity algorithm. Magn Reson Imag 5:345 352
6. Elvins TT (1992) A survey of algorithm for volume visualization. Comput Graph 26(3):194 201
7. Fox SH (1997) A review of available solid state CT detector materials. General Electric Comp Publ 97 5175, Milwaukee, WI
8. Fuchs T, Kachelrieß M, Kalender WA (2000) Direct comparison of a xenon and a solid state CT detector system: measurements under working conditions. IEEE Trans Med Imag 19(9):941 948
9. Gonzalez RC, Woods RE (1992) Digital image processing. Addison Wesley, Reading
10. Greskovich CD, Cusano D, Hoffman D et al (1992) Ceramic scintillators for advanced, medical X ray detectors. Am Ceramic Soc Bull 71:1120 1130
11. Greskovich CD, Cusano D (1997) Ceramic scintillators. Annu Rev Mater Sci 27:69 88
12. Haar T, Klingenbeck Regn K, Hupke R (1998) Improvement of CT performance by UFC detector technology. In: Krestin GP, Glazer GM (eds) Advances in CT. In: Proceedings of 4th international Somatom Plus CT sci user conference, Rotterdam
13. Hahn G, Hupke R, Kohl G et al (1997) Ultra fast detector for computed tomograph. Res Innov 1:15 22
14. Heuscher DJ, Lindstrom WW, Tuy HK (1996) Multiple detector ring spiral scanner with relatively adjustable helical paths. U.S. Patent No. 5,485,492
15. Hsieh J, Gurmen OE, King KF (2000) Investigation of a solid state detector for advanced computed tomography. IEEE Trans Med Imag 19(9):930 940
16. Jain AK (1989) Fundamentals of Digitals Image Processing. Prentice Hall, Englewood Cliffs
17. Kak AC, Slanley M (1988) Principles of computerized tomographic imaging. IEEE Press, New York
18. Kalender WA (2009) Computed tomography: fundamentals, system technology. Image quality. Wiley, New York
19. King KF, Crawford CR (1993) Compensation of computed tomograpfy data for X ray detector afterglow artifacts. U.S. Patent 5,265,013
20. Kopp AF, Klingenbeck Regn K, Heuschmid M et al (2000) Multislice computed tomography: Basic principles and clinical applications. Electromed 68(2):94 105
21. Kudo H, Noo F, Defrise M (1998) Cone beam filtered backpropagation algorithm for truncated helical data. Phys Med Biol 43:2885 2909
22. Lakshminarayanan AV (1975) Reconstruction from divergent ray data. Tech Rep TR 92, Department of Computer Science, State University of New York, Buffalo, New York
23. Langmuir I (1913) Phys Rev 2:450
24. Magnusson M, Lez R, Danielsson P E (1991) Evoluation of methods for shaded Surface Display of CT volumes. Comput Med Imag Graph 15(4):247 225
25. Nishimura H, Miyazaki O (1988) CT system for spirally scanning subject on a movable bed synchronized to X ray tube revolution. U.S. Patent No. 4,789,929
26. Ohnesorge B, Flohr T, Schaller S (1999) Technische Grundlagen und Anwendungen der Mehrschicht CT. Radiology 39:923 931
27. Peschmann KR, Couch JL, Parker DL (1981) New developments in digital X ray detection. SPIE 314:50 54
28. Peschmann KR (1981) Xeneon gas ionization detectors. In: Newton TH, Potts DG (eds) Radiology of the scull and brain: technical aspects of computed tomography. Mosby, Saint Louis
29. Rontó G, Tarjan I (1999) An introduction to biophysics with medical orientation. Akademiai Kiado, Budapest
30. Rossner W, Bödinger H, Leppert J et al (1993) The conversion of high energy radiation to visible light by luminescent ceramics. IEEE Trans Nucl Sci NS 40:376 379
31. Schaller S, Flohr T, Klingenbeck K et al (2000) Spiral interpolation algorithms for multislice spiral CT Part I: Theory. IEEE Trans Med Imag 19(9):822 834

32. Schwierz G, Lichtenberg W, Fuhrere K (1980) Influence of the focal spot on CT Image quality. Electromed 4:134 139
33. Taguchi K (1975) U.S. Patent No. 5,825,842
34. Wilson O, Gelder van A, Wilhelms J (1994) Direct volume rendering via 3D textures. Tech Rep USCS CRL 94 19

Chapter 4
The Physics of Data Acquisition

The chance discovery of X-rays, followed by deeper understanding of their nature, properties and methods of generation led not only to the creation of devices to perform standard X-ray photographs (see Fig. 4.1) and mammograms but also to the creation of radiotherapy devices and the development of computed tomography.

4.1 X-ray Propagation Through Matters

In order to help us to understand the nature of X-rays let us assume that we have a beam of monoenergetic photons. One of the fundamental quantities associated with radiation is its intensity I, which is defined as the amount of photon energy passing through unit area in unit time:

$$I = \frac{\text{number\_of\_photons} \cdot hv}{\mathrm{S} \cdot \mathrm{t}} \left[\frac{1}{\mathrm{cm}^2 \cdot \mathrm{s}}\right] \tag{4.1}$$

where h is Planck's constant, v is the frequency of the photon of radiation emitted, S is area, and t is time.

When an X-ray beam of intensity $I(0)$ is directed at an object, certain physical processes take place within the object. These processes are responsible for the attenuation of the radiation, its loss of energy and the consequent raising of the object's temperature. The mechanisms involved include

- the photoelectric effect (absorption),
- incoherent and coherent scattering.

In the case of the photoelectric effect, the X-ray photons interact with the electron shells of the atoms in the irradiated sample [1]. Some of the incident photon energy is used to overcome the binding energy of electrons that are ejected;

R. Cierniak, *X Ray Computed Tomography in Biomedical Engineering*,
DOI: 10.1007/978 0 85729 027 4 4, © Springer Verlag London Limited 2011

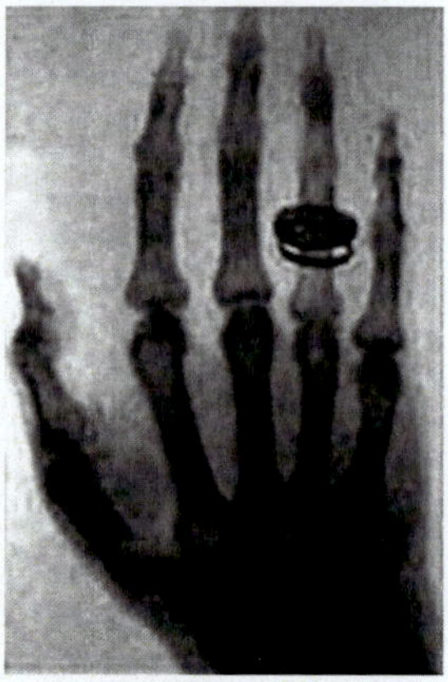

Fig. 4.1 The hand of Professor Albert von Kölliker, the first publicly performed X ray, 23 January 1896

the rest of the energy is transferred to the photoelectrons in the form of kinetic energy

$$E_i = E_b + E_k, \tag{4.2}$$

where E_b is the electron binding energy, E_k is the kinetic energy transferred to the photoelectron, $E_i = h\nu$ is the energy of the incident photon.

The vacancies in lower electron shells cause other electrons from higher shells to move into them. The energy difference between the electron that was removed and the electron brought from the higher shell is emitted as a quantum of secondary X-ray energy. In each element, only certain transitions between shells are permitted and so the quanta of secondary radiation emitted will have well-defined characteristic wavelengths.

Another effect that influences the attenuation of the radiation is scattering, both coherent (Rayleigh) and incoherent (Compton) scattering [1]. In the first case, the X-ray photons incident on the sample change direction without loss of energy. In the second case, the radiation quanta both change their direction and lose energy during their interaction with the electrons. The remaining energy of a scattered quantum can be expressed by

$$E_n = \frac{h\nu}{1 + \zeta(1 - \cos \xi)}, \tag{4.3}$$

where ζ is the ratio of the incident quantum energy to the rest energy of the target electron with which the quantum interacts, ξ is the angle of scattering, $E_n = h\nu'$ is the energy of the scattered quantum, and ν' is the frequency of the scattered quantum.

All of the factors mentioned above are responsible, in varying degrees, for the attenuation of X-rays as they pass through an object. If we accept that each of the three factors mentioned above has an influence on the radiation passing through the sample then we should be able to determine the total value of the factor attenuating this radiation. This is called the *mass attenuation coefficient* [17, 19] or alternatively the *linear attenuation coefficient* [4] (for the sake of simplicity the linear attenuation coefficient will in future be referred to as the attenuation coefficient):

$$\mu = \mu_a + \mu_c + \mu_n, \tag{4.4}$$

where μ_a is the true absorption coefficient caused by the photoelectric effect (absorption), μ_c is the scattering coefficient for coherent scattering, μ_n is the scattering coefficient for incoherent scattering.

The value of the attenuation coefficient is a characteristic of a particular substance and is given in tables of physical constants.

It should be stressed that the attenuation coefficient is the link between the physical processes occurring inside a substance as X-rays pass through and the mathematical relationships allowing us to quantify the interaction.

To define the basic mathematical relationships describing the passage of X-rays through matter, let us consider a beam of radiation of intensity $I(0)$ directed at a uniform object of cross-sectional area 1 m^2, as shown in Fig. 4.2.

Let us assume that in 1 m^3 of the irradiated material there are N centres of interaction, which cause the incident radiation to undergo attenuation, and that after passing through a distance u the radiation intensity has a value $I(u)$. In an extremely thin layer of width du there will be $N \cdot \mathrm{d}u$ centres of interaction. The total reduction of X-ray intensity d$I(u)$ in this layer is proportional to the number of incident photons per unit time and to the number of centres of interaction in the layer:

$$\mathrm{d}I(u) = -\sigma \cdot I(u) \cdot N\mathrm{d}u, \tag{4.5}$$

where σ (m^2) is the constant of proportionality (dependent on the type of material) known as the total cross-section.

This relationship is only valid for isotropic scattering of photons or ejected electrons, where the total cross-section $\sigma(\phi, \psi)$ is constant, i.e. not dependent on the direction of scattering (the angles ϕ and ψ are directions in the spherical coordinate system). Dividing both sides of Eq. 4.5 by $I(u)$ and integrating both sides over the thickness of the sample U, as in the equation below:

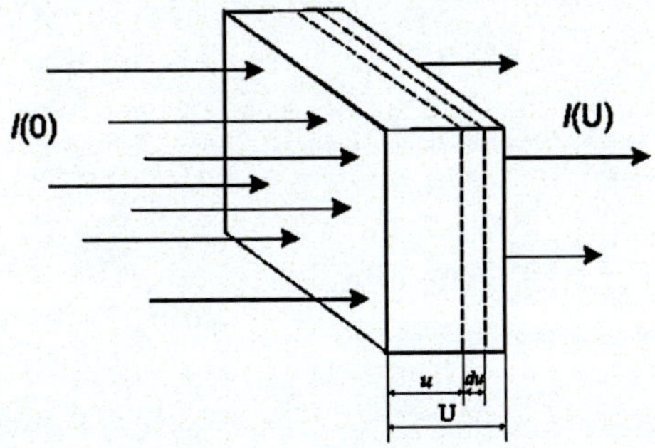

Fig. 4.2 The attenuation of X rays as they pass through matter

$$\int_{0}^{U} \frac{dI(u)}{I(u)} = -\sigma \cdot N \int_{0}^{U} du, \tag{4.6}$$

we obtain the relationship [17, 19]:

$$I(U) = I(0) \cdot e^{\sigma N U} = I(0) \cdot e^{\mu_{const} U}, \tag{4.7}$$

where $\mu_{const} = \sigma N$ (m^{-1}) is the attenuation coefficient (dependent on the material).

If we have a heterogeneous sample of material (such as the human body), we should replace the attenuation coefficient in Eq. 4.7 with the integral of the attenuation coefficient over the path through which the radiation passes (see Fig. 4.3). So for a one-dimensional path, the equation takes the following form:

$$I(U) = I(0) \cdot e^{\int_{0}^{U} \mu(u) du}, \tag{4.8}$$

where $\mu(u)$ is the function defining the attenuation coefficient distribution along the path of the radiation.

The determination of $\mu(u)$ allows us to define the spatial structure of the human body in terms of the ability of its individual layers to attenuate radiation. This will allow us to distinguish the body tissues in a tomographic image, characterised as

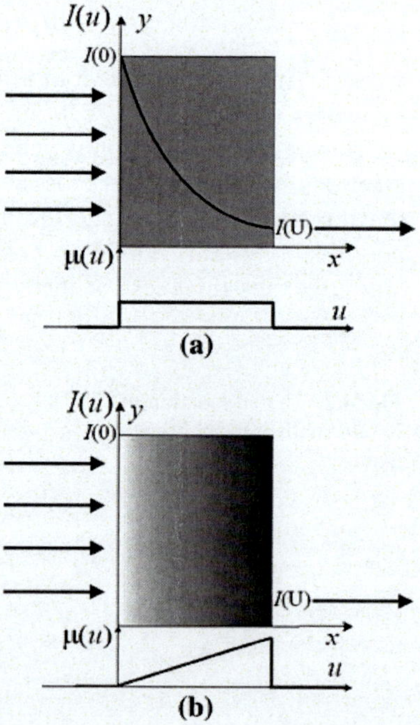

Fig. 4.3 The transmission of radiation through matter. **a** A homogeneous attenuation coefficient, **b** a linearly increasing attenuation coefficient

Table 4.1 The proportions of some elements in selected tissues (in the case of blood given in mg/dm^3, for the remaining tissues in μg/g of dry mass ppm)

Element	Blood	Brain	Liver	Lungs	Muscles
Sodium (Na)	1,970.00	10,000.00	5,500.00	1,200.00	4,000.00
Potassium (K)	1,620.00	11,600.00	7,400.00	8,600.00	10,500.00
Mercury (Hg)	0.0078		0.0220	0.03	0.02
Calcium (Ca)	61.00	320.00	140.00	480.00	105.00
Gold (Au)	0.0002	0.50	0.0001	0.30	0.40
Iron (Fe)	447.00	200.00	520.00	1,300.00	140.00

they are by the distinct properties of their constituent elements and compounds, e.g. calcium and water. Table 4.1 shows the proportions of certain elements in selected tissues.

For convenience during diagnosis, the Hounsfield scale has been introduced [11] to define the degree of attenuation of radiation by various substances. The so-called Hounsfield number for a particular tissue is defined relative to the attenuation properties of water, as follows:

$$HU_{\text{tissue}} = 1{,}000\frac{\mu_{\text{tissue}} - \mu_{\text{H}_2 0}}{\mu_{\text{H}_2 0}}, \qquad (4.9)$$

where μ_{tissue} is the resultant X-ray attenuation coefficient for the tissue, $\mu_{\text{H}_2 0}$ is the X-ray attenuation coefficient for water.

Hounsfield numbers can range from −1,000 for gases up to a maximum of 3,000 for bone. We can, therefore, express the range of Hounsfield numbers as follows:

$$HU \in [-1{,}000, 3{,}000] \subset \mathbb{R}. \qquad (4.10)$$

Hydrated body tissues have a Hounsfield numbers that varies in the region of $HU = 0$. The Hounsfield numbers for various tissues are given in Table 4.2.

Table 4.2 Hounsfield numbers for selected tissues

Tissue	Before the application of contrast	After the application of contrast
Brain	35	45
Fresh blood in the brain	65	
Liver	50	80 90
Kidneys	27 30	100
Spleen	50	70 80
Pancreas	20 30	50
Muscles	40	
Fat	70 to 110	
Bone	300 1,300	

4.2 The Radon Transform

Equation 4.8 is fundamental for X-ray imaging techniques and provides a starting point for considering the physical processes involved. It is, therefore, worth looking at this relationship once more, this time from the point of view of the transmission of an X-ray beam through a sample with specific attenuation characteristics:

$$I(\mathrm{U}) = I(0) \cdot \mathrm{e}^{\int_0^{\mathrm{U}} \mu(x,y)\mathrm{d}u}, \tag{4.11}$$

where $I(0)$ is the initial X-ray intensity, $I(\mathrm{U})$ is the X-ray intensity after passing through a distance U, $\mu(x, y)$ is the function defining the spatial distribution of the attenuation coefficient in the sample.

In the rest of this chapter, we assume that the object being X-rayed is a patient's body, whose form depends on its anatomical structure. Knowledge of the spatial distribution of the attenuation coefficient $\mu(x, y)$ allows us, in most cases, to get a picture of the arrangement of various organs inside the body and makes it possible to diagnose the location of possible injuries. In the next chapters, we will discuss the image reconstruction algorithms that are used to obtain information about the form of $\mu(x, y)$ anywhere in the body from these X-ray projections.

Finding the logarithm of both sides of Eq. 4.11, we obtain a quantity that has fundamental significance for image reconstruction algorithms:

$$p \triangleq \ln\left(\frac{I(0)}{I(\mathrm{U})}\right) = \int_0^{\mathrm{U}} \mu(x,y)\mathrm{d}u, \tag{4.12}$$

In a projection system consisting of an X-ray tube, the patient's body and a photographic film, the quantity p can be interpreted as the ratio of the X-ray intensity directed at a given point in the body to the radiation intensity after passing through the body. In practice, this means less darkening of the photographic film in those places where there has been more attenuation of the radiation as it passes through the various tissues (i.e. there is a negative image on the X-ray film). Figure 4.4 illustrates this effect for a spherical object.

To obtain a picture of the inside of an object, it is necessary to collimate the stream of X-rays to create a suitably shaped beam with which to obtain the projection. Here, by "projection", we mean the image produced on the screen by the X-rays falling on it after they have passed through the patient's body. If the radiation is collimated into a very narrow parallel beam, then we need only use a screen in the form of a thin strip, as shown in Fig. 4.5.

To obtain an image of the cross-section of an object in the plane of the projection, we need to identify parameters for the quantity p, as shown in Fig. 4.6. Here the first parameter is the variable s, describing the axis perpendicular to the direction of the incident X-ray. The value $s = 0$ defines the principal axis of

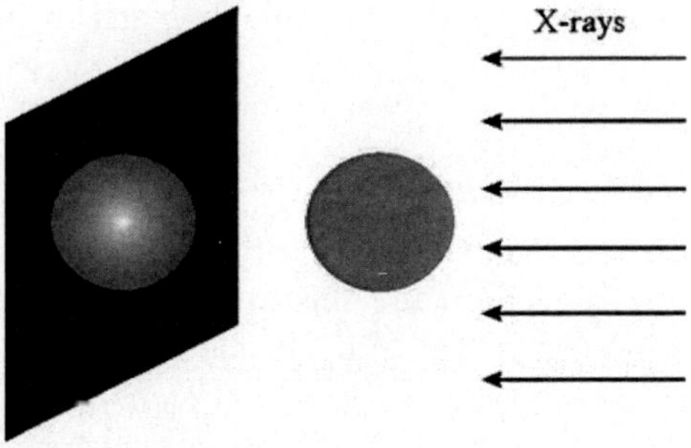

Fig. 4.4 Darkening of a photographic film by X rays

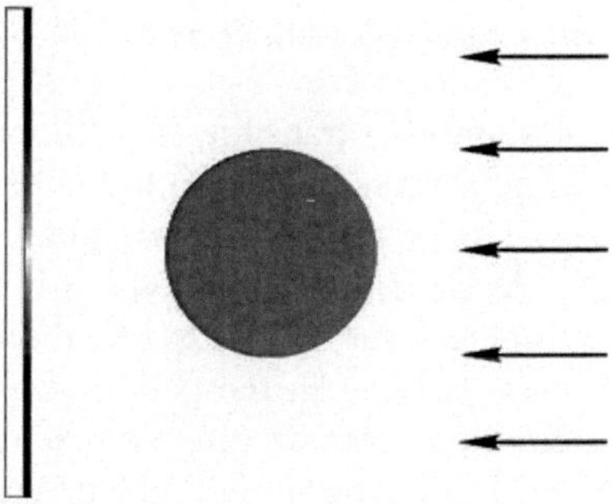

Fig. 4.5 Obtaining projections using a parallel beam of X rays

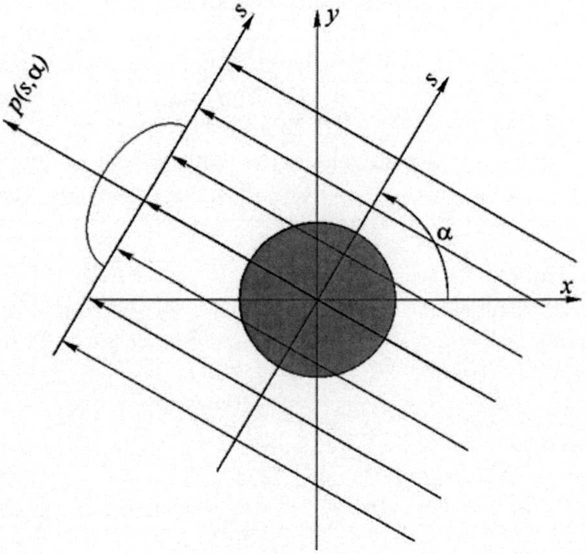

Fig. 4.6 Projections carried out at an angle α

projection. The second parameter is the angle α at which, at any given moment, the projection is made. This is measured relative to the principal projection axis. The point about which the scanner rotates lies on the principal projection axis and for practical reasons is located inside the test object.

We can write the variable p and its parameters as follows:

$$p(s,\alpha) = \int_u \mu(x,y)\mathrm{d}u, \tag{4.13}$$

where the parameters vary within the ranges: $-\infty < s < \infty$, $0 \leq \alpha < \pi$.

In the literature, this equation is often called the Radon transform [9, 11, 14, 16] and is represented mathematically by

$$R : \mu(x,y) \in \mathbb{HU} \xrightarrow{R} p(s,\alpha) \in \mathbb{R}. \tag{4.14}$$

In computed tomography, the Radon transform is performed physically by the attenuation of the X-rays as they pass through the tissues. The task of the apparatus is simply to transmit an appropriately collimated beam of radiation, and then, using sensors placed on the screen, to record the intensity of the radiation after it has passed through the sample.

As shown in Fig. 4.7, the X-ray intensity at a point on the screen corresponds to a single value of $p(s, \alpha)$. As the radiation is in the form of a parallel beam, only material lying in the path of the ray arriving at that point is responsible for the attenuation of the radiation. It follows from Eq. 4.13 that the attenuation takes place along the straight line defined by the parameter u, where the total path length is U.

There is, however, a problem with the use of relationship (4.13). The problem lies in the dependence of the attenuation function on the spatial variables (x, y). The integration with respect to variable u takes place along a line at a distance s from the projection axis. This means that we need to find a formula for converting from the fixed coordinate system (x, y) into the moving system (s, u), which is rotated by an angle α with respect to the (x, y) system. The geometry of

Fig. 4.7 The geometry of the parallel beam scanner

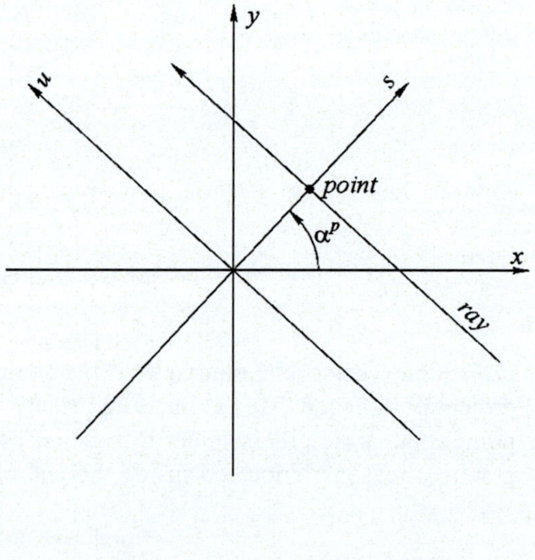

Table 4.3 Trigonometric relationships between the moving coordinate system (*s*, *u*) and the fixed system (*x*, *y*)

$(x, y) \rightarrow (s, u)$		$(s, u) \rightarrow (x, y)$	
s	$x\cos\alpha + y\sin\alpha$	x	$s\cos\alpha \quad u\sin\alpha$
u	$x\sin\alpha + y\cos\alpha$	y	$s\sin\alpha + u\cos\alpha$

the situation is illustrated in Fig. 4.7. This helps to identify the line along which the incident ray lies.

Using Fig. 4.7, we can derive the trigonometric relationships given in Table 4.3. These relationships allow us to convert the coordinates of any point in the fixed coordinate system into coordinates in the moving system and vice versa.

Proof Figure 4.8 illustrates the trigonometric relationships in a parallel-beam scanner.

// Combining the elements $s \quad s' + s''$	Based on Fig. 4.8
// The x relationship in the fixed coordinate // system (x, y) $\frac{s'}{x} \quad \cos\alpha$	Based on Fig. 4.8
// The y relationship in the fixed coordinate // system (x, y) $\frac{s''}{y} \quad \cos(\frac{\pi}{2} \quad \alpha) \quad \sin\alpha$	Based on Fig. 4.8
$s \quad x\cos\alpha + y\sin\alpha$	Substituting into the equation given in step 1 of this proof

and

// Combining the elements $u \quad u' + u''$	Based on Fig. 4.8
// The x relationship in the fixed coordinate // system (x, y) $\frac{u'}{y} \quad \cos\alpha$	Based on Fig. 4.8
// The y relationship in the fixed coordinate // system (x, y) $\frac{u''}{x} \quad \cos(\frac{\pi}{2} \quad \alpha) \quad \sin\alpha$	Based on Fig. 4.8
$u \quad x\sin\alpha + y\cos\alpha$	Substituting into the equation given in step 1 of this proof

Using the trigonometric conversions given in Table 4.3, we can modify Eq. 4.13 as follows:

$$p(s,\alpha) = \int_{\infty}^{\infty}\int_{\infty}^{\infty} \mu(x,y)\delta(x\cos\alpha + y\sin\alpha - s)\mathrm{d}x\mathrm{d}y. \tag{4.15}$$

The equation above means that in order to determine the projection function for a particular point s on the screen and a particular angle of rotation α of the scanner, we simply need to sum the values of the attenuation coefficients of the patient's body along the path of the ray that strikes that point on the screen.

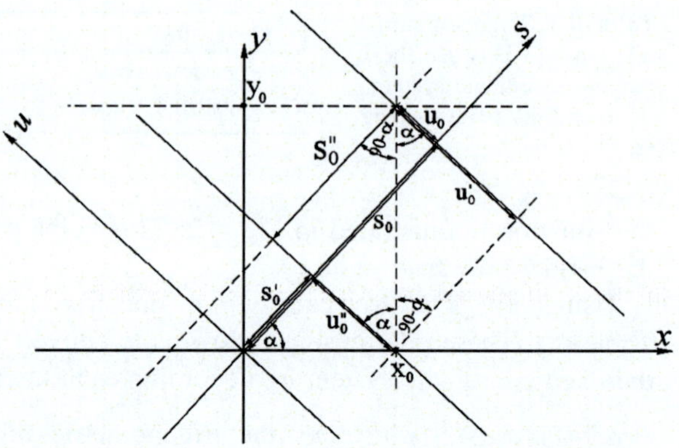

Fig. 4.8 Details of the trigonometric relationships in a parallel beam scanner

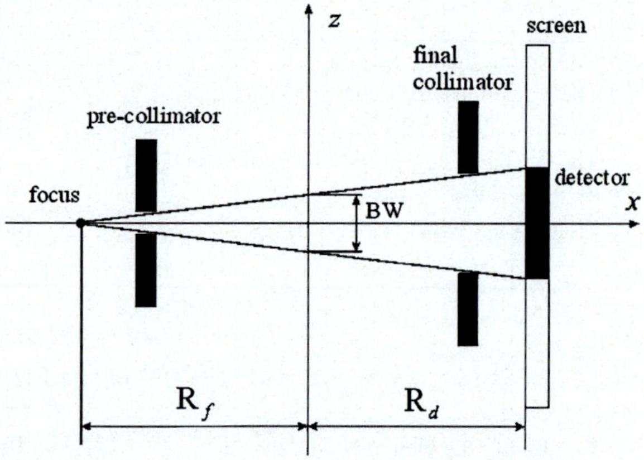

Fig. 4.9 An X ray collimator

4.3 X-ray Collimators

The acquisition of projection values in any CT scanner requires an appropriate projection system (construction details can be found in Chaps. 5, 6 and 7). One of the defining characteristics of a projection system is the shape of X-ray beam used to determine the individual projection values. To obtain a useful beam of the desired shape, the X-rays need to be collimated. A drawing of an X-ray collimator is given in Fig. 4.9.

For convenience, in our theoretical discussions, we will replace the X-ray tube as the source of radiation with a single point situated at the focus of the tube. The beam of radiation produced by the tube is first constrained spatially by the initial collimator (called a pre-collimator). In different designs of CT scanner, collimators with different aperture shapes are used to obtain beams such as those shown schematically in Fig. 4.10.

Figure 4.9 shows the basic layout of a collimator system in which the radiation beam gradual widens as it passes through the irradiated space where the test object is placed. However, when considering reconstruction algorithms we often make a

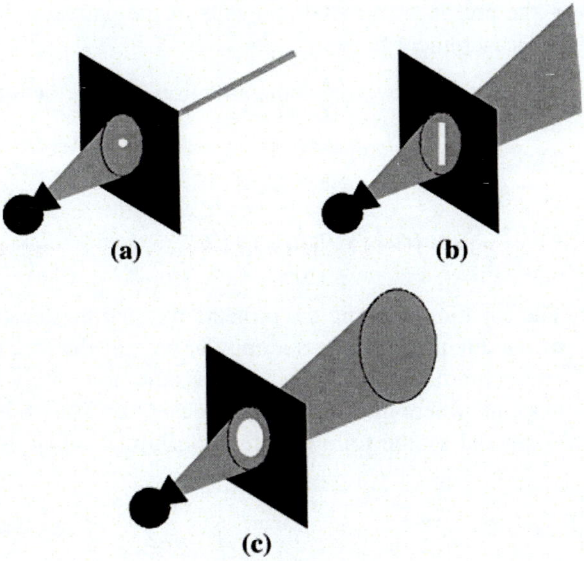

Fig. 4.10 Shapes of X ray beams used in CT scanner projection systems: **a** a parallel beam of radiation, **b** a fan beam of radiation, **c** a beam in the form of a cone

simplification; we define the thickness of the *radiation beam* BW (beam width) as the width of the beam as it crosses the principal projection axis. Before the beam formed in this way reaches the radiation detectors however, further, final collimation takes place. This is to limit the effect of scattering on the measurements.

In Fig. 4.9, the symbol R_d represents the distance of the screen from the main projection axis (the middle of the (x, y) coordinate system) and R_f represents the distance of the focus from the main projection axis. It is worth mentioning that in practice we use the following X-ray beam widths, for example: bones 1 mm, lungs, blood vessels 2 3 mm, kidneys, pancreas 5 mm, chest, liver 8 mm.

4.4 Physical Causes of Artefacts in the Reconstructed Image

All image reconstruction methods produce post-scanning distortions, mainly due to simplifications made during signal processing. We can deal with these kinds of distortions to a limited extent using algorithms. However, there are some artefacts whose causes are not related to the reconstruction method used but result from the physical conditions in which the projections were made. Technical and design limitations of the projection system can have a negative impact on the image quality obtained by computed tomography techniques. Some of the more serious physical factors affecting image quality include:

- the polychromatic nature of the X-ray beam,
- the non-zero thickness of the beam,
- shortcomings in the collimator,

- the presence of metal elements in the patient's body,
- measurement noise.

It is worth devoting some attention to these factors, and to methods of reducing their impact.

4.4.1 Spectral Nonlinearities

The equation defining the projection function, the Radon transform, is the integral of the attenuation values along the path of the ray, but only when the radiation is monochromatic. However, this assumption rarely holds true in real projection systems where the radiation intensity measured by the individual detectors is expressed by the following relationship [11, 14]:

$$I = \int I_0(E) \cdot \mathrm{e}^{\int_0^{\mathrm{U}} \mu(x,y,E)\mathrm{d}u} \mathrm{d}E, \tag{4.16}$$

where $I_0(E)$ is the energy spectrum of the radiation source, U is the distance that the ray travels from the source to the detector, $\mu(x, y, E)$ is the attenuation of radiation with quantum energy E at a specific point in the test object.

Assumptions about the monochromatic nature of the radiation can be expressed as follows:

$$I(E) = I_0 \cdot \delta(E - E^*). \tag{4.17}$$

If we use assumption (4.17) in Eq. 4.16 we get back to Eq. 4.11, defining the intensity of monochromatic X-rays after they have passed through a sample of thickness U. However, we cannot just forget about the realities of the practical situation, so we have take into account the polychromatic nature of the radiation source. As we can see, for example, in Fig. 3.17, the energy spectrum of a radiation source has an upper limit. This allows us to derive an equation to define the projection function for polychromatic radiation in a way similar to that for the monochromic case:

$$p(s, \alpha) = \int_u \mu(x, y, E)\mathrm{d}u, \tag{4.18}$$

where $\mu(x, y, E)$ is the attenuation coefficient, at a point in the test object with coordinates (x, y), of a ray of average energy E.

We can evaluate the integral in Eq. 4.18, which defines the projection $p(s, \alpha)$ for a polychromatic beam, using the following relationship:

$$\int \mu(x,y,E)\mathrm{d}u = \frac{\int I_0(E) \cdot \mathrm{e}^{\int_0^U \mu(x,y,E)\mathrm{d}u} \mathrm{d}E}{\int I_0(E)\mathrm{d}E}. \tag{4.19}$$

Here, the estimator of the integral of the attenuation coefficient distribution is biased, since it depends on the form of the X-ray energy spectrum. Furthermore, the dependence of the estimator on the attenuation value (in turn dependent on the quantum energy) indicates the presence of strong nonlinearities. These arise during the passage of polychromatic radiation because the various components of its energy spectrum are not attenuated uniformly. This happens because of the so-called beam hardening effect. Thus, we cannot express the value of Eq. 4.19 as a linear relationship with the integral of the attenuation coefficient distribution. However, we can use its expansion [2, 5, 14]:

$$\ln\left(\frac{I_0(E)}{I}\right) = a_0 + a_1 \cdot \int \mu(x,y,\overline{E})\mathrm{d}u + a_2\left(\int \mu(x,y,E)\mathrm{d}u\right)^2 + \cdots. \tag{4.20}$$

When the X-ray source is monochromatic or the attenuation coefficient does not depend on the energy of the incident radiation, the above equation can be reduced to the single component with the coefficient a_1. The contributions of the remaining components of the expansion depend on the distribution of $I_0(E)$ and on the strength of the dependence of $\mu(x, y)$ on E. Artefacts caused by the nonlinearities discussed here appear in the reconstructed image especially when a low energy beam is used. This is because in the low energy range $\mu(x, y)$ is strongly dependent on E.

Artefacts resulting from the polychromatic nature of the X-ray beam can be eliminated in many ways [3, 6, 12, 14, 15]. One of the early correction methods was to use a compensating bag of water, which surrounded the test object during a scan [12, 14]. This reduced the degree of variation of the attenuation coefficients of the tissues and corrected for the nonlinearity in Eq. 4.19.

Another way to correct for this kind of nonlinearity is to linearize the exponential function, using the following relationship [14]:

$$\mathrm{e}^{\int \mu(x,y)\mathrm{d}u} \cong 1 - \int \mu(x,y)\mathrm{d}u. \tag{4.21}$$

By substituting this into Eq. 4.19, we can obtain a formula defining the projection integral free of nonlinearities. Unfortunately, the linearization (4.21) is only valid for projection values satisfying the condition:

$$\int \mu(x,y)\mathrm{d}u < 1, \tag{4.22}$$

which for many regions of the human body restricts the use of such methods far too severely.

In computed tomography, the most popular method of reducing the effect of the X-ray spectral distribution is to use special phantoms, which, in structure, size and type of material, resemble the parts of the human body being examined [14]. In this method, the projection is first made with the phantom placed in the scanner at a location corresponding to the position in the body of the part selected for examination. In this way, we obtain the radiation intensity after passage of the radiation along the path U from source to detector as follows:

$$I(\mathrm{U}) = I_0 \cdot \mathrm{e}^{\int_0^{\mathrm{U}} \mu(x,y)\mathrm{d}u} = I_0 \cdot \mathrm{e}^{\mu_{\text{phantom}}\mathrm{U}}, \tag{4.23}$$

which, for the phantom, can be summarized as $\mu(x, y) = \text{const} = \mu_{\text{phantom}}$.

In the next stage of the procedure, projections are carried out on the actual part of the patient's body. The difference between the measurement of radiation intensity made during the actual examination and the measurement made using the phantom is defined by the following Eq. 4.23:

$$I(\mathrm{U}) - I_{\text{phantom}}(\mathrm{U}) = I_0 \cdot \mathrm{e}^{\int_0^{\mathrm{U}} \mu(x,y)\mathrm{d}u} - I_0 \cdot \mathrm{e}^{\mu_{\text{phantom}}\mathrm{U}}. \tag{4.24}$$

After suitable mathematical manipulation, we can represent this difference by:

$$I(\mathrm{U}) - I_{\text{phantom}}(\mathrm{U}) = I_0 \cdot \mathrm{e}^{\mu_{\text{phantom}}\mathrm{U}} \cdot \left(\mathrm{e}^{\left(\int_0^{\mathrm{U}} \mu(x,y)\mathrm{d}u \quad \mu_{\text{phantom}}\mathrm{U}\right)} - 1 \right). \tag{4.25}$$

Assuming a structural similarity between the phantom and the test object, we can say that in all probability:

$$\int_0^{\mathrm{U}} \mu(x, y)\mathrm{d}u - \mu_{\text{phantom}} \cdot \mathrm{U} \ll 1, \tag{4.26}$$

which allows us to use the linearization expressed by Eq. 4.21. So, we now have a linear version of the relationship defining the radiation intensity measured by the detector, after the radiation has passed through the test area of the human body:

$$I(\mathrm{U}) = I_0 \cdot \mathrm{e}^{\mu_{\text{phantom}}\mathrm{U}} \cdot \left(\mu_{\text{phantom}} \cdot \mathrm{U} - \int_0^{\mathrm{U}} \mu(x, y)\mathrm{d}u \right) + I_{\text{phantom}}(\mathrm{U}). \tag{4.27}$$

This method reduces the effect that nonlinearities, caused by the use of polychromatic X-rays, have on the quality of the reconstructed image obtained by computed tomography.

4.4.2 Beam-width Nonlinearities

The next source of non-linear distortion in practical projection systems is related to the fact that the beam width of the collimated X-rays is non-zero with respect to the z axis. For the sake of simplicity, we will assume that the beam is parallel and has an angle of projection of zero, i.e. $\alpha = 0$. This means that the rays making up the beam will be parallel to the y axis of the projection system. We can therefore formulate the relationship defining the projection function measured by the radiation sensors on the screen [6, 14] as follows:

$$I(\mathrm{U}) = \int\int dist(x,z)\mathrm{e}^{\int \mu(x,y,z)\mathrm{d}y}\mathrm{d}x\mathrm{d}z, \tag{4.28}$$

where $dist(x, z)$ is a function defining the radiation distribution in the test layer.

Of course, if the thickness of the body layer irradiated by the beam is very small, then we can omit that dimension from the formula above and so eliminate the problem. In practice, however, it is necessary to take the whole of Eq. 4.28 into account, especially in cases where, within the irradiated layer, there are sudden changes in the coefficient $\mu(x, y, z)$ along the z axis. In that situation, the presence of the exponential term in Eq. 4.28 causes stratification of various parts of the radiation beam, as far as its attenuation along the z axis is concerned. So, as with the nonlinear distortion discussed previously, we can now expand Eq. 4.28 as follows:

$$\ln\left(\frac{I_0(E)}{I}\right) = a_0 + a_1 \cdot \int \mu(x,y,z)\mathrm{d}y + a_2\left(\int \mu(x,y,z)\mathrm{d}y\right)^2 + \cdots, \tag{4.29}$$

where $\mu(x,y,z)$ is the mean value of the attenuation coefficient along the z axis.

Faced with such strong nonlinearities, the most effective way to eliminate these artefacts is to use narrow beams of radiation.

Alternatively, we can minimise this distortion with a technical solution using an array of small detectors in place of a single large one. Assuming that each detector l in the array is very small, we can modify Eq. 4.28 as follows:

$$I_l(\mathrm{U}) = \int\int dist_l(x,z)\mathrm{e}^{\int \mu(x,y,z)\mathrm{d}y}\mathrm{d}x\mathrm{d}z = I_l(0)\mathrm{e}^{\int \mu(x,y)\mathrm{d}y}, \tag{4.30}$$

where $I_l(0) = \iint dist_l(x,z)\mathrm{d}x\mathrm{d}z$ is a function defining the radiation distribution in the test layer.

Each sensor in the array makes its contribution to the measurement of the intensity and the average value of the projection function recorded by the sensors is defined by the relationship:

$$p(s,\alpha_0) = p(x,\alpha_0) = \int \mu(x,y,z)\mathrm{d}u = \frac{1}{\mathrm{L}} \cdot \sum_{l=1}^{\mathrm{L}} \ln\left(\frac{I_l(0)}{I_l(\mathrm{U})}\right). \tag{4.31}$$

This use of the average value of the radiation intensities as measured by the individual detectors of the matrix, results in the elimination of the non-linear distortions caused by the non-zero thickness of the radiation beam.

4.4.3 Scatter Nonlinearities

X-rays scattered by the test object during a CT scan (especially as a result of incoherent or Compton scattering) cause additional components to appear in the individual intensity measurements [8, 10]. Figure 4.11 shows the result of radiation intensity measurements made at the screen and shows a combination of two phenomena absorption (I) and scattering (I_s).

The radiation intensity recorded is the sum of these two components:

$$I_{sum} = I + I_s, \tag{4.32}$$

and after appropriate modification takes the following form:

$$\ln(I_{sum}) = \ln I \cdot \left(1 + \frac{I_s}{I}\right). \tag{4.33}$$

If the term $\frac{I_s}{I}$ is small compared to one, we can say:

$$-\ln(I_{sum}) \approx -\ln I - \frac{I_s}{I}. \tag{4.34}$$

After subtracting $\ln(I_0)$ from both sides of Eq. 4.34, we obtain:

$$-\ln\left(\frac{I_{sum}}{I_0}\right) \approx -\ln\left(\frac{I}{I_0}\right) - \frac{I_s}{I}. \tag{4.35}$$

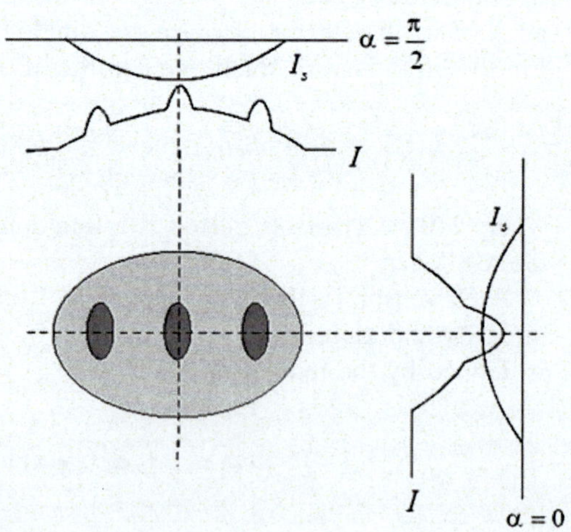

Fig. 4.11 Components of radiation intensity measurements made at angles 0° and 90°

Bearing in mind the definition of a projection given in Eq. 4.12, the equation above leads to the following:

$$p_{\text{sum}} \approx p - \frac{I_s}{I}. \tag{4.36}$$

where $p_{\text{sum}} \equiv -\ln\left(\frac{I_{\text{sum}}}{I_0}\right)$.

From Eq. 4.36, we can assume that a reduction of the measured radiation intensity I corresponds to rays passing through areas with high absorption coefficient. This implies an increase in the value of $\frac{I_s}{I}$, that is an increase in the influence of the scattering effect on the measurements (as can be seen in Fig. 4.11, the influence of the term $\frac{I_s}{I}$ is greater at an angle of projection $\alpha = 0°$ than at an angle $\alpha = 90°$). The artefacts produced in this way appear as black stripes in the reconstructed image of the object's cross-section. We can counteract distortions caused by the scattering effect in two ways: by increasing the precision of the collimator and using an algorithm to correct the radiation intensity measurements. The first of these methods relies on designing the collimator in such a way as to eliminate as many as possible of the X-ray photons that do not strike the radiation detectors perpendicularly. In the second method, the simplest correction algorithm relies on pre-determining the value of $\frac{I_s}{I}$ for each detector at all projection angles, using an appropriate phantom. The correction parameters, established in this way, are then added to each of the projection values obtained by the scanner.

4.4.4 Metal Artefacts

From a physical point of view, metallic elements in the body form regions of very strong X-ray attenuation when compared to the surrounding soft tissue or even when compared to bones. This is due to the high atomic number of metallic elements. However, from a mathematical point of view, metal fillings, plates or fragments of bullets lodged in the body are simply treated as opaque areas. In a reconstructed tomographic image, the artefacts created by the presence of such objects appear in the form of streaks radiating out from the location of the metal element.

In most publications, the problem of reducing distortions caused by the presence of metallic elements is reduced to solving the reconstruction problem from incomplete projections [7, 13, 18, 20]. The variety of possible approaches and the limited scope of this book do not allow for a deeper analysis of algorithms developed to eliminate this kind of artefact. It is worth mentioning, however, that the most popular practical approaches are based on determining the missing projection values using measurements from the immediate neighbourhood of the pieces of metal.

4.4.5 Measurement Noise

In contrast to techniques using electromagnetic waves in the radio waveband, where the quantum energy is relatively low, the X-radiation used in computed tomography operates with highly energetic quanta. In radio wave applications, the main form of noise is Gaussian noise from thermal sources. In the case of X-rays, the level of noise is determined by the number of incident quanta per information unit, e.g. per image pixel. This means a strong dependence of the signal to noise ratio (SNR) on the irregularity of the density of radiation quanta in the beam incident on the test object. When using reconstruction methods by convolution and back-projection, we can use the following relationship to define the level of variance σ_μ^2 of the estimated value of the attenuation coefficient μ [14]:

$$\sigma_\mu^2 = \frac{\Psi}{\upsilon \cdot z_{\mathrm{th}}} \int_{\infty}^{\infty} h^2(s)\mathrm{d}s, \tag{4.37}$$

where Ψ is the number of projections carried out, υ is the mean photon density of the X-ray beam, z_{th} is the thickness of the beam of radiation, $h(s)$ is the convolution kernel, used in the convolution and back projection method.

Using Eq. 4.37, we can derive an equation for the SNR in the reconstructed image:

$$\mathrm{SNR} = \frac{\Delta\mu}{\sigma_\mu} = \varsigma \cdot \Delta\mu \cdot s_{\mathrm{det}} \cdot \sqrt{\upsilon_{\mathrm{det}}} \cdot \Psi, \tag{4.38}$$

where $\Delta\mu$ is the change in attenuation coefficient in the region of interest, ς is a constant of order unity which depends on the kernel used, υ_{det} is the mean number of photons incident on the radiation detector; s_{det} is the width of the radiation detector perpendicular to the direction of the radiation.

In contrast to other methods of determining the SNR for projections, in the reconstruction method using convolution there is a strong dependence of SNR on the size of the detector s_{det}. Thus, an attempt to increase the resolution of CT scanners by reducing the size of the radiation detectors reduces the SNR in Eq. 4.38. This is easy to see, if we realise that:

$$\upsilon_{\mathrm{det}} \sim s_{\mathrm{det}}^2, \tag{4.39}$$

hence,

$$\mathrm{SNR} = \frac{\Delta\mu}{\sigma_\mu} \sim \varsigma \cdot \Delta\mu \cdot s_{\mathrm{det}} \cdot \sqrt{s_{\mathrm{det}}^2} \cdot \Psi \sim \varsigma s_{\mathrm{det}}^2. \tag{4.40}$$

The dependence of the SNR on the parameter ς, defining the effect of the convolution kernel, is evident in the reconstructed image by the different noise levels in different areas of the scan. This occurs especially when the part of the body under investigation includes oval structures. The combination of such rounded structures and the radial nature of the convolution kernels causes the rays passing through the middle of the structures to be more affected by noise than the rays passing through their edges.

References

1. Agarwal BK (1979) X ray spectroscopy. Springer, Berlin
2. Alvarez RE, Macovski A (1976) Energy selective reconstructions in X ray computer tomography. Phys Med Biol 21:733 744
3. Brooks RA, DiChiro G (1976) Principles of computer assisted tomography (CAT) in radiographic and radioisotopic imaging. Phys Med Biol 21:689 732
4. Cullity BD, Stock SR (2001) Elements of X ray diffraction, 3rd edn. Addison Wesley, Reading
5. Duerinckx AJ, Macovski A (1978) Polychromatic streak artifacts in computed tomography images. J Comp Assist Tomogr 2:481 487
6. Glover GH, Pelc NJ (1980) Nonlinear partial volume artifacts in X ray computed tomography. Med Phys 7(3):238 248
7. Glover GH, Pelc NJ (1981) An algorithm fot the reduction of metal clip artifacts in CT reconstructions. Med Phys 8:799 807
8. Glover GH (1982) Compton scatter effects in CT reconstructions. Med Phys 9(6):860 867
9. Jain AK (1989) Fundamentals of digitals image processing. Prentice Hall, Englewood Cliffs
10. Joseph PM (1982) The effects of scatter in X ray computed tomography. Med Phys 9(4): 464 472
11. Kak AC, Slanley M (1988) Principles of computerized tomographic imaging. IEEE Press, New York
12. Kijewski PK, Bjärngard BE (1978) Correction for beam hardening in computer tomography. Med Phys 5(3):209 214
13. Lonn AHR, Crawford CR (1988) Reduction of artifacts caused by metallic objects in CT. Radiology 169(P):116
14. Macovski A (1983) Physical problems of computer tomography. Proc IEEE 71(3):373 378
15. McDavid WD, Waggener RG, Payne WH et al (1975) Spectral effects on three dimentional reconstruction from X rays. Med Phys 2:321 324
16. Radon J (1917) Über die Bestimmung von Funktionen durch ihre Integralwerte längs gewisser Mannigfaltigkeiten. Berichte Sächsische Akademie der Wissenschaften (Leipzig) 69:262 277
17. Rontó G, Tarjan I (1999) An introduction to biophysics with medical orientation. Akademiai Kiado, Budapest
18. Snyder DL, O'Sullivan JA, Whiting BR et al (2001) Deblurring subject to nonnegativity constraints when known functions are present with application to object constrained computerized tomography. IEEE Trans Med Imaging 20(10):1009 1017
19. Suryanarayana C, Grant Norton M (1998) X ray diffraction: a practical approach. Plenum Press, New York
20. Wang G, Snyder DL, O'Sullivan JA et al (1996) Iterative deblurring for CT metal artifact reduction. IEEE Trans Med Imaging 15(5):657 664

Chapter 5
Reconstruction from Parallel-beam Projections

Because of the performance limitations of scanners that used parallel beams of X-rays, engineers were obliged to modify the design of this system. However, the fact remains that all new generation CT scanners are based on parallel-beam image reconstruction algorithms. So, rather than algorithms dictated by the actual geometry of their projection systems, in most new image reconstruction techniques we use parallel beam methods.

This means that in order to understand fully the construction and algorithms of the current generations of CT scanners, it is essential to have an in-depth knowledge of all aspects of the operation of scanners that use parallel-beam X-ray projection systems. It is also necessary to indicate the differences between the actual cross-section of the patient's body and the image obtained by projection and back-projection, to show what causes these differences and to show how to describe them mathematically.

This will allow us to get to the core of the process of using parallel X-ray projections to obtain information about the structure of an organism's internal tissues. The solution of this problem for parallel-beam systems was fundamental for the development of the first generation CT devices.

5.1 Geometry of the Parallel-beam Scanner

Figure 5.1 shows schematically a method of carrying out a parallel-beam projection [5 7] irrespective of the type and generation of CT device.

As can be seen in Fig. 5.1a, the moveable part of the scanner, consisting of an emitter of X-rays and a screen on which radiation detectors are placed, revolves around the body being examined. The body remains motionless the whole time the system rotates. During this rotation, radiation is emitted from the source, is collimated into a very narrow parallel beam, penetrates the object and reaches the detectors. The detectors measure the intensity of the radiation as it arrives at the

R. Cierniak, *X Ray Computed Tomography in Biomedical Engineering*,
DOI: 10.1007/978 0 85729 027 4 5, © Springer Verlag London Limited 2011

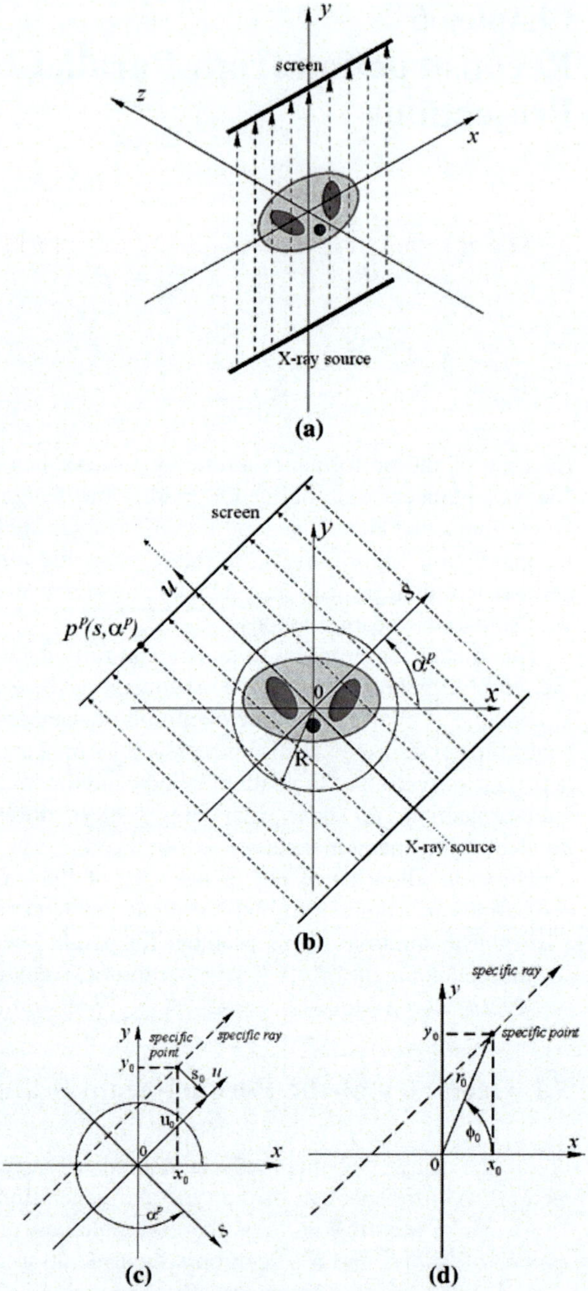

Fig. 5.1 The geometry of a parallel beam scanner: **a** a pictorial view; **b** a view in the x, y plane; **c** the geometrical relationships; **d** the polar coordinate system

screen. Each measurement of radiation intensity at the screen is evaluated relative to the original radiation intensity as defined by (4.12). This is the value of the projection function and is represented by $p^p(s, \alpha^p)$, where the parameters of the rays originating from the emitter and reaching the screen are represented in this system by:

α^P the angle at which the projection is carried out, i.e. the angle between the x-axis and the s-axis of the rotated scanner;

s the position of a particular place on the screen, with respect to the axis of the moving scanner, at the time the projection is made.

The distribution of the radiation intensity observed on the screen varies with the angle through which the scanner is rotated.

This method of scanning only allows us to obtain the image of the attenuation coefficient distribution for one cross-section of the body under examination. The width of this slice is determined by the capacity of the projection system and is one of the basic parameters of CT scanners. If required, the next cross-section can be obtained by repeating the scan-reconstruction procedure at another position on the z-axis.

Figure 5.1b shows the scanner geometry in the plane of the x and y coordinates, that is in the plane perpendicular to the z-axis. The coordinate system (s, u) is also shown in the diagram. This indicates the situation after rotation of the scanner through an angle α^P. The relationships between the coordinates in these two systems have been shown earlier, in Table 4.3. Using these relationships, we can modify 4.15, describing the Radon transform, into a form more convenient for further consideration:

$$p^P(s, \alpha^P) = \int_{\infty}^{+\infty} \mu(s \cos \alpha^P - u \sin \alpha^P, s \sin \alpha^P + u \cos \alpha^P) du, \quad (5.1)$$

where $-\infty < s < \infty$, $0 \leq \alpha^P < \pi$.

The projection function defined in this way allows for easy physical interpretation. Its value at each point on the screen (a distance s from the origin of the (x, y) coordinate system) is the sum of all the values of attenuation coefficient $\mu(x, y)$ encountered by the ray on its way to that point. This equation only applies to a scan carried out at a particular angle α^P.

Often, when considering image reconstruction problems, we use a polar coordinate system (r, ϕ) [5] as shown in Fig. 5.1d. The most important relationships between this coordinate system and the two coordinate systems encountered earlier are given in Table 5.1.

Figure 5.1b illustrates another, practical consideration concerning the scans, namely the limited space in which they take place. Because of the geometry of the scanner's rotational movement, during the scan, the data acquisition takes place

Table 5.1 Relationships between coordinate system (r, ϕ) and coordinate systems (x, y) and (s, u)

$(r, \phi) \rightarrow (x, y)$		$(r, \phi) \rightarrow (s, u)$	
x	$r \cos \phi$	s	$r \cos(\alpha^P \quad \phi)$
y	$r \sin \phi$	u	$r \sin(\alpha^P \quad \phi)$

inside the circle of radius R. The cross-section of the patient's body must be contained entirely within this circle. Furthermore, the table on which the patient lies is positioned in the space so that his body fits comfortably inside the scanner's gantry. The remaining space in the tunnel is filled with air of minimal value of attenuation coefficient $\mu(x, y)$ ($\mu_{air} = -1{,}000$ on the Hounsfield scale). It should be mentioned that no function limited in space, including this function describing projection $p^p(s, \alpha^p)$, can possess a finite spectrum [8, 15], represented here by $P(f, \alpha^p)$, where

$$P(f, \alpha^p) = F_1\{p^p(s, \alpha^p)\} = \int_{\infty}^{+\infty} p^p(s, \alpha^p) e^{\ j2\pi fs} ds. \tag{5.2}$$

This fact has substantial implications for the selection of filters for some reconstruction methods. This will be discussed later.

5.2 Geometry of the Discrete Parallel-beam Scanner

For various reasons, problems arise in practical projection systems in adapting the image reconstruction algorithm to the discrete nature of the projections. The projections are discrete with respect to both the angle at which they are obtained and the finite number of places on the screen at which their values are measured. There is also a fundamental difference between the approach to the question of discretisation in a system with one detector and one with a matrix of detectors. However, in both systems we have to take into consideration the distribution function characterising the way in which the individual detectors respond to the radiation reaching them. That function will be represented by $d(s)$, and an example of its form is shown in Fig. 5.2.

In first generation CT scanner, which had only one detector, carrying out the projections more closely resembled what we understand by a process of "scanning" across the object. It depended on the simultaneous lateral displacement of the X-ray tube and detector on opposite sides of the object and the continuous measurement of the radiation during the whole exposure. This procedure was repeated for each discrete value of projection angle. The arrangement for the acquisition of a single projection is shown diagrammatically in Fig. 5.3. Taking into account the distribution function of a particular detector, the projection

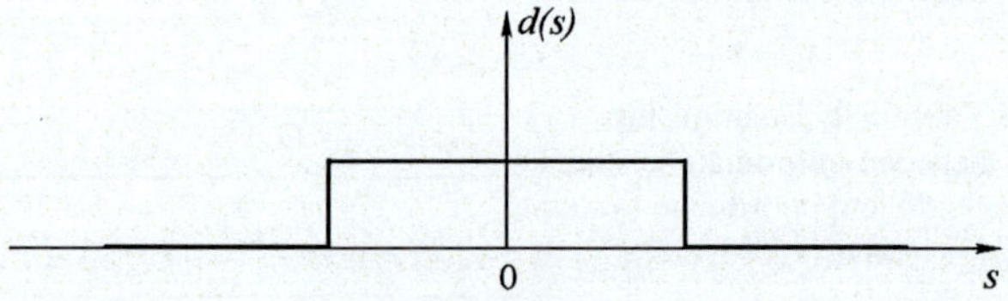

Fig. 5.2 An example of a distribution function of an X ray detector

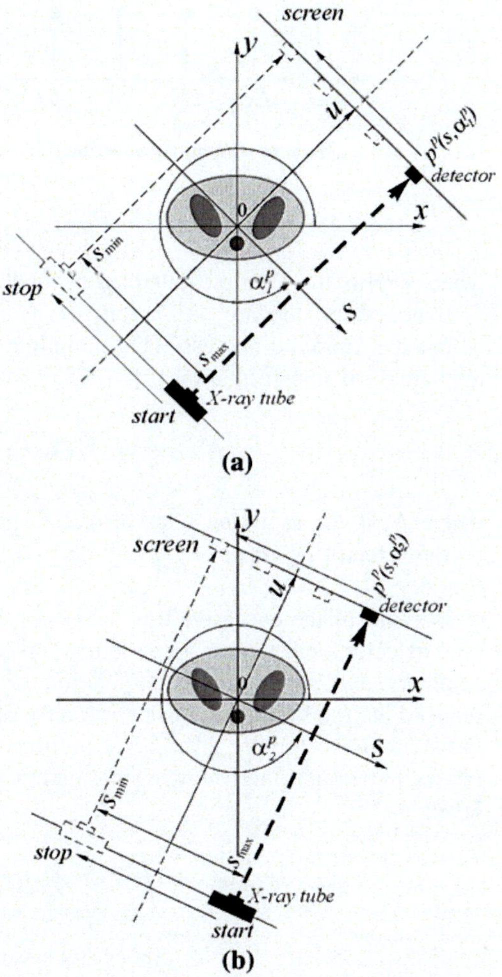

Fig. 5.3 The scanning process in a system with one radiation detector: **a** the projection at angle $\alpha^p{}_1$; **b** the projection at angle $\alpha^p{}_2$

function value obtained at the aperture of the detector can be described using the following formula [9]:

$$\tilde{p}^p(s,\alpha^p) = \int p^p(\dot{s},\alpha^p)d(\dot{s}-s)\mathrm{d}\dot{s} = p^p(s,\alpha^p)\bigstar d(s), \tag{5.3}$$

where $p^p(s, \alpha^p)$ is the original projection function; $\tilde{p}^p(s,\alpha^p)$ is the projection function registered by the detector; $d(s)$ is the distribution function of the detector; $\bigstar$ is the cross-correlation operator.

It should be noted that, in this case, it is the hardware that is carrying out the low-pass filtering of projection $p^p(s, \alpha^p)$, using the following frequency domain relationship:

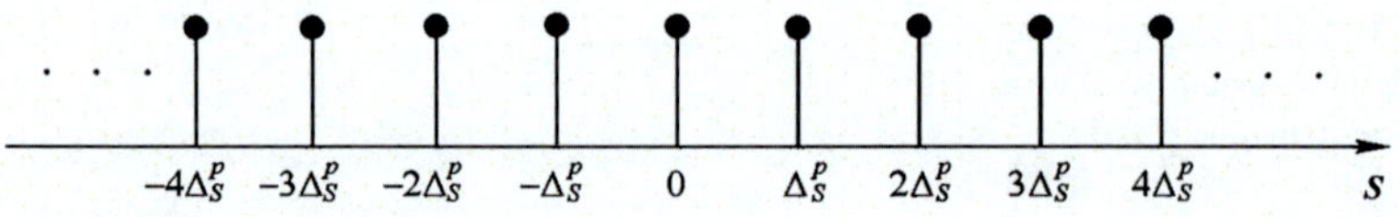

Fig. 5.4 An example of a sampling function

$$\tilde{P}(f,\alpha^p) = P(f,\alpha^p)D(-f), \tag{5.4}$$

where $D(f)$ is the Fourier transform of function $d(s)$.

If necessary, the projection function (5.3) can be subjected to filtering even before the sampling process. This sampling process is described by the following mathematical transformation [9]:

$$\hat{\tilde{p}}^p(s,\alpha^p) = \tilde{p}^p(\dot{s},\alpha^p)\cdot comb\left(\frac{s}{\Delta_s^p}\right), \tag{5.5}$$

where Δ_s^p is the sampling interval (the distance between the individual detectors on the screen); $comb(x) = \sum_{l=-\infty}^{\infty}\delta(x-l)$ is the sampling function, as shown in Fig. 5.4; $l \in \mathbb{I}$.

Because of the excessive time taken for each projection in a system with only one detector, subsequent generations of scanners used a complex matrix of detectors and simultaneous acquisition of projections. This arrangement also reduced the total radiation dose needed for a projection at a particular angle. If, as in the previous case, we take into account the particular distribution of the detector matrix, we obtain the following projection function [9] sampled at the hardware level:

$$\begin{aligned} \hat{\tilde{p}}^p(s,\alpha^p) &= \int p^p(\dot{s},\alpha^p)d(s-\dot{s})\mathrm{d}\dot{s}\cdot comb\left(\frac{s}{\Delta_s^p}\right) \\ &= \left(p^p(s,\alpha^p) * d(s)\right)\cdot comb\left(\frac{s}{\Delta_s^p}\right), \end{aligned} \tag{5.6}$$

where * is the convolution operator.

In the frequency domain, this relationship is expressed as:

$$\hat{\tilde{P}}(f,\alpha^p) = \Delta_s^p\left(P(f,\alpha^p)D(f)\right) * \mathrm{COMB}\left(\Delta_s^p\cdot f\right), \tag{5.7}$$

which, assuming the projection function has an infinite spectrum$P(f, \alpha^p)$, represents a spectrum with overlapping segments, as shown in Fig. 5.5.

This overlapping of the individual components of spectrum $\hat{\tilde{P}}(f,\alpha^p)$ (known as aliasing) occurs least when the width of the individual detectors in the matrix is a maximum [9], that is, when:

$$d(s) = rect\left(\frac{s}{\Delta_s^p}\right). \tag{5.8}$$

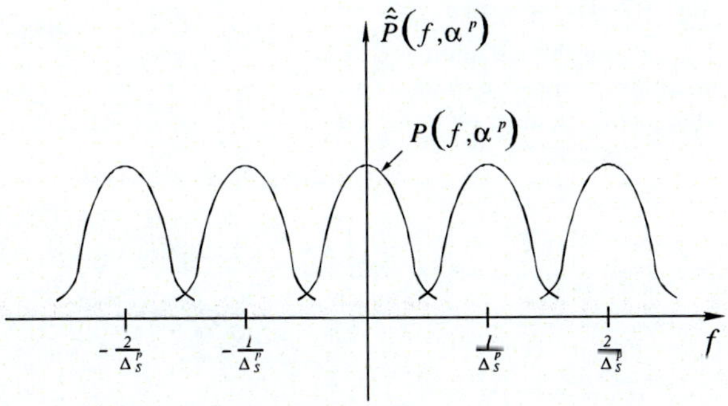

Fig. 5.5 The spectrum of the sampled projection function $\hat{\hat{P}}(f, \alpha^p)$, obtained at the aperture of the detector matrix

This form of detector distribution means that the surface of the screen is completely covered by a homogeneously active surface of detectors, as shown in Fig. 5.6.

A further consequence of using the detector matrix distribution (5.8) is the fact that the spectrum of this function:

$$D(f) = \Delta_s^p \cdot sinc\left(\Delta_s^p \cdot f\right) \tag{5.9}$$

has its first zero at:

$$f = \pm\frac{1}{\Delta_s^p}, \tag{5.10}$$

which causes repeating segments of spectrum $\hat{\hat{P}}(f, \alpha^p)$ at equal frequency intervals:

$$\Delta f = \frac{1}{\Delta_s^p}. \tag{5.11}$$

As can be seen from Fig. 5.7, this results in a reduction of the overlapping effect of the individual segments of spectrum $\hat{\hat{P}}(f, \alpha^p)$ because in this case Δf is twice as large as the cut-off frequency of the hypothetically band-limited spectrum $\tilde{P}(f, \alpha^p)$.

Clearly, the use of a low-pass filter does not completely eliminate the effect of the overlapping individual segments of the spectrum.

However, a mechanical solution has been suggested [10], which, thanks to the use of a suitably designed projection system, has improved this situation. In this approach, rotating the system through 180° about the object is accompanied by a smooth displacement of the detector panel by a distance $\frac{\Delta_s^p}{2}$ with respect to its

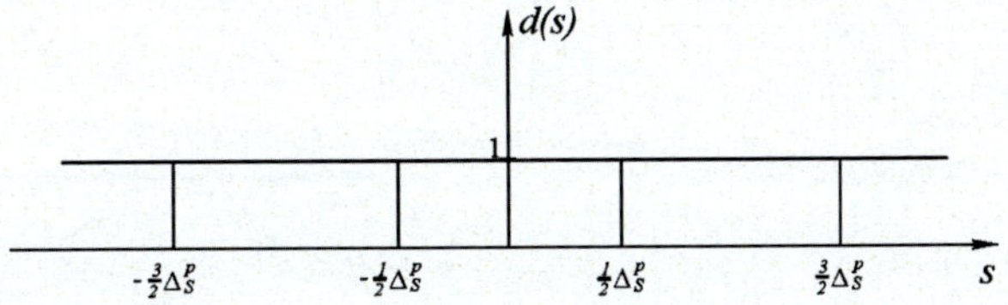

Fig. 5.6 The screen distribution, assuming the detector distribution from (5.8)

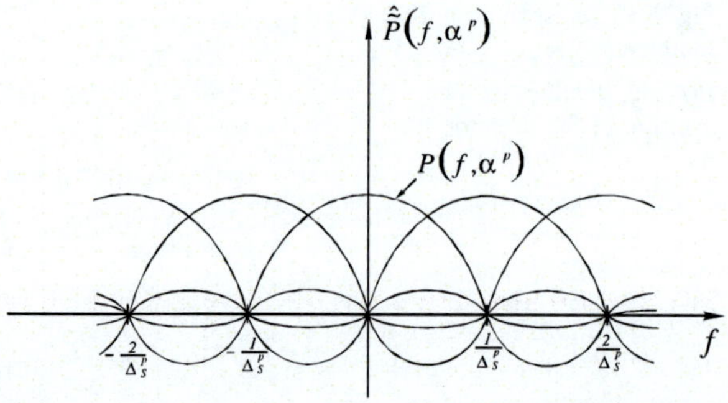

Fig. 5.7 The spectrum $\hat{\hat{P}}(f,\alpha^p)$ for the radiation detector arrangement with a distribution defined by (5.8)

starting position. In this way, we get an effective shortening of the sampling interval to $\frac{\Delta_s^p}{2}$, and thereby an increase of the separation along the frequency axis of spectrum $\hat{\hat{P}}(f,\alpha^p)$ to:

$$\Delta f = \frac{2}{\Delta_s^p}. \tag{5.12}$$

This is a great improvement in comparison with the cases considered previously. The spectrum $\hat{\hat{P}}(f,\alpha^p)$ obtained using this technique is illustrated in Fig. 5.8.

In practice however, we only have a few projection function values available: i.e. those measured at the places on the screen where the radiation sensors are located. The number of sensors is limited and represented by the symbol L. There are two cases concerning this number, which we should take into consideration: the odd and the even case. This condition has an influence on the deployment of the sensors with respect to the main axis of the moving projection system. If the number of detectors in the matrix is represented by l, then the range of possible values of this parameter is specified in the following way:

$$l \in \left[L^{\downarrow},\ldots,L^{\uparrow}\right]. \tag{5.13}$$

where [8]:

$$L^{\downarrow} = \begin{cases} -\frac{(L\ 1)}{2} & \text{for l even} \\ -\frac{L}{2} & \text{for l odd} \end{cases}, \tag{5.14}$$

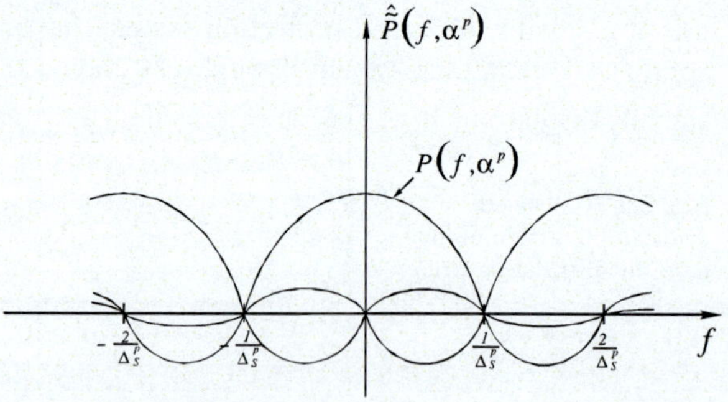

Fig. 5.8 The spectrum $\hat{\hat{P}}(f,\alpha^p)$ obtained using a mechanical technique to shorten the sampling interval

$$\mathrm{L}^{\uparrow} = \begin{cases} \frac{(\mathrm{L}\ 1)}{2} & \text{for l even} \\ \frac{\mathrm{L}}{2} - 1 & \text{for l odd} \end{cases}. \tag{5.15}$$

Taking into account the geometry of the moving projection system, the location of the individual radiation sensors when a particular projection is carried out can be defined by:

$$s_l = l \cdot \Delta_s^p. \tag{5.16}$$

It follows from the Kotelnikov Shannon sampling theorem that if the cut-off frequency of the Fourier distribution spectrum of the object's projection function is f_0 then the distance between the individual detectors should fulfil the condition:

$$\Delta_s^p \leq \Delta_{s,0}^p, \tag{5.17}$$

where $\Delta_{s,0}^p = \frac{1}{2f_0}$ is the Nyquist interval.

The number of detectors on an annular screen of radius R, enabling the reconstruction of a limited image, is therefore:

$$\mathrm{L} \geq 4f_0R. \tag{5.18}$$

In addition, we can assume that the resolution of the detectors is equal to the resolution of the reconstructed image obtained:

$$\Delta_s^p = \Delta_x = \Delta_y, \tag{5.19}$$

where Δ_x is the horizontal raster discretisation of the digital image; Δ_y is the vertical raster discretisation of the digital image.

It now remains for us to establish the relationships concerning the limited number of projections made during one full revolution of the scanner. The individual projections made at discrete angles α^p are indexed using $\psi = 0,\ldots,\Psi$, where Ψ is the maximum number of projections made during one half-turn.

Because of the symmetry property of the Radon transform, projections can only be carried out during one half-turn, that is:

$$\Delta_\alpha^p = \frac{\pi}{\Psi}, \tag{5.20}$$

where Δ_α^p is the angle through which the tube-screen system is rotated after making each projection.

We can therefore state that the exposure to X-rays and the collection of information about the radiation intensity reaching the screen after passing through the patient's body occurs when:

$$\alpha_\psi^p = \psi \cdot \Delta_\alpha^p. \tag{5.21}$$

The angle Δ_α^p represents the sampling interval during the rotation of the projection system. The only way to reduce distortion in the reconstructed image, caused by too small an angular sampling frequency, is to reduce the interval Δ_α^p.

For example, in the methods to be described in Sect. 5.4 the number of projections made should be greater than the cut-off value [1, 8]:

$$\Psi_{\min} = \frac{\pi L}{2} + 1. \tag{5.22}$$

The geometrical relationships of the discrete projection system described above are illustrated in Fig. 5.9.

In order to simplify matters later in the text, we will assume that the detector distribution of each individual detector in the matrix has the following form:

$$d(s) = \delta(s). \tag{5.23}$$

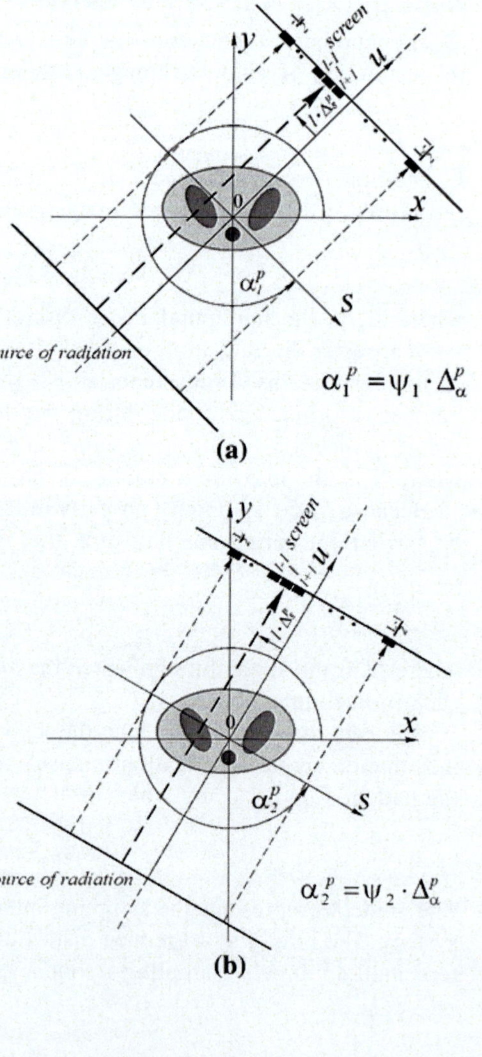

Fig. 5.9 The geometry of a discrete projection system: **a** the projection at angle α_1^p; **b** the projection at angle α_2^p

In view of this, each projection value in a parallel-beam system at angle α^p_ψ, determined at a point s_l on the screen will be represented by the discrete form of the projection function as follows:

$$\hat{p}^p(l,\psi) = p^p\left(l\cdot\Delta^p_s, \psi\cdot\Delta^p_\alpha\right), \tag{5.24}$$

where ψ is the projection number; l is the detector number, in the matrix.

A significant problem in discrete implementations of image reconstruction methods however, is the effect of the overlapping of the segments of the spectrum arising after the sampling process. It follows from sampling theory that the discrete version of the Fourier transform, represented by $\hat{P}^p(f,\alpha^p)$ is a quantity defined by the following relationship [8]:

$$\hat{P}(f,\alpha^p) = \sum_{i=\ \infty}^{\infty} P\left(f + \frac{i}{\Delta^p_s}, \alpha^p\right), \tag{5.25}$$

which can also be written as:

$$\hat{P}(f,\alpha^p) = \Delta^p_s \sum_{i=\ \infty}^{\infty} p^p\left(i\Delta^p_s, \alpha^p\right)\mathrm{e}^{\ j2\pi i\Delta^p_s}, \tag{5.26}$$

where $\hat{P}(f,\alpha^p) = P(f,\alpha^p)$, when the range of index i is limited to the case of $i = 0$.

This means that for projection functions $p^p(s, \alpha^p)$ limited in space, for which the frequency spectrum is infinite, the component spectra $P(f, \alpha^p)$ in spectrum $\hat{P}(f,\alpha^p)$ overlap when $i \neq 0$. This represents a serious source of distortion in reconstructed images.

5.3 Image Reconstruction from Projections: Problem Formulation

When trying to devise a way of determining the distribution of function $\mu(x, y)$ defining the internal structure of a patient's body, we make use of the concept of the Radon transform described in Chap. 4. We can justify the use of the Radon transform in medical imaging because it is identical to the projection function whose values are measured by a parallel-beam scanner.

The next step towards obtaining a diagnostically useful tomographic image is to apply the idea of back-projection to the Radon transform as follows [5, 6, 8]:

$$B(x,y) = \int_0^\pi p^p(x\cos\alpha^p + y\sin\alpha^p, \alpha^p)\,\mathrm{d}\alpha^p. \tag{5.27}$$

Equation (5.27) allows us to assign to each point in space (x, y), the sum of all the projection function values, which correspond to the rays going through each point in the course of obtaining the projections.

Assuming that every point in the object has an influence on the projection function value at the place on the screen reached by the ray passing through the point, we can say that summation (5.27) contains information about the attenuation coefficient at that point. At the same time however, it would be mistaken to believe that we could obtain the true attenuation coefficient distribution simply by carrying out back-projection directly after the acquisition process. Such an attempt would produce an indistinct image. Hopes of easy success would turn out to be unfounded because back-projection is not the same as the inverse Radon transform and the image defined by function $\tilde{\mu}(x, y) = B(x, y)$, obtained in this way, would be distorted so much as to make any medical interpretation impossible. The process of obtaining the image $\mu(x, y)$ by projection and back-projection is shown in Figure 5.10.

Because of its fundamental significance for computed tomography, the relationship between the attenuation function $\tilde{\mu}(x, y)$, obtained by projection and back-projection, and the actual attenuation function $\mu(x, y)$ of the cross-section of the object, is worth analysing in some detail. The equation defining this relationship is as follows [5, 6, 8]:

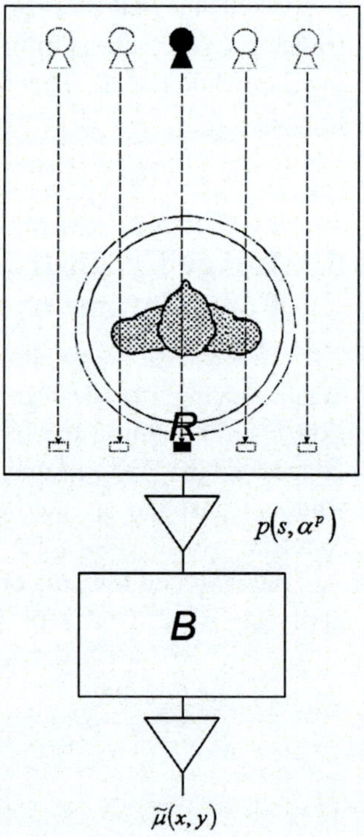

Fig. 5.10 Obtaining an image by projection and back projection

$$\tilde{\mu}(x,y) = \mu(x,y) * \left(x^2 + y^2\right)^{\frac{1}{2}} = \int_{\infty}^{+\infty} \int_{\infty}^{+\infty} \mu(\dot{x},\dot{y}) \frac{1}{\sqrt{\left((x-\dot{x})^2 + (y-\dot{y})^2\right)}} \quad (5.28)$$

where this equation is defined with the exception of points $(\dot{x},\dot{y})$, for which $x = \dot{x} \wedge y = \dot{y}$.

Proof

//Let $\tilde{\mu}(x,y) \quad B(x,y)$

$$\tilde{\mu}(x,y) \quad \int_0^{\pi} p^p(x\cos\alpha^p + y\sin\alpha^p, \alpha^p)\mathrm{d}\alpha^p$$

Follows from the definition of back projection

//Substituting the expression for the projection
//values $p^p(s, \alpha^p)$

$$\int_0^{\pi}\left(\int_{-\infty}^{+\infty}\int_{-\infty}^{+\infty} \mu(\dot{x},\dot{y}) \cdot \delta(\dot{x}\cos\alpha^p + \dot{y}\sin\alpha^p \quad s)\mathrm{d}\dot{x}\mathrm{d}\dot{y}\right)\mathrm{d}\alpha^p$$

Coordinates $(\dot{x},\dot{y})$ refer to all points in the reconstructed image, variable s only to those points which, for a particular projection, lie on the same straight line as the reconstructed image point specified by coordinates (x, y)

//Substituting the formula for the distance s of the reconstructed image point
//(x, y) from the main axis of the scanner (see Table 4.3)

$$\int_0^{\pi}\left(\int_{-\infty}^{+\infty}\int_{-\infty}^{+\infty} \mu(\dot{x},\dot{y}) \cdot \delta(\dot{x}\cos\alpha^p + \dot{y}\sin\alpha^p \quad x\cos\alpha^p \quad y\sin\alpha^p)\mathrm{d}\dot{x}\mathrm{d}\dot{y}\right)\mathrm{d}\alpha^p$$

//Simplifying the expression

$$\int_0^{\pi}\left(\int_{-\infty}^{+\infty}\int_{-\infty}^{+\infty} \mu(\dot{x},\dot{y}) \cdot \delta((\dot{x} \quad x)\cos\alpha^p + (\dot{y} \quad y)\sin\alpha^p)\mathrm{d}\dot{x}\mathrm{d}\dot{y}\right)\mathrm{d}\alpha^p$$

//Changing the order of the integration

$$\int_{-\infty}^{+\infty}\int_{-\infty}^{+\infty} \mu(\dot{x},\dot{y})\left(\int_0^{\pi} \delta((\dot{x} \quad x)\cos\alpha^p + (\dot{y} \quad y)\sin\alpha^p)\right)\mathrm{d}\alpha^p\mathrm{d}\dot{x}\mathrm{d}\dot{y}$$

//Using the substitution:
//$\delta((\dot{x} \quad x)\cos\alpha^p + (\dot{y} \quad y)) \quad \frac{1}{\sqrt{\left((\dot{x}-x)^2+(\dot{y}-y)^2\right)}}$

$$\int_{-\infty}^{+\infty}\int_{-\infty}^{+\infty} \mu(x,y)\frac{1}{\sqrt{\left((x-\dot{x})^2+(y-\dot{y})^2\right)}}\mathrm{d}\dot{x}\mathrm{d}\dot{y}$$

Proof of the substitution used is given in Appendix A, in the discussion of the properties of the $\delta(x, y)$ function

//Final form

$$\mu(x,y) * (x^2 + y^2)^{-\frac{1}{2}}.$$

□

If the attenuation coefficient distribution is to be considered in polar coordinates, then we could write the polar equivalent of (5.28) as:

$$\tilde{\mu}(r,\phi) = \mu(r,\phi) * \frac{1}{|r|} \quad (5.29)$$

We can conclude from inspection of (5.28) that the image obtained by back-projection does carry information about the actual form of the attenuation function,

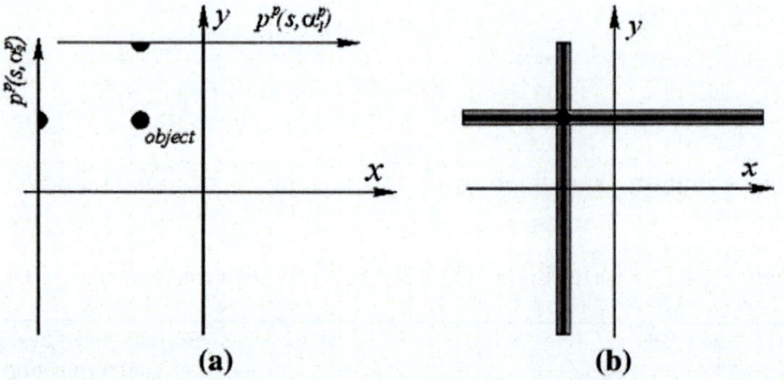

Fig. 5.11 The formation of image distortions obtained after back projection: **a** a sequence of two projections; **b** the image showing the artefacts formed after the process of back projection

but distorted by the geometrical factor $(x^2 + y^2)^{\frac{1}{2}}$. The principle behind the formation of these distortions is explained in Fig. 5.11, for the simplified case when only two projections are performed.

A result of the interaction of this geometrical distorting factor on the original attenuation function is the appearance of artefacts (elements of the image that do not exist in reality). They take the form of a line lying along the path of the ray as can be seen in Fig. 5.11. Obviously, this only happens when, in the course of a particular projection, the ray passing through the distorted points of the image encounters somewhere else an element of non-zero value of $\mu(x, y)$. In other words, as a result of back-projection, the ray passing through that point of non-zero value of $\mu(x, y)$ transmits this value to all the image points lying in its path. When data acquisition is carried out continuously, it is convenient to assume that the object consists of one non-zero point at its centre, as follows:

$$\mu(x,y) = \delta(x - x_0, y - y_0), \tag{5.30}$$

where $(x - x_0, y - y_0)$ is the coordinates of the centre of the object's cross-section.

As a result of carrying out projections followed by the process of back-projection, the image obtained could be represented as in Fig. 5.12.

In the frequency domain, the geometrical distorting function $fun(x,y) = (x^2 + y^2)^{\frac{1}{2}}$ is represented by:

$$FUN(f_1,f_2) = (f_1^2 + f_2^2)^{\frac{1}{2}}. \tag{5.31}$$

The Fourier equivalent of relationship (5.29) is:

$$\tilde{M}(f) = \frac{1}{|f|} M(f), \tag{5.32}$$

where

$$|f| = \sqrt{f_1^2 + f_2^2}. \tag{5.33}$$

Expression (5.32) forms a convenient starting point for a whole class of analytical image reconstruction methods, which will be the subject of the following sections of the chapter.

5.4 Reconstruction Methods by Convolution/Filtration and Back-Projection

At this point, we will introduce the most popular and most often used family of image reconstruction algorithms, especially as far as medical computed tomography is concerned. Underlying this type of algorithm is the assertion that at each angle, every individual result streaming into the computer may be adapted to the reconstruction task in an appropriate way. To help us in our task we will use the projection-slice theorem, which relates a projection to a cross-section of the reconstructed image [5, 8]. This can be expressed by the following equation:

$$P(f,\alpha^p) = M(f\cos\alpha^p, f\sin\alpha^p). \tag{5.34}$$

Proof

$P(f,\alpha^p) \quad \int_{-\infty}^{\infty} p^p(s,\alpha^p)e^{-j2\pi fs}ds$	Follows from the definition of the Fourier transform
//The projection for one particular s is the integral //over all points lying in one straight line $P(f,\alpha^p) \quad \int_{-\infty}^{+\infty}\int_{-\infty}^{+\infty} \mu(x,y)\delta(x\cos\alpha^p + y\sin\alpha^p \quad s)e^{-j2\pi fs}dsdu$	Follows from the definition of the Radon transform (4.15)
//Modifying the above (see (5.1) and Table 4.3) $\int_{-\infty}^{+\infty}\int_{-\infty}^{+\infty} \mu(s\cos\alpha^p \quad u\sin\alpha^p, s\sin\alpha^p + u\cos\alpha^p)e^{-j2\pi fs}dsdu$	
//Converting this to the (x, y) coordinate system (see Table 5.1) $\int_{-\infty}^{+\infty}\int_{-\infty}^{+\infty} \mu(x,y)e^{-j2\pi f(x\cos\alpha^p + y\sin\alpha^p)}dxdy$	
//Modifying the above (see Table 4.3) $\int_{-\infty}^{+\infty}\int_{-\infty}^{+\infty} (\mu(s\cos\alpha^p \quad u\sin\alpha^p, s\sin\alpha^p + u\cos\alpha^p)\cdot e^{-j2\pi fx\cos\alpha^p + y\sin\alpha^p}dx)e^{-j2\pi fy\sin\alpha^p}dy$	
//Final form $M(f\cos\alpha^p, f\sin\alpha^p)$.	Follows from the definition of the two dimensional Fourier transform

□

From relationship (5.34) it follows that the frequency spectrum $P(f, \alpha^p)$ of a projection carried out at an angle α^p is equal to a section of the two dimensional spectrum $M(f_1,f_2)$ of the original image. The points making up this section fulfil two conditions: $f_1 = f\cos\alpha^p$ and $f_2 = f\sin\alpha^p$, which means that they lie in a straight line at an angle α^p with respect to the f_1 axis. Figure 5.13 explains this relationship (5.34) graphically.

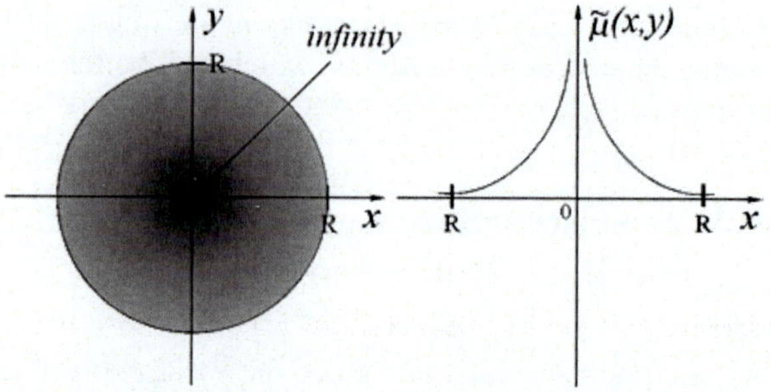

Fig. 5.12 Image of a point object obtained after projection followed by back projection

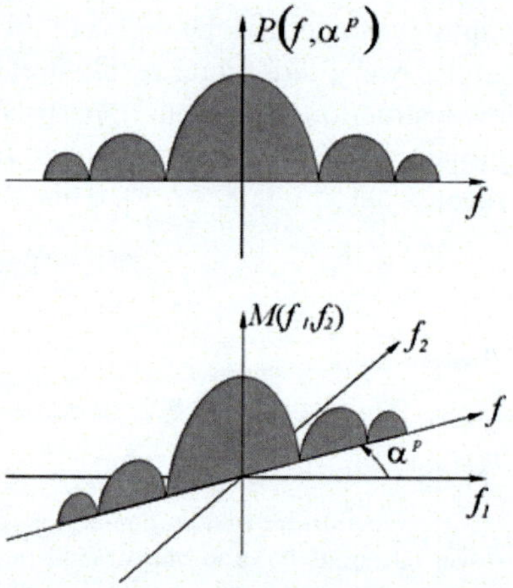

Fig. 5.13 The relationship between the one dimensional Fourier transform of projection $p(s, \alpha^P)$ and a section of the two dimensional spectrum of the original image $\mu(x, y)$

In practice, this means that instead of filtering the whole image in two dimensions, it is enough to filter all projections $p(s, \alpha^P)$ in one dimension, using the familiar filter form $|f|$. It is only after the filtering of the individual projections that they take part in the process of back-projection. This resembles a sort of pre-processing carried out on the projections, in order to prevent them from introducing distortion in the subsequently reconstructed image. By treating the results streaming into the computer system in this way, we can also significantly reduce the calculation time needed to reconstruct the image. A general flowchart for reconstruction methods based on relationship (5.34) is given in Fig. 5.14.

Up to now, we have aimed to show that instead of filtering the image obtained after back-projection in two dimensions, we can filter each projection separately and only later carry out the back-projection. Before we do this however, we need to determine how to carry out the one-dimensional filtering of the individual projections. We can accomplish this by establishing the form of the inverse Radon transform $R^{-1}\{p(s,\alpha^P)\}$. This transform should not be confused with the idea of back-projection $B\{p(s, \alpha^P)\}$, which only allows us to obtain an image with geometric distortions. The following rule shows how we can obtain the reconstructed image from the inverse Radon transform:

$$\mu(x,y) = R^{\;1}\{R\{\mu(x,y)\}\}. \tag{5.35}$$

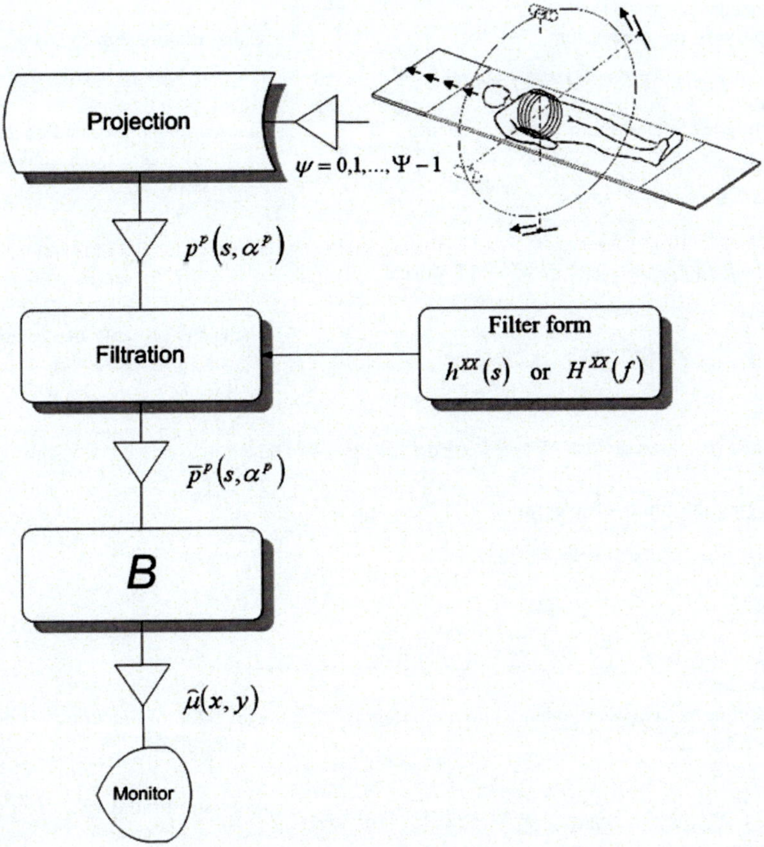

Fig. 5.14 Flowchart for reconstruction methods using one dimensional filtration

The following equation fulfils the requirements of (5.35) and is proved below [5]:

$$\mu(x, y) = R\ ^{1}(p(s, \alpha^p)) = \frac{1}{2\pi^2}\int\limits_{0}^{\pi}\int\limits_{\infty}^{+\infty}\frac{\frac{\partial p^p(s,\alpha^p)}{\partial s}}{x\cos\alpha^p + y\sin\alpha^p - s}\mathrm{d}s\mathrm{d}\alpha^p. \qquad (5.36)$$

Proof

//The inverse Fourier transform

$$\mu(x, y) \quad \int\limits_{-\infty}^{+\infty}\int\limits_{-\infty}^{+\infty} M(f_1, f_2)e^{j2\pi(f_1x+f_2y)}\mathrm{d}f_1\mathrm{d}f_2$$

//Converting to polar coordinates — Changing the limits of integration

$$= \int\limits_{0}^{2\pi}\int\limits_{0}^{+\infty} M(f\cos\alpha^p, f\sin\alpha^p)$$

$$e^{j2\pi f(x\cos\alpha^p + y\sin\alpha^p)}\begin{vmatrix}\cos\alpha^p & f\sin\alpha^p\\ \sin\alpha^p & f\cos\alpha^p\end{vmatrix}\mathrm{d}f\mathrm{d}\alpha^p =$$

(continued)

(continued)

//Simplifying the expression

$$\int_0^{2\pi}\int_0^{\infty} P(f,\alpha^P)e^{j2\pi f(x\cos\alpha^P + y\sin\alpha^P)} f\,\mathrm{d}f\,\mathrm{d}\alpha^P$$

Using relationship (5.34)

//Splitting the integral into two components

$$\int_0^{\pi}\int_0^{\infty} P(f,\alpha^P)e^{j2\pi f(x\cos\alpha^P + y\sin\alpha^P)} f\,\mathrm{d}f\,\mathrm{d}\alpha^P + \int_0^{\pi}\int_0^{\infty} P(f,\alpha^P+\pi)e^{j2\pi f(x\cos\alpha^P + y\sin\alpha^P)} f\,\mathrm{d}f\,\mathrm{d}\alpha^P$$

One component considers angles of rotation $\alpha^P \in [0,\pi]$ and the other $\alpha^P \in [\pi, 2\pi]$

$$\int_0^{\pi}\int_0^{\infty} P(f,\alpha^P)e^{j2\pi f(x\cos\alpha^P + y\sin\alpha^P)} f\,\mathrm{d}f\,\mathrm{d}\alpha^P + \int_0^{\pi}\int_0^{\infty} P(\ f,\alpha^P)e^{j2\pi f(x\cos\alpha^P + y\sin\alpha^P)} f\,\mathrm{d}f\,\mathrm{d}\alpha^P$$

Using the property of the Fourier transform: $P(f, \alpha^P + \pi)$ $P(\ f, \alpha^P)$

//Changing the limits of integration

$$\int_0^{\pi}\int_0^{\infty} P(f,\alpha^P)e^{j2\pi f(x\cos\alpha^P + y\sin\alpha^P)} f\,\mathrm{d}f\,\mathrm{d}\alpha^P + \int_0^{\pi}\int_{-\infty}^{0} P(f,\alpha^P)e^{j2\pi f(x\cos\alpha^P + y\sin\alpha^P)} (\ f)\,\mathrm{d}f\,\mathrm{d}\alpha^P$$

//Combining the two components into one integral

$$\int_0^{\pi}\left(\int_{-\infty}^{\infty} |f|\cdot P(f,\alpha^P)\cdot e^{j2\pi f(x\cos\alpha^P + y\sin\alpha^P)}\mathrm{d}f\right)\mathrm{d}\alpha^P$$

The value of function $|f|$ is never negative

$$\int_0^{\pi}\left(\int_{-\infty}^{\infty} P(f,\alpha^P)\cdot f\cdot sign(f)\cdot e^{j2\pi f(x\cos\alpha^P + y\sin\alpha^P)}\mathrm{d}f\right)\mathrm{d}\alpha^P$$

After substituting: $|f|$ $f \cdot \mathrm{sign}(f)$

$$\int_0^{\pi}\left(F_1^{-1}(P(f,\alpha^P)\cdot f\cdot sign(f))\right)\mathrm{d}\alpha^P$$

After applying the definition of the inverse Fourier transform

$$\int_0^{\pi}\left(F_1^{-1}(f\cdot P(f,\alpha^P)) * F_1^{-1}(sign(f))\right)\mathrm{d}\alpha^P$$

The product of the functions in the frequency domain is equal to their convolution in the s domain (see Appendix A)

$$\int_0^{\pi}\left(\left(\left(\frac{1}{j2\pi^2}\right)\frac{\partial p^P(s,\alpha^P)}{\partial s}\right) * \left(\frac{-1}{j\pi s}\right)\right)\mathrm{d}\alpha^P$$

After determining the inverse Fourier transform of both functions

$$\int_0^{\pi}\int_{-\infty}^{\infty} \frac{1}{j2\pi^2}\frac{\partial p^P(\dot{s},\alpha^P)}{\partial \dot{s}}\cdot\frac{-1}{j\pi(s-\dot{s})}\mathrm{d}\dot{s}\,\mathrm{d}\alpha^P$$

Follows from the definition of convolution

//Simplifying the expression

$$\frac{1}{2\pi^2}\int_0^{\pi}\int_{-\infty}^{\infty} \frac{\partial p^P(\dot{s},\alpha^P)}{\partial \dot{s}}\cdot\frac{1}{(s-\dot{s})}\mathrm{d}\dot{s}\,\mathrm{d}\alpha^P$$

//Final form

$$\frac{1}{2\pi^2}\int_0^{\pi}\int_{-\infty}^{\infty} \frac{\partial p^P(s,\alpha^P)}{\partial s}\cdot\frac{1}{(x\cos\alpha^P + y\sin\alpha^P - s)}\mathrm{d}s\,\mathrm{d}\alpha^P$$

□

For practical reasons, another form of (5.36) is often used:

$$\mu(x, y) = \int_{0}^{\pi} p^{p}(x \cos \alpha^{p} + y \sin \alpha^{p}, \alpha^{p}) \mathrm{d}\alpha^{p}, \tag{5.37}$$

where

$$p^{p}(x \cos \alpha^{p} + y \sin \alpha^{p}, \alpha^{p}) = \int_{\infty}^{\infty} |f| \cdot P(f, \alpha^{p}) e^{j2\pi f (x \cos \alpha^{p} + y \sin \alpha^{p})} \mathrm{d}f \tag{5.38}$$

is the projection after the filtering process.

It is necessary to stress that (5.37) defines the inverse Radon transform [4, 5, 7], that is, quite simply it is the process reversing the Radon transform. This fact will be used next to develop two competing methods of reconstructing the image:

- the convolution and back-projection method,
- the filtration and back-projection method.

In both of these methods, which follow from (5.37), the main aim is to obtain filtered projection values $p^{p}(s, \alpha^{p})$. These methods will be the subject of later sections of this chapter, but first we will analyse some of the filters that could be used.

5.4.1 Choice of the Filter Forms

The image reconstruction methodology formulated in the previous section relies for its operation on the appropriate preparation (i.e. filtering) of each projection individually. Irrespective of the domain in which this process occurs, the design of filters relies on an equation appearing in the proof of relationship (5.36) [5]:

$$\mu(x, y) = \int_{0}^{\pi} \int_{\infty}^{\infty} |f| \cdot P(f, \alpha^{p}) e^{j2\pi f (x \cos \alpha^{p} + y \sin \alpha^{p})} \mathrm{d}f \mathrm{d}\alpha^{p}. \tag{5.39}$$

At this point, it is worth reminding ourselves of the geometry of the moving projection system of the CT scanner and emphasizing the restricted space in which the projections $p^{p}(s, \alpha^{p})$ are carried out. No function limited in space can have a finite frequency spectrum, in this case represented by $P(f, \alpha^{p})$. Because at some stage of the reconstruction process, function $p^{p}(s, \alpha^{p})$ is always subjected to sampling, the conditions will be such as to cause overlapping of the components of the frequency spectrum $\hat{P}(f, \alpha^{p})$. The source of this effect is the form of the frequency spectrum $\hat{P}(f, \alpha^{p})$ of the sampled function $p^{p}(s, \alpha^{p})$. This spectrum consists of a series of spectra $P(f, \alpha^{p})$ displaced with respect to each other on the frequency axis (see Fig. 5.5 and Eq. 5.25). Since function $P(f, \alpha^p)$ is unbounded, parts of the components of the total spectrum $\hat{P}(f, \alpha^p)$ would overlap each other causing distortion in the reconstructed image (so-called aliasing) [2]. In considering this problem further, we will distinguish two cases [9]:

- a projection system with one scanning detector,
- a projection system with a matrix of detectors.

By using a projection system with one scanning detector, we can significantly limit the effect discussed above. As already mentioned during our discussion of the design limitations of this generation of scanner (see Sect. 5.2), a process of low-pass filtering of the individual projections already occurs at the hardware level, in accordance with (4). This limits the bandwidth of the spectrum $P(f, \alpha^p)$ of the individual projections. It is most important that this process take place before the sampling of the projection function so as to minimise the incidence of the phenomenon of the overlapping components of spectrum $\hat{P}(f, \alpha^p)$. If necessary, we can also carry out further remedial low-pass filtering by using signal processing. Both of these procedures result in a preventative limiting of the bandwidth of spectrum $P(f, \alpha^p)$ and a significant reduction in the number of artefacts appearing in the reconstructed image.

During the development of computed tomography, a design emerged which used a matrix of detectors. This significantly reduced the time taken to acquire the projection values. In such a system, the sampling is carried out by the array of detectors at the same time as the value of the projection function is being determined. Because of this, preliminary limiting of the frequency bandwidth of the projection becomes impossible. This lack of a finite frequency spectrum causes overlapping of the individual components of the spectrum $\hat{P}(f, \alpha^p)$ of the sampled projection function and so is a direct cause of distortion in the reconstructed image.

In each of the two cases discussed above it is necessary to apply filters permitting partial rejection of the components of spectrum $\hat{P}(f, \alpha^p)$ [8], other than the first component, which is identical to spectrum $P(f, \alpha^p)$. However, we need to reconcile ourselves with the real threat of interference in the reconstructed image.

The filtering of spectrum $P(f, \alpha^p)$ takes place with the aid of a suitably well-matched window function and the process can be represented by the following operation [5]:

$$\breve{P}(f, \alpha^p) = P(f, \alpha^p) W(f), \tag{5.40}$$

where $\breve{P}(f, \alpha^p)$ is the filtered spectrum of the projection function $p^p(s, \alpha^p)$; $W(f)$ is the window function, defining the part of the spectrum of projection $P(f, \alpha^p)$ under consideration.

We also need to be aware that, in practice, minimising the side effects of the sampling process by filtering also applies to the sampled projection function $\hat{p}(l, \psi)$. The following equation defines the filtering process as applied to the combined frequency spectrum $\hat{P}(f, \alpha^p)$:

$$\hat{\hat{P}}(f,\alpha^p) = \hat{P}(f,\alpha^p)W(f), \tag{5.41}$$

where $\hat{\hat{P}}(f,\alpha^p)$ is the filtered spectrum of the sampled projection function $\hat{p}(l,\psi)$. The basic condition imposed on the form of the applied window function is that:

$$W(f) = 0 \quad \text{for } |f| \geq f_0, \tag{5.42}$$

where f_0 is the cut-off frequency of the filter.

For the unbounded frequency spectrum $P(f, \alpha^p)$, f_0 has the value:

$$f_0 = \frac{1}{2\Delta_s^p}, \tag{5.43}$$

where Δ_s^p is the sampling interval.

The most straightforward form of window function is a function with the following properties [5, 6, 8]:

$$W^{RL} = \begin{cases} 1 & \text{for } |f| \leq f_0 \\ 0 & \text{for } |f| > f_0 \end{cases}, \tag{5.44}$$

the graph of which is shown in Fig. 5.15.

The window function defined in (5.44) can also be represented in the following, equivalent way:

$$W^{RL} = rect\left(\frac{f}{2f_0}\right). \tag{5.45}$$

Taking into consideration the bandwidth limitation of function $P(f, \alpha^p)$ introduced in relationship (41), we can modify (5.39) as follows:

$$\breve{\mu}(x,y) = \int_0^{\pi} \int_{\infty}^{+\infty} |f| W^{RL}(f) P(f,\alpha^p) e^{j2\pi f(x\cos\alpha^p + y\sin\alpha^p)} df\, d\alpha^p. \tag{5.46}$$

The application of the window function forces us to accept the fact that the reconstructed function $\breve{\mu}(x,y)$ describing the image will only be a band-limited

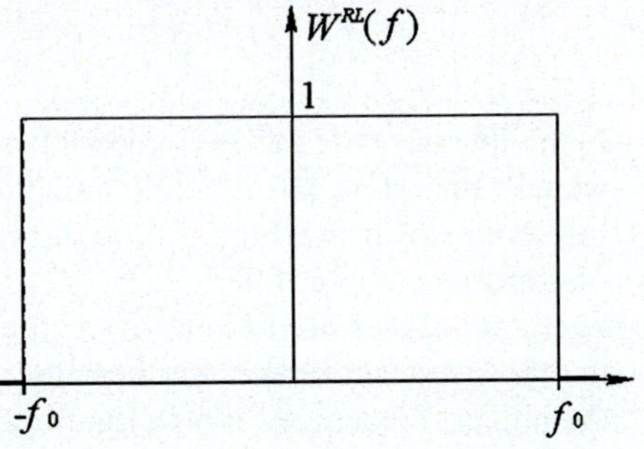

Fig. 5.15 The window function defined by (5.44)

approximation of $\mu(x, y)$. In view of this, (5.46) can be converted into the following form:

$$\breve{\mu}(x,y) = \int_{0}^{\pi} \int_{f_0}^{f_0} |f| W^{\mathrm{RL}}(f) P(f, \alpha^p) e^{j2\pi f(x\cos\alpha^p + y\sin\alpha^p)} df d\alpha^p. \tag{5.47}$$

Applying the product theorem of the frequency function to formula (5.47) (obtained by restricting the limits of integration), we obtain:

$$\breve{\mu}(x,y) = \int_{0}^{\pi} \int_{\mathrm{R}}^{\mathrm{R}} p^p(s, \alpha^p) h(x\cos\alpha^p + y\sin\alpha^p - s) ds d\alpha^p, \tag{5.48}$$

where

$$h(s) = h^{\mathrm{RL}}(s) = \int_{f_0}^{f_0} |f| W^{\mathrm{RL}}(f) e^{j2\pi fs} df. \tag{5.49}$$

Equation (5.48) resembles relationship (5.47) in its relevance to the convolution and back-projection reconstruction method. In the back-projection process, each projection $p^p(s, \alpha^p)$ is filtered before the summation process, as shown below:

$$\breve{\mu}(x,y) = \int_{0}^{\pi} p^p(s, \alpha^p) d\alpha^p, \tag{5.50}$$

where

$$p^p(s, \alpha^p) = \int_{\mathrm{R}}^{\mathrm{R}} p^p(\dot{s}, \alpha^p) \cdot h(s - \dot{s}) d\dot{s}. \tag{5.51}$$

Equation (5.49) defines the filter $h(s)$ in the spatial domain. The equivalent function in the frequency domain is:

$$H^{\mathrm{RL}}(f) = |f| W^{\mathrm{RL}}(f) = |f| rect\left(\frac{f}{2f_0}\right). \tag{5.52}$$

In the literature, this filter is known by an abbreviation of the names of its authors, namely Ram Lak [11, 12] (a contraction of the Indian names Ramachandran and Lakshminarayanan). Figure 5.16 shows the frequency graph of this filter.

Unfortunately a filter such as this, with the acute gradients apparent in Fig. 5.16, causes oscillations in the filtered signal $p^p(s, \alpha^p)$, and thus distortions in the reconstructed image. Furthermore, this filter has a natural tendency to prefer the higher frequencies, which due to the low signal-to-noise ratio (SNR) (or high

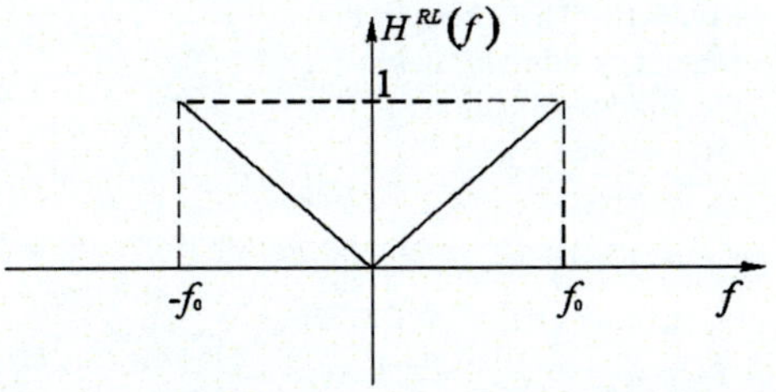

Fig. 5.16 The Ram Lak filter in the frequency domain

level of noise compared to the signal) of the images causes an intensification of the noise. In order to eliminate these undesirable properties a different filter form was proposed, as defined by the formula:

$$H(f) = |f|W(f), \tag{5.53}$$

in which [8]:

$$W(f) = \begin{cases} 1 - \frac{\varepsilon \cdot |f|}{f_0} & \text{for} \quad |f| \leq f_0 \\ 0 & \text{for} \quad |f| > f_0 \end{cases}, \tag{5.54}$$

where f_0 is the cut-off frequency of the filter; ε is a value in the range [0,1].

Figure 5.17 shows the window function expressed by (5.54), for selected values of ε.

A graphical interpretation of the filters resulting from the window function as defined in the equation above, for the same selected values of ε, is found in Fig. 5.18.

Currently, in commonly applied reconstruction procedures such as the convolution and back-projection algorithm, filters defined in the s-domain are used. In the s-domain, in order to determine the filter form from relationship (5.53) we need to determine the inverse Fourier transform, as follows:

$$h(s) = F_1^{\ 1}\{H(f)\} = F_1^{\ 1}\{|f|W(f)\} = \int_{\infty}^{\infty} |f|W(f)e^{j2\pi fs}df. \tag{5.55}$$

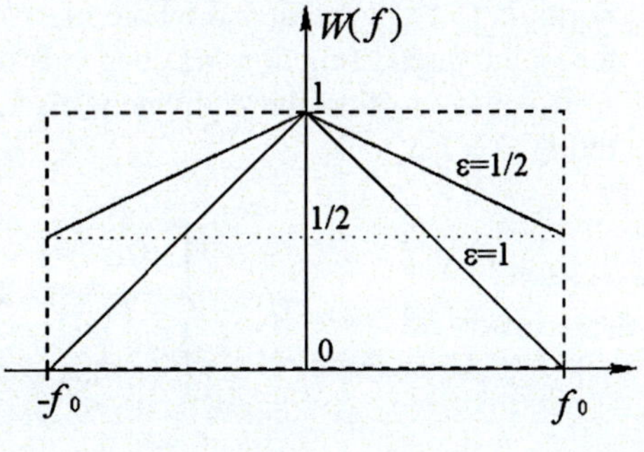

Fig. 5.17 The window function $W(f)$ defined by (5.54)

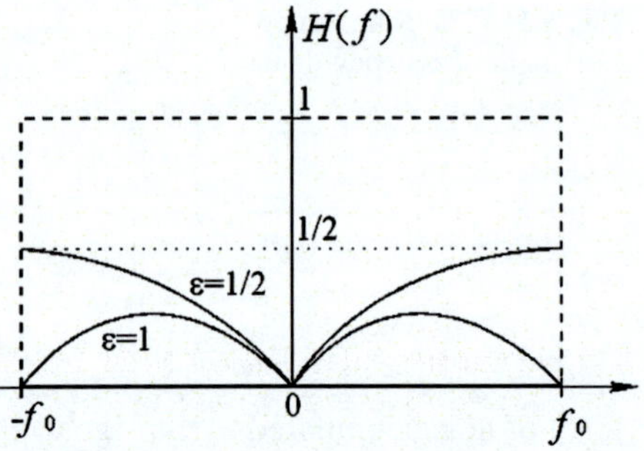

Fig. 5.18 The filters in the frequency domain, based on the window function $W(f)$ defined by (5.54)

Using the window function (5.54) with a cut-off frequency of $f_0 = \frac{1}{2\Delta_s^p}$, we can express the above relationship in the following way:

$$h(s) = F_1^{\ 1}\{H(f)\} = \int_{f_0}^{f_0} |f| \cdot \left(1 - \frac{\varepsilon|f|}{f_0}\right) e^{j2\pi fs} \mathrm{d}f. \tag{5.56}$$

The greatest problem in establishing the final form of (5.56) is the determination of the inverse Fourier transform for a function containing the factor $|f|$. If we apply the approximation [6, 13]:

$$|f| \cong \lim_{\eta \to 0} \left(|f| \mathrm{e}^{\ \eta|f|} \right), \tag{5.57}$$

we can prove (the proof of the inverse Fourier transform of function $|f|$ is found in Appendix A, Sect. A.2) that the solution of (5.56) is the following formula defining the frequency form of this filter (proof in Appendix A, Sect. A.2):

$$h(s) = \frac{1}{2\left(\Delta_s^p\right)^2} \frac{\sin\left(\frac{\pi s}{\Delta_s^p}\right)}{\frac{\pi s}{\Delta_s^p}} + \\ - \frac{1}{4\left(\Delta_s^p\right)^2} \left(\sin\left(\frac{\pi s}{2\Delta_s^p}\right) \frac{\pi s}{2\Delta_s^p} \right)^2 - \varepsilon \left(\frac{\sin\left(\frac{\pi s}{\Delta_s^p}\right)}{2\pi s \Delta_s^p} + \frac{\cos\left(\frac{\pi s}{\Delta_s^p}\right)}{(\pi s)^2} - \frac{\Delta_s^p \sin\left(\frac{\pi s}{\Delta_s^p}\right)}{(\pi s)^3} \right). \tag{5.58}$$

Formula (5.58) generates a whole class of filters, for which the particular form of the point spread function $h(s)$ depends on the value of ε.

It is easy to find the equivalent discrete version [8] of this formula by substituting $s = l \cdot \Delta_s^p$:

$$\hat{h}(l) = \begin{cases} \frac{3\ \ 2\varepsilon}{12\left(\Delta_s^p\right)^2} & \text{for } l = 0 \\ -\frac{\varepsilon}{\left(\pi l \Delta_s^p\right)^2} & \text{for } l \text{ even and } l \neq 0 \\ -\frac{1\ \ \varepsilon}{\left(\pi l \Delta_s^p\right)^2} & \text{for } l \text{ odd} \end{cases}. \tag{5.59}$$

If we then assume that $\varepsilon = 0$, we obtain a form of the aforementioned Ram Lak filter:

$$h^{\mathrm{RL}}(s) = \frac{1}{2\left(\Delta_s^p\right)^2} \frac{\sin\left(\frac{\pi s}{\Delta_s^p}\right)}{\frac{\pi s}{\Delta_s^p}} - \frac{1}{4\left(\Delta_s^p\right)^2} \left(\frac{\sin\left(\frac{\pi s}{2\Delta_s^p}\right)}{\frac{\pi s}{2\Delta_s^p}} \right)^2, \tag{5.60}$$

while in the discrete version

$$\hat{h}^{\mathrm{RL}}(l) = \begin{cases} \frac{1}{\left(2\Delta_s^p\right)^2} & \text{for } l = 0 \\ 0 & \text{for } l \text{ even and } l \neq 0\,. \\ -\frac{1}{\left(\pi l \Delta_s^p\right)^2} & \text{for } l \text{ odd} \end{cases} \tag{5.61}$$

Figure 5.19 shows a Ram Lak filter in the s-domain, in a continuous as well as a discrete form. Other filters of this type, assuming values $\varepsilon = \frac{1}{2}$ and $\varepsilon = 1$, have also been considered to see how useful they could be for application in the convolution and back-projection reconstruction method [8]. However, until now, they have not found wider application and so will not be discussed any further here. Because of the limited space in CT scanners, the spectrum of their images is infinitely wide. Under these conditions, the use of filters which have a sudden drop in the transmission bandwidth at relatively low cut-off frequency f_0 (as is the case with

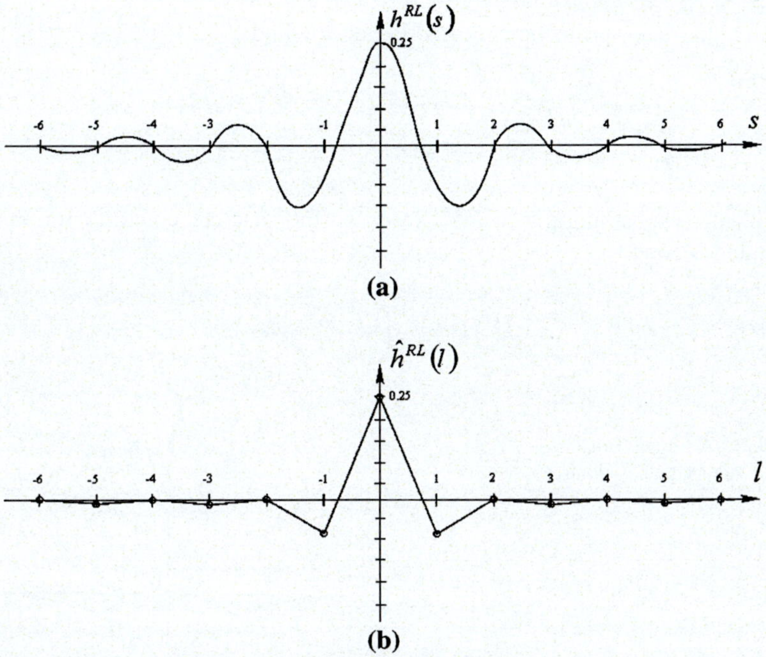

Fig. 5.19 A Ram Lak filter in the s domain: **a** in a continuous form; **b** in a discrete form

Ram Lak filters) causes oscillations, which lead to distortions in the reconstructed image. However, because of the adverse signal-to-noise ratio at high frequencies too large a value of f_0 causes an increase in noise. In the light of such serious disadvantages, new, alternative solutions to this type of filter are still being sought.

In practical applications, the Shepp Logan filter [8, 14] (so-called by combining the names of its creators) is of great significance. The formula for this type of window function is:

$$W^{SL}(f) = \begin{cases} \left| \dfrac{\sin\left(\frac{\pi f}{2f_0}\right)}{\frac{\pi f}{2f_0}} \right| & \text{for } |f| \leq f_0 \\ 0 & \text{for } |f| > f_0 \end{cases}, \tag{5.62}$$

where f_0 is the cut-off frequency of the filter.

The complete frequency form of the Shepp Logan filter, obtained from the window function described by relationship (5.62), is given by the formula below and is shown graphically in Fig. 5.20:

$$H^{SL}(f) = |f| W^{SL}(f) = \left| \frac{\sin\left(\frac{\pi f}{2f_0}\right)}{\frac{\pi f}{2f_0}} \right| \operatorname{rect}\left(\frac{f}{2f_0}\right). \tag{5.63}$$

By substituting formula (5.63) into (5.55) and taking the value of the cut-off frequency to be $f_0 = \frac{1}{2\Delta_s^p}$, we obtain an s-domain filter that is useful for the convolution and back-projection reconstruction method:

$$h^{SL}(s) = -\left(\frac{\sqrt{2}}{\pi \Delta_s^p}\right)^2 \frac{1 - 2\frac{s}{\Delta_s^p} \sin\left(\frac{\pi s}{\Delta_s^p}\right)}{4\left(\frac{s}{\Delta_s^p}\right)^2 - 1}, \tag{5.64}$$

which, after substituting $s = l \cdot \Delta_s^p$, leads to the discrete equation for this filter presented below:

$$\hat{h}^{SL}(l) = -\left(\frac{\sqrt{2}}{\pi \Delta_s^p}\right)^2 \frac{1}{4l - 1}. \tag{5.65}$$

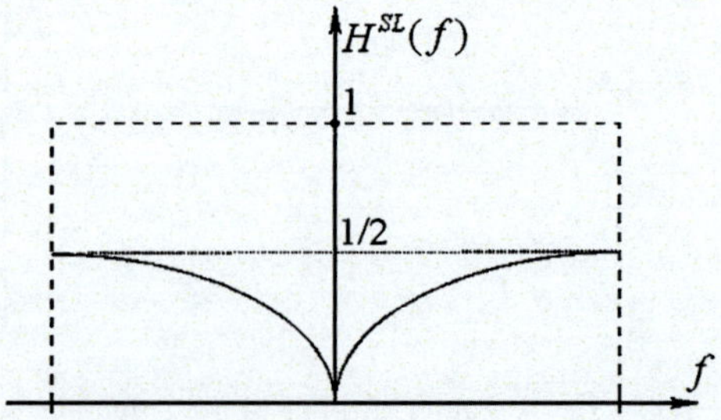

Fig. 5.20 A Shepp Logan filter in the frequency domain

As we did in the case of the Ram Lak filter, we can also show the function devised by Shepp and Logan both in its continuous and its discrete form (see Fig. 5.21).

Tables 5.2, 5.3 and 5.4 include a survey of the more popular implementations of filters [5], which owing to the role that they play in the reconstruction problem bear the name convolution kernels. As well as the two filter forms introduced above, the tables also contain the well-known Low-pass cosine and the generalised Hamming filters.

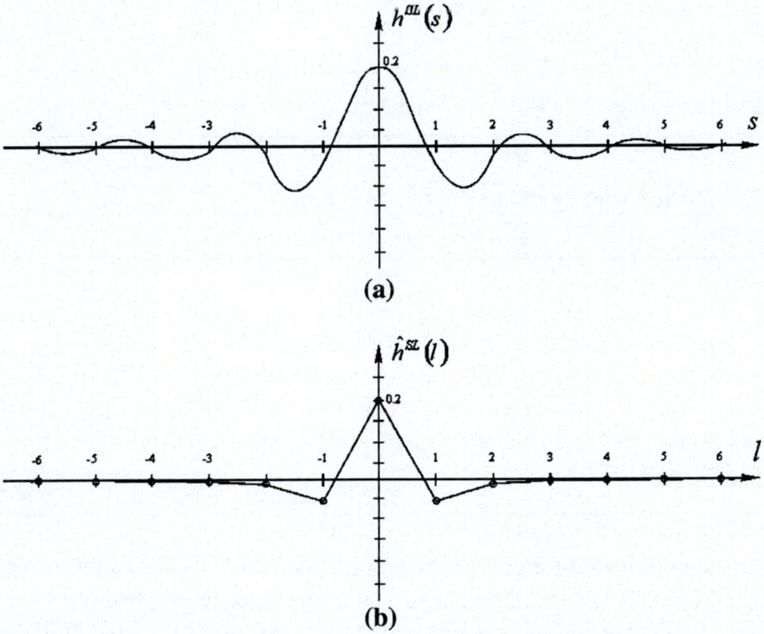

Fig. 5.21 A Shepp Logan filter in the s domain: **a** in the form of a continuous function; **b** in its discrete form

Table 5.2 Examples of convolution kernels in the frequency domain

Type of filter	Response in the frequency domain $H(f)$
Shepp Logan (Shepp and Logan)	$H^{SL}(f) \quad \lvert f\rvert W^{SL}(f) \quad \left\lvert \frac{\sin\left(\frac{\pi f}{2f_0}\right)}{\frac{\pi f}{2f_0}} \right\rvert rect\left(\frac{f}{2f_0}\right)$
Ram Lak (Ramachandran and Lakshminarayanan)	$H^{RL}(f) \quad \lvert f\rvert rect\left(\frac{f}{2f_0}\right)$
Low pass cosine	$H^{LC}(f) \quad \lvert f\rvert \cos\left(\frac{\pi f}{2f_0}\right) rect\left(\frac{f}{2f_0}\right)$
Generalised Hamming	$H^{GH}(f) \quad \lvert f\rvert \left(\eta + (1 \quad \eta)\cos\left(\frac{\pi f}{2f_0}\right)\right) rect\left(\frac{f}{2f_0}\right)$ η parameter

Table 5.3 Point spread functions of the convolution kernels

Type of filter		Point spread function $h(s)$
Shepp Logan	$h^{SL}(s)$	$\left(\frac{\sqrt{2}}{\pi\Delta_s^p}\right)^2 \frac{1-2\frac{s}{\Delta_s^p}\sin\left(\frac{\pi s}{\Delta_s^p}\right)}{4\left(\frac{s}{\Delta_s^p}\right)^2-1}$
Ram Lak	$h^{\mathrm{RL}}(s)$	$\frac{1}{2(\Delta_s^p)^2}\frac{\sin\left(\frac{\pi s}{\Delta_s^p}\right)}{\frac{\pi s}{\Delta_s^p}}\quad\frac{1}{4(\Delta_s^p)^2}\left(\frac{\sin\left(\frac{\pi s}{2\Delta_s^p}\right)}{\frac{\pi s}{2\Delta_s^p}}\right)^2$
Low pass cosine	$h^{LC}(s)$	$\frac{1}{2}\left(h^{\mathrm{RL}}\left(s\quad\frac{\Delta_s^p}{2}\right)+h^{\mathrm{RL}}\left(s+\frac{\Delta_s^p}{2}\right)\right)$
Generalised Hamming	$h^{GH}(s)$	$\eta h^{\mathrm{RL}}(s)+\frac{1-\eta}{2}\left(h^{\mathrm{RL}}(s\quad\Delta_s^p)+h^{\mathrm{RL}}(s+\Delta_s^p)\right)$ η parameter

Table 5.4 Discrete implementation of convolution kernels

Type of filter		Discrete point spread function $\hat{h}(l)$
Shepp Logan	$\hat{h}^{SL}(l)$	$\left(\frac{\sqrt{2}}{\pi\Delta_s^p}\right)^2\frac{1}{4l-1}$
Ram Lak	$\hat{h}^{\mathrm{RL}}(l)$	$\begin{cases}\frac{1}{(2\Delta_s^p)^2} & \text{for } l\quad 0\\ 0 & \text{for } l \text{ even and } l\ /\ 0\\ \frac{1}{(\pi l\Delta_s^p)^2} & \text{for } l \text{ odd}\end{cases}$
Low pass cosine	$\hat{h}^{LC}(l)$	$\frac{1}{2\Delta_s^p}\left(\hat{h}^{\mathrm{RL}}(l\quad\frac{1}{2})+\hat{h}^{\mathrm{RL}}(l+\frac{1}{2})\right)$
Generalised Hamming	$\hat{h}^{GH}(l)$	$\frac{\eta}{\Delta_s^p}\hat{h}^{\mathrm{RL}}(l)+\frac{1-\eta}{2\Delta_s^p}\left(\hat{h}^{\mathrm{RL}}(l\quad 1)+\hat{h}^{\mathrm{RL}}(l+1)\right)$ η parameter

The Shepp Logan filter gives better results than the Ram Lak in the presence of low-level noise. However, the general Hamming filter, whose parameter η can be optimised for the noise content, gives good results in the presence of high-level noise.

Other possible forms of filters such as Hann, Parzen and Blackman filters are presented, for example, in book [3].

5.4.2 Reconstruction Method by Convolution and Back-Projection

Among the methods for obtaining reconstructed images in modern CT scanners, the one that deserves particular attention is that using convolution and back-projection [4 6, 8]. Thanks to the simplicity of its implementation, it has virtually cornered the market for reconstruction software and despite a huge number of rival algorithms, this method occupies the leading position.

In the convolution and back-projection method, filtering takes place in the s-domain using the following equation derived in the proof of relationship (5.36) above:

$$\mu(x,y)=\int_0^{\pi}\left(F_1^{\ 1}(P(f,\alpha^p)\cdot f\cdot sign(f))\right)\mathrm{d}\alpha^p. \tag{5.66}$$

By applying the Fourier transform of the product function (see Appendix A), (5.66) can be converted into the following form:

$$\mu(x,y) = \int_{0}^{\pi} \left(F_1^{\ 1}(P(f,\alpha^p)) * F_1^{\ 1}(f \cdot sign)\right) d\alpha^p, \qquad (5.67)$$

and hence eventually:

$$\mu(x,y) = \int_{0}^{\pi} \left(p^p(s,\alpha^p) * F_1^{\ 1}(f \cdot sign(f))\right) d\alpha^p. \qquad (5.68)$$

By comparing this with (5.37) we obtain:

$$p^p(x\cos\alpha^p + y\sin\alpha^p, \alpha^p) = p^p(s,\alpha^p) * F_1^{\ 1}(f \cdot sign(f)). \qquad (5.69)$$

It is now worth looking at equations that describe this method from the point of view of the application of the Hilbert transform. This transform is defined as:

$$H(fun) \equiv fun(s) * \frac{1}{\pi s} = \frac{1}{\pi} \int_{\infty}^{\infty} \frac{fun(\dot{s})}{s - \dot{s}} d\dot{s}. \qquad (5.70)$$

By suitably selecting *fun*(*s*), we can state that [5, 6]:

$$\tilde{H}\left(\frac{1}{2\pi}\frac{\partial p^p(s,\alpha^p)}{\partial s}\right) = \frac{1}{2\pi^2} \int_{\infty}^{\infty} \frac{\partial p^p(\dot{s},\alpha^p)}{\partial s} \frac{1}{s - \dot{s}} d\dot{s} = p^p(s,\alpha^p). \qquad (5.71)$$

In this way, we obtain $p^p(s,\alpha^p)$ from the original projection $p^p(s, \alpha^p)$ and so we can write:

$$p^p(s,\alpha^p) = \tilde{H}\left(\frac{1}{2\pi} D(p^p(s,\alpha^p))\right), \qquad (5.72)$$

where

$$D(p^p(s,\alpha^p)) = \frac{\partial p^p(s,\alpha^p)}{\partial s}. \qquad (5.73)$$

The values $p^p(s,\alpha^p)$ obtained in this way, according to (5.37), need only be subjected to the process of back-projection in order to reconstruct the final image. The whole process can be reduced to the following:

$$\mu(x,y) = B\left(\tilde{H}\left(\frac{1}{2\pi}(p^p(s,\alpha^p))'\right)\right) = \frac{1}{2\pi} B\left(\tilde{H}(D(p^p(s,\alpha^p)))\right) \qquad (5.74)$$

or to the equivalent form:

$$\mu(x,y) = B\left(p^P(s,\alpha^P) * F_1^{-1}\{|f|\}\right). \tag{5.75}$$

Figure 5.22 illustrates the image reconstruction process as expressed by (5.75).

At this point, it is worth looking at the effect of limiting the space in which the projections $p^P(s, \alpha^P)$ are carried out in the s-domain, that is to say, the physical boundaries of the space in which we can place the patient undergoing tomographic examination. If we assume that $\breve{\mu}(x,y)$ is a function with a finite spectrum approximating to $\mu(x, y)$, then (5.46) assumes the following form:

$$\breve{\mu}(x,y) = \int_0^{\pi}\left(\int_{\infty}^{+\infty} W(f)\cdot rect\left(\frac{f}{2f_0}\right)\cdot P(f,\alpha^P)\cdot f\cdot sign(f)e^{j2\pi fs}df\right)d\alpha^P, \tag{5.76}$$

where f_0 is the cut-off frequency of function $p^P(s, \alpha^P)$.

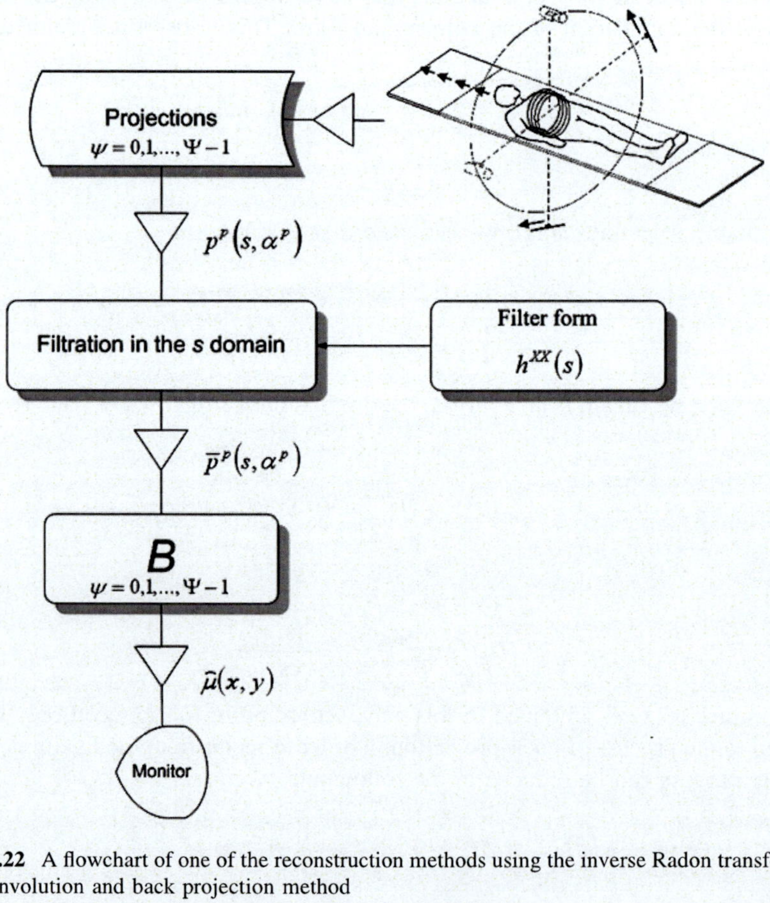

Fig. 5.22 A flowchart of one of the reconstruction methods using the inverse Radon transform the convolution and back projection method

Because the value of the window function is $W(f) = 0$ for $|f| > f_0$, we can make the following transformation:

$$\breve{\mu}(x,y) = \int_{0}^{\pi} \left(\int_{\infty}^{+\infty} P(f,\alpha^p) e^{j2\pi fs} \mathrm{d}f \right. \\ \left. * \int_{f_0}^{f_0} W(f) \cdot rect\left(\frac{f}{2f_0}\right) \cdot f \cdot sign(f) e^{j2\pi fs} \mathrm{d}f \right) \mathrm{d}\alpha^p. \tag{5.77}$$

From a comparison of (5.77) and (5.37), it follows that in this case:

$$\breve{\mu}(x,y) = \int_{0}^{\pi} \breve{p}^p(s,\alpha^p) \mathrm{d}\alpha^p, \tag{5.78}$$

where

$$\breve{p}^p(x\cos\alpha^p + y\sin\alpha^p, \alpha^p) = p^p(s,\alpha^p) * \int_{f_0}^{f_0} W(f) \cdot f \cdot sign(f) e^{j2\pi fs} \mathrm{d}f \tag{5.79}$$

and bearing in mind our earlier consideration of convolution kernels, that is the convolving functions, we can finally write:

$$\breve{\mu}(x,y) = \int_{0}^{\pi} p^p(s,\alpha^p) * h^{XX}(s) \mathrm{d}\alpha^p, \tag{5.80}$$

where $h^{XX}(s)$ is the point spread function of the selected convolution kernel.

The conversion of this reconstruction method into its discrete form is given below.

5.4.3 Discrete Implementation of the Reconstruction Method by Convolution and Back-Projection

The limited number of projections carried out during each revolution of the X-ray tube and the limited resolution at which the radiation intensities are measured have been given earlier by (5.16) and (5.21) and their associated descriptions. According to these equations, the angles at which the individual discrete projections are carried out are represented by $\alpha^p_\psi = \psi \Delta^p_\alpha$; $\psi = 0, \ldots, \Psi - 1$ and at each of these angles, we use radiation detectors placed at equal intervals at locations $s_l = l \cdot \Delta_s^p$ on the screen, where the index variable is $l = -(L-1)/2, \ldots, 0, \ldots, (L-1)/2$. It is therefore only the projection values $\hat{p}^p(l, \psi)$, obtained at these defined angles and these selected points, that are available to the reconstruction algorithm.

The procedure for obtaining a reconstructed image from projection values defined in this way is outlined in the steps shown below, which are based on the sequence of operations set out in the formula [5]:

$$\breve{\mu}(x,y) = B\{p^p(s,\alpha^p) * h^{XX}(s)\}. \tag{5.81}$$

Step I In order to carry out the subsequent steps in this image reconstruction method, we need to begin by performing convolution operations on each projection delivered in turn by the scanner, using a suitably well-matched convolution kernel representing the filter. Bearing in mind the factors involved in the discrete implementation of the algorithm, we need to consider what conditions must be fulfilled in order for the filtered projection function $p^p(s, \alpha^p)$ (having the form (5.79) in the continuous version) to reduce to the following, discrete form:

$$\hat{p}^p(l,\psi) = \Delta_s^p \sum_{\dot{l}=\ \infty}^{\infty} \hat{p}^p(\dot{l},\psi)\hat{h}(l-\dot{l}). \tag{5.82}$$

The proof of relationship (5.82) is based on the discrete approximation of the convolution theorem assuming a band-limited function $p^p(s, \alpha^p)$. For now, it will be enough to restrict the summation limits to the values $-(L-1)/2 \leq l \leq (L-1)/2$ and to choose an appropriate discrete form of filter for this application. Table 5.4 includes the discrete formulas of four of the most popular filters, obtained by the substitution of $\hat{h}(l) = h(l \cdot \Delta_s^p)$ into the corresponding continuous versions presented in Table 5.3. Using the selected convolution kernel, the final discrete filtering takes place according to the following equation:

$$\hat{p}^p(l,\psi) = \Delta_s^p \sum_{\dot{l}=\ (L\ 1)/2}^{(L\ 1)/2} \hat{p}^p(\dot{l},\psi)\hat{h}^{XX}(l-\dot{l}), \tag{5.83}$$

where *XX* is the symbol representing the selected convolution kernel (e.g. 'RL').

If the frequency spectrum of the discrete projection function $\hat{p}^p(l,\psi)$ is represented by $\hat{P}(f,\psi)$, then after carrying out the projection method $\hat{p}^p(l,\psi)$ described above, we obtain the frequency characteristic $\hat{P}(f,\psi)$. Obviously, the form of spectrum $\hat{P}(f,\psi)$ depends on the type of filter applied. These operations are performed with the aim of preventing geometrical distortions in the projections.

Step II Although as a result of carrying out the previous phase of the reconstruction algorithm we obtain the projection function $\hat{p}^p(l,\psi)$ devoid of geometrical distortions, these projection values most often relate to a line of travel which does not go through the discrete points (i, j) needed for (5.88). It then becomes necessary to apply yet another step in the processing of projection $\hat{p}^p(l, \psi)$: interpolation based on the projections made by the rays passing nearest to the point (i, j) under consideration. An illustration of the application of linear interpolation is given in Fig. 5.23.

The interpolation operation carried out on the values of projection function $\hat{p}^p(l, \psi)$ can be written mathematically as follows:

$$\dot{p}^p\left(i\Delta_x \cos\psi\Delta_\alpha^p + j\Delta_y \sin\psi\Delta_\alpha^p, \psi\Delta_\alpha^p\right) = \Delta_s^p \sum_l \hat{p}^p(l, \psi) \cdot I\left(i\Delta_x \cos\psi\Delta_\alpha^p + j\Delta_y \sin\psi\Delta_\alpha^p - l\Delta_s^p\right), \tag{5.84}$$

where $I(\Delta s)$ is the interpolation function, defining the dependence of the value of $\dot{p}^p(s, \psi\Delta_\alpha^p)$ at any point on the screen on the value $\hat{p}^p(l, \psi)$ at a measured point, as a function of the distance between the two points.

If we apply a linear interpolation function of the following form [5]:

$$I^L = \begin{cases} \frac{1}{\Delta_s^p}\left(1 - \frac{|\Delta s|}{\Delta_s^p}\right) & \text{for } |\Delta s| \le \Delta_s^p \\ 0 & \text{for } |\Delta s| > \Delta_s^p \end{cases}, \tag{5.85}$$

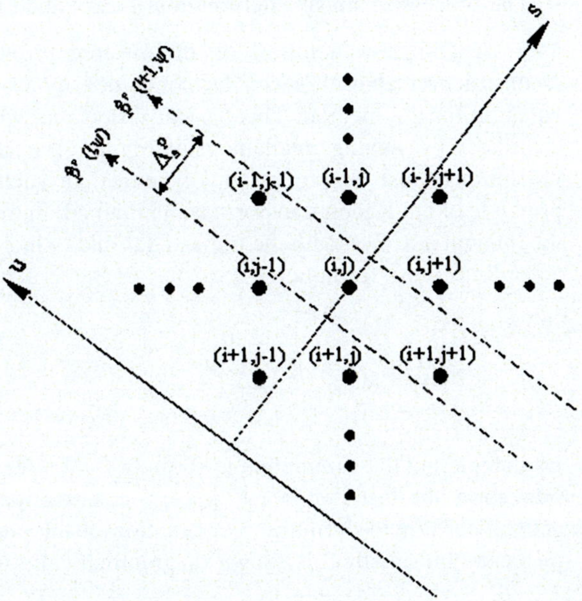

Fig. 5.23 The interpolation of projection values at a point of interest based on values obtained from neighbouring projection lines

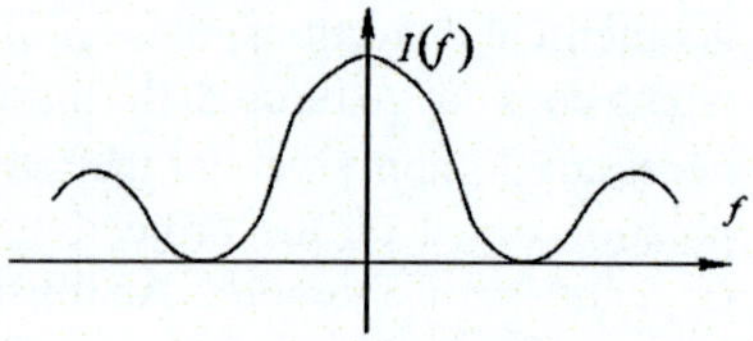

Fig. 5.24 The frequency spectrum of the interpolation function from (5.85)

where $\Delta s = i\Delta_x \cos\psi\Delta^p_\alpha + j\Delta_y \sin\psi\Delta^p_\alpha - l\Delta^p_s$, then formula (5.84) becomes:

$$\dot{p}^p\left(s_{ij}, \psi\Delta^p_\alpha\right) \cong \hat{\tilde{p}}^p\left(l^\downarrow, \psi\right) + \left(\frac{s_{ij}}{\Delta^p_s} - l^\downarrow\right)\left(\hat{\tilde{p}}^p\left(l^\uparrow, \psi\right) - \hat{\tilde{p}}^p\left(l^\downarrow, \psi\right)\right), \tag{5.86}$$

where $s_{ij} = i\Delta_i \cos\Delta^p_\alpha + j\Delta_j \sin\Delta^p_\alpha$ is the coordinate defining the position of point (i, j) on the screen, during a projection carried out at angle $\alpha^p_\psi = \psi\Delta^p_\alpha$; $l^\downarrow = \text{Trunc}(s_{ij}, \Delta^p_s)$ is the position of the first of the rays passing in the vicinity of point (i,j); $l^\uparrow = l^\downarrow + 1$ is the position of the second of the neighbouring rays.

The frequency form of the interpolation function obtained from (5.85) is given by this formula:

$$I^L(f) = \left(\frac{\sin\left(\frac{\pi f}{2f_0}\right)}{\frac{\pi f}{2f_0}}\right)^2, \tag{5.87}$$

and is shown in Fig. 5.24.

The process of linear interpolation is explained in more detail by Fig. 5.25.

Step III Our consideration of the discrete convolution and back-projection reconstruction algorithm can be concluded by re-stating (5.78), a fundamental equation for the method. This basically says that we can reconstruct the image of an object by having available suitably pre-prepared projections. The original projections must be processed, of course, in such a way that the inversibility principle of the Radon transform is maintained. In the discrete case, we can replace the integral in (5.78) with the trapezoidal rule (which approximates to the integral), according to the formula:

$$\hat{\mu}(i,j) \cong \Delta^p_\alpha \cdot \sum_{\psi=0}^{\Psi - 1} \dot{p}^p\left(i\Delta_x \cos\psi\Delta^p_\alpha + j\Delta_y \sin\psi\Delta^p_\alpha, \psi\Delta^p_\alpha\right). \tag{5.88}$$

By completing the summation in formula (5.88), we complete the process of back-projection, the last step in the image reconstruction process. An overview of the actions performed during implementation of the convolution and back-projection reconstruction method is shown diagrammatically in Fig. 5.26.

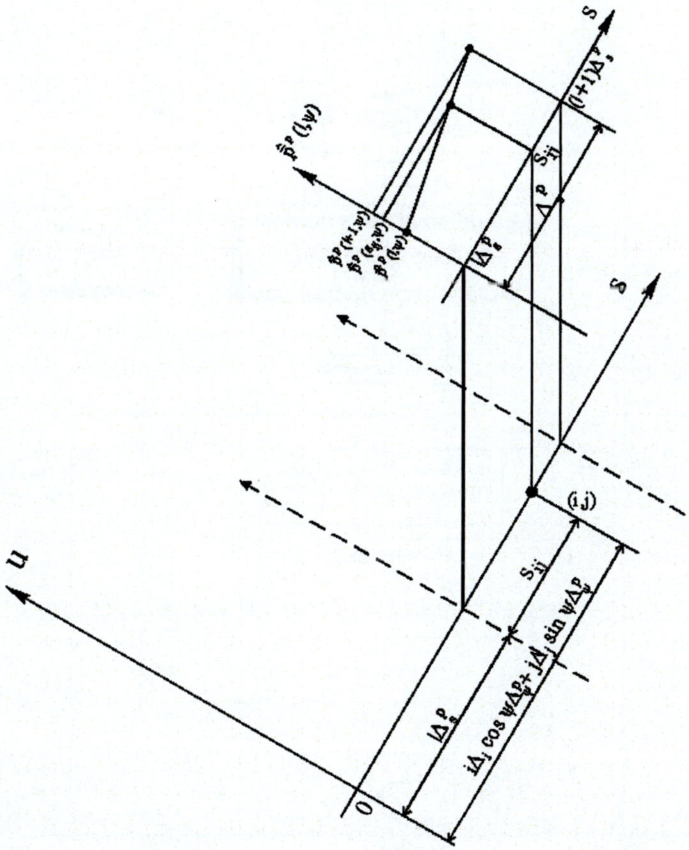

Fig. 5.25 The linear interpolation of projection values at points through which the rays do not pass

5.4.4 Reconstruction Method by Filtration and Back-Projection

In contrast to the previous convolution and back-projection approach to the reconstruction problem, in this algorithm filtering takes place in the frequency domain [5]. In order to derive a formula for this method, we need to make use of the following equation again (introduced in the proof of (5.36)):

$$\mu(x,y) = \int_{0}^{\pi} \left(F_1^{-1}(P(f,\alpha^p)) \cdot f \cdot sign(f)\right) \mathrm{d}\alpha^p. \tag{5.89}$$

In this case, after applying the Fourier transform to the individual projections we obtain:

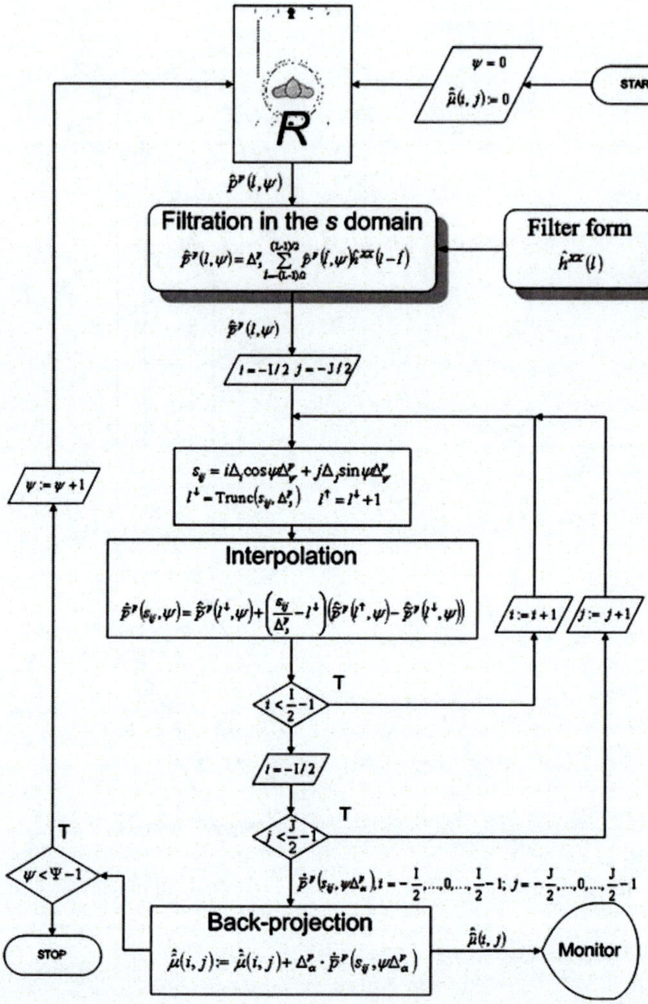

Fig. 5.26 A flowchart of the discrete convolution and back projection algorithm

$$\mu(x,y) = \int_0^{\pi} \left(F_1^{-1}(F_1(p^p(s,\alpha^p))) \cdot f \cdot sign(f)\right) d\alpha^p, \tag{5.90}$$

which means that, with reference to (5.37), we can apply the following substitution:

$$p^p(x\cos\alpha^p + y\sin\alpha^p, \alpha^p) = F_1^{-1}(F_1(p^p(s,\alpha^p)) \cdot f \cdot sign(f)). \tag{5.91}$$

As we already know how to prevent distortion of the projections in this algorithm, we can write:

$$p^p(s, \alpha^p) = F_1^{-1}(|f| \cdot F_1(p^p(s, \alpha^p))). \tag{5.92}$$

Using (5.92) and (5.90) and assuming unlimited space, we can express the filtration and back-projection reconstruction method in the following way:

$$\mu(x, y) = B\left(F_1^{-1}(|f| \cdot F_1(p^p(s, \alpha^p)))\right). \tag{5.93}$$

Figure 5.27 shows a flowchart of the actions performed in this reconstruction method, based on formula (5.93).

If however we take into account the physical constraint of the space available as well as the effect of sampling on the projection spectrum, then we should include the window function in (5.89) as we did with the convolution and back-projection

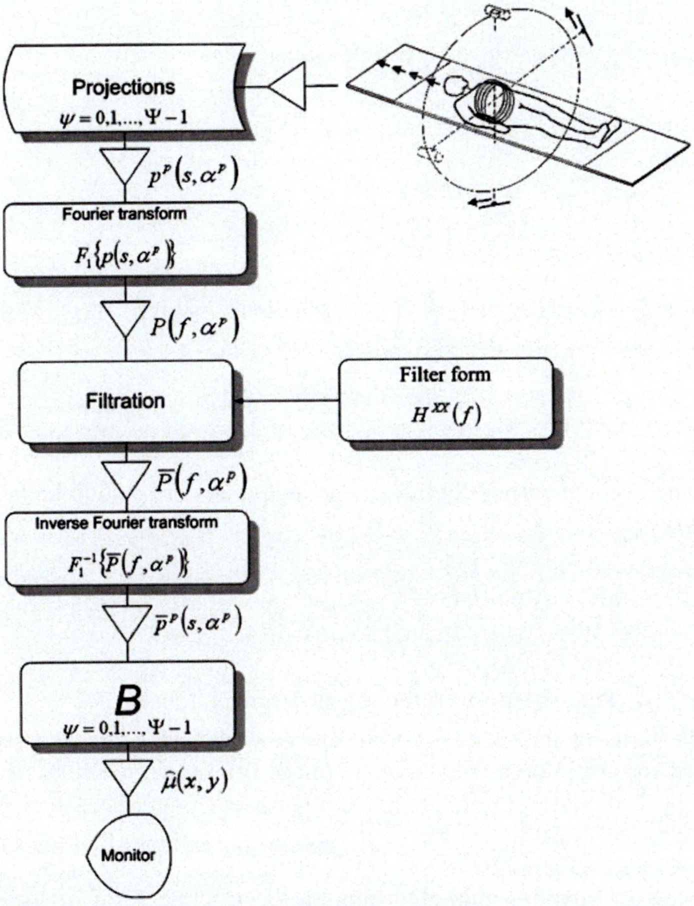

Fig. 5.27 A flowchart for the filtration and back projection reconstruction method

method. This entails the following modification of the reconstructed attenuation function with band-limited spectrum:

$$\breve{\mu}(x,y) = \int_0^{\pi}\left(\int_{\infty}^{+\infty} W(f)\cdot rect\left(\frac{f}{2f_0}\right)\cdot P(f,\alpha^p)\cdot f\cdot sign(f)\mathrm{e}^{j2\pi fs}\mathrm{d}f\right)\mathrm{d}\alpha^p, \quad (5.94)$$

where f_0 is the cut-off frequency of function $p^p(s, \alpha^p)$.

By considering the value of the window function $W(f)$ for $|f| > f_0$ to be equal to zero, the above relationship takes the form:

$$\breve{\mu}(x,y) = \int_0^{\pi}\int_{\infty}^{+\infty}\left(\int_{\infty}^{+\infty} p^p(s,\alpha^p)\mathrm{e}^{\ j2\pi fs}\mathrm{d}s\right)W(f)rect\left(\frac{f}{2f_0}\right)f\cdot sign(f)\mathrm{e}^{j2\pi fs}\mathrm{d}f\,\mathrm{d}\alpha^p. \quad (5.95)$$

By comparing (5.95) and (5.37), it follows that:

$$\breve{\mu}(x,y) = \int_0^{\pi}\breve{p}^p(s,\alpha^p)\mathrm{d}\alpha^p, \quad (5.96)$$

where

$$\breve{p}^p(x\cos\alpha^p + y\sin\alpha^p,\alpha^p) = \int_{\infty}^{+\infty}\left(\int_{\infty}^{+\infty} p^p(s,\alpha^p)\mathrm{e}^{\ j2\pi fs}\mathrm{d}s\right)\cdot W(f)\cdot rect\left(\frac{f}{2f_0}\right)\cdot f \cdot sign(f)\mathrm{e}^{j2\pi fs}\mathrm{d}f. \quad (5.97)$$

Taking into account earlier considerations regarding convolution kernels, we can finally write:

$$\breve{\mu}(x,y) = \int_0^{\pi}\left(\int_{\infty}^{+\infty} P(f,\alpha^p)\cdot H^{XX}(f)\mathrm{e}^{j2\pi fs}\mathrm{d}f\right)\mathrm{d}\alpha^p, \quad (5.98)$$

where $H^{XX}(f)$ is the spectrum of the selected convolution kernel.

On the basis of formula (5.98) we are now able to define the sequence of operations for obtaining a reconstructed image from the projections as:

$$\breve{\mu}(x,y) = B\left\{F_1^{\ 1}\left\{F_1\{p^p(s,\alpha^p)\}\cdot H^{XX}(f)\right\}\right\}. \quad (5.99)$$

The process of adapting this algorithm to the discrete form of the projection function is discussed next.

5.4.5 Discrete Implementation of the Reconstruction Method by Filtration and Back-Projection

In the practical implementation of this reconstruction algorithm, as in the previous method, projections are only carried out at specific angles α^p, i.e. only at angles $\alpha^p_\psi = \psi \cdot \Delta^p_\alpha$; $\psi = 0,\ldots, \Psi - 1$, where Δ^p_α represents the angle through which the source-screen system is rotated after each projection. While these projections are being carried out at angles α^p_ψ, the X-ray intensity is measured by radiation detectors placed on a screen at accurately determined positions s, fulfilling the condition $s_l = l \cdot \Delta^p_s$; $l = -\mathrm{L}/2, \ldots, 0,\ldots, (\mathrm{L}/2) - 1$. Here, L is the number of detectors on the screen, while Δ^p_s is the distance between detectors. Bearing in mind the future use of FFT algorithms, the quantity L is chosen to be equal to a positive integer power of 2.

Taking these circumstances into account, the filtration and back-projection reconstruction method is implemented in the following sequence [5]:

Step I Since in this reconstruction approach we use discrete forms of projection (represented by $\hat{p}^p(l,\psi); l = -\mathrm{L}/2,\ldots,0,\ldots,(\mathrm{L}/2) - 1;\ \psi = 0,\ldots, \Psi - 1$) and especially since their spectra are obtained using FFT algorithms, it becomes necessary to change the sample index of the projection function. The value of L is increased to a multiple of itself and is then represented by $\acute{\mathrm{L}}$. So the new sequence $\acute{l}$ becomes $\acute{l} = 1,\ldots,\acute{\mathrm{L}}$. The relationship between L and $\acute{\mathrm{L}}$ determines the sampling resolution of the spectrum and might have a value of say $\acute{\mathrm{L}} = 2\mathrm{L}$. The new range of the sample index is increased to $\acute{\mathrm{L}}$ according to the following pattern:

$$\acute{\hat{p}}^p(\acute{l},\psi) = \begin{cases} \hat{p}^p\left(\acute{l} - 1, \psi\right) & \text{for } \acute{l} = 1,\ldots,\mathrm{L}/2 \\ 0 & \text{for } \acute{l} = \mathrm{L}/2 + 1,\ldots,\acute{\mathrm{L}} - \mathrm{L}/2 \cdot \\ \hat{p}^p\left(\acute{l} - \acute{\mathrm{L}} - 1, \psi\right) & \text{for } \acute{\mathrm{L}} - \mathrm{L}/2 + 1,\ldots,\acute{\mathrm{L}} \end{cases} \tag{5.100}$$

This procedure is illustrated in Fig. 5.28.

Step II In this step, the individual projections $\acute{\hat{p}}^p(\acute{l},\psi); \psi = 0,\ldots,\Psi - 1$ are transferred to the frequency domain using an FFT algorithm (an implementation of one of the FFT algorithms is found in Appendix B). In other words, this stage determines the spectra of the individual projections $\acute{\hat{P}}(\acute{l},\psi); \acute{l} = 1,\ldots,\acute{\mathrm{L}}$; for $\psi = 0,\ldots, \Psi - 1$.

The change in the sample index is applied to the discrete spectrum of the selected filter $\acute{\hat{H}}^{XX}(\acute{l})$; where $\acute{l} = 1,\ldots,\acute{\mathrm{L}}$. Obviously, this action is performed only once, at the beginning of the reconstruction process, using one of the possible filters presented in Table 5.2. The spectrum of the chosen filter is prepared according to the following transformation:

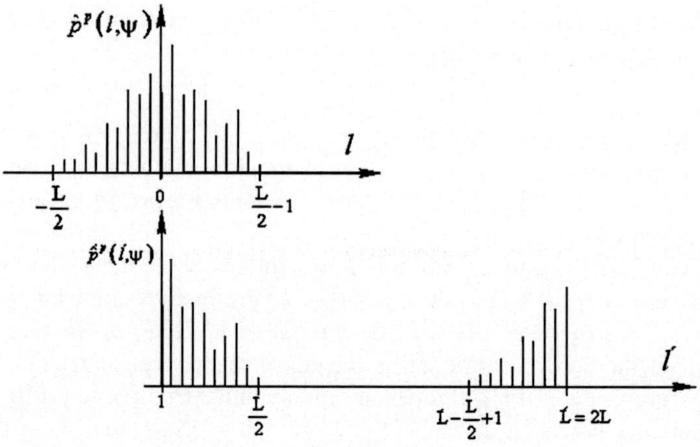

Fig. 5.28 The shift of sampling sequence needed for the implementation of FFT algorithms

$$\acute{H}^{XX}\left(\acute{l}\right) = \begin{cases} H^{XX}\left(\left(\acute{l}-1\right)\cdot\Delta_f\right) & \text{for } \acute{l} = 1,\ldots,\acute{L}/2 \\ H^{XX}\left(\left(\acute{l}-\acute{L}-1\right)\cdot\Delta_f\right) & \text{for } \acute{l} = \acute{L}/2+1,\ldots,\acute{L} \end{cases}, \tag{5.101}$$

in which Δ_f is the spectrum sampling interval, where

$$\Delta_f = \frac{1}{\acute{L}}\Delta_s^p. \tag{5.102}$$

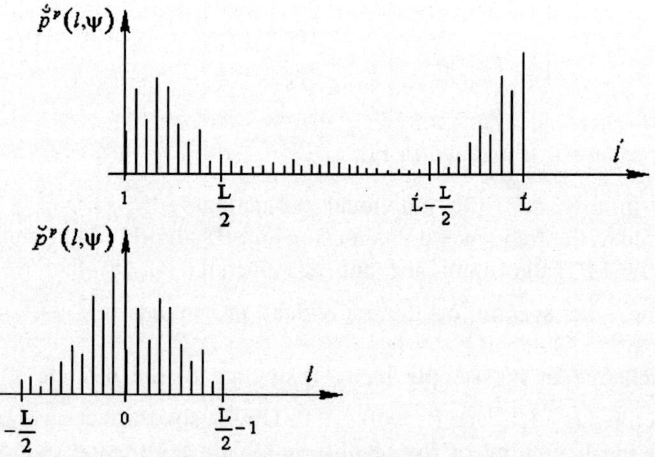

Fig. 5.29 The filtered projection after the sequence of operations carried out in the frequency domain

Step III As outlined by relationship (5.98), it is necessary here to multiply the discrete values of the frequency function $\acute{\hat{P}}\left(\acute{l},\psi\right)$ of the individual projections $\psi = 0,\ldots, \Psi - 1$ by the sampled values of the spectrum of the selected filter $\acute{\hat{H}}^{XX}\left(\acute{l}\right)$:

$$\acute{\hat{P}}\left(\acute{l},\psi\right) = \acute{\hat{P}}\left(\acute{l},\psi\right) \cdot \acute{\hat{H}}^{XX}\left(\acute{l}\right), \tag{5.103}$$

for each $\acute{l} = 1,\ldots,\acute{L}$.

Step IV The result of each of these multiplications for $\psi = 0,\ldots, \Psi - 1$ is subjected to inverse Fourier transformation (IFFT) to obtain $\acute{\hat{p}}^{p}(\acute{l},\psi)$, where $\acute{l} = 1,\ldots,\acute{L}$; $\psi = 0,\ldots,\Psi - 1$. An implementation of one of the IFFT algorithms can be found in Appendix B.

Step V In this step, the projection values $\acute{\hat{p}}^{p}(\acute{l},\psi); \acute{l} = 1,\ldots,\acute{L}$ need to be indexed, in a way which is the reverse of the process in *Step I*, to obtain values $\hat{p}^{p}(l,\psi)$ arranged in the order $l = -L/2, \ldots, 0, \ldots, (L/2) - 1$, as follows:

$$\hat{p}^{p}(l,\psi) = \begin{cases} \acute{\hat{p}}^{p}(l+1,\psi) & \text{for } l = 0,\ldots,(L/2)-1 \\ \acute{\hat{p}}^{p}(\acute{L}+l+1,\psi) & \text{for } l = -L/2,\ldots,-1 \end{cases}. \tag{5.104}$$

The process of obtaining projection $\hat{p}^{p}(l,\psi)$, defined in this way, is shown in Fig. 5.29.

Step VI The paths of the projections $\hat{p}^{p}(l,\psi)$, obtained as described in previous stages of the reconstruction process, can often miss discrete points (i, j) of the image, as expressed in (5.88). It is therefore necessary to interpolate the projection values $\dot{p}^{p}(s_{ij},\psi)$ going through point (i, j), based on the values of function $\hat{p}^{p}(l,\psi)$. Equation (5.84) shows the formal notation for this operation. We usually consider the two lines directly neighbouring the line in question $\dot{p}^{p}(s_{ij},\psi)$, applying the principle of linear interpolation defined by formula (5.85). Thus, the values of this projection $\dot{p}^{p}(s_{ij},\psi)$ assigned to the individual discrete points of the image $i = I/2,\ldots, 0,\ldots, I/2 - 1$; $j = J/2,\ldots, 0,\ldots, J/2 - 1$ can now be written down in a similar way to (5.86).

Step VII After obtaining projection values $\dot{p}^{p}(s_{ij},\psi)$ for all angles $\psi = 0,\ldots, \Psi - 1$, we can use (5.88) to carry out the summation that completes the discrete version of the back-projection operation. Combining the projections in this way, at the individual points (i, j) of the image, concludes the reconstruction process.

An overview of all the operations performed in the course of image reconstruction using the filtration and back-projection algorithm is shown in the flowchart in Fig. 5.30.

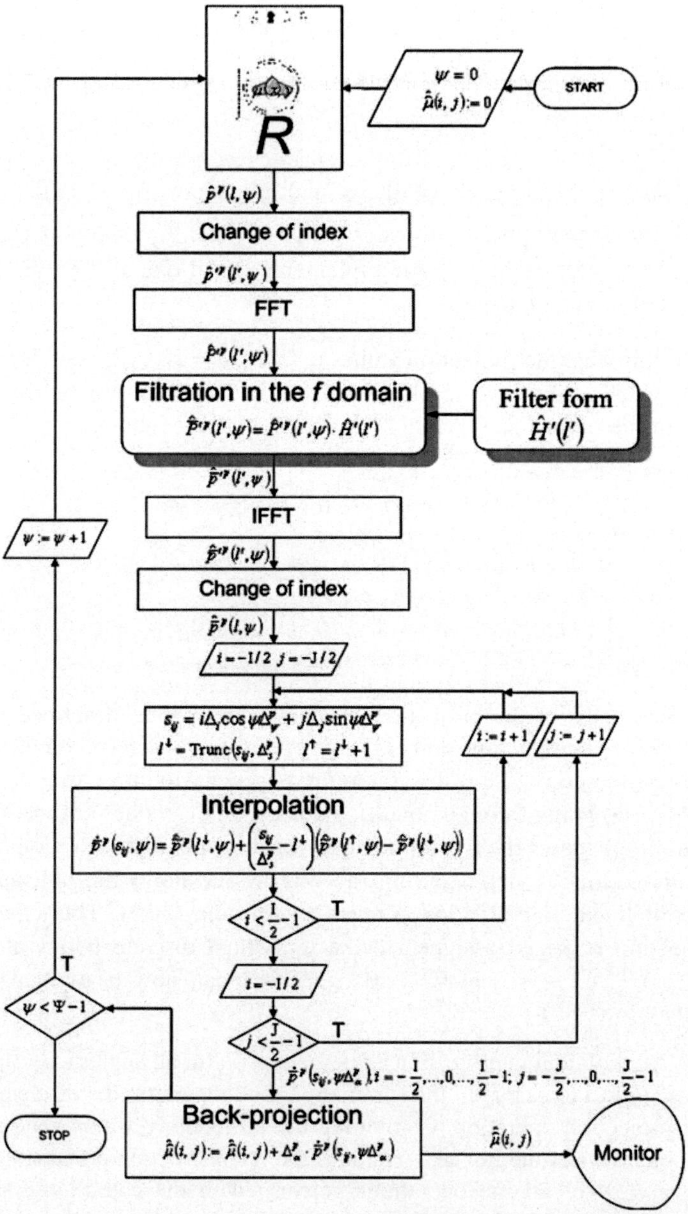

Fig. 5.30 A flowchart of the discrete version of the filtration and back projection algorithm

References

1. Abramowitz M, Stegun IA (1968) Handbook of mathematical functions. US Government Print Office, Dover
2. Crawford CR, Kak AC (1979) Aliasing artifacts in computerized tomography. Appl Opt 18:3704 3711
3. Hamming RW (1989) Digital filters. Prentice Hall, Englewood Cliffs
4. Herman GT (1981) Image reconstruction form projections: the fundamentals of computerized tomography. Academic Press, New York
5. Jain AK (1989) Fundamentals of digitals image processing. Prentice Hall, Englewood Cliffs
6. Kak AC, Slanley M (1988) Principles of computerized tomographic imaging. IEEE Press, New York
7. Ludwig D (1966) The Radon transform on Euclidean space. Commun Pure Appl Math 19:49 81
8. Lewitt RM (1983) Reconstruction algorithms: transform methods. Proc IEEE 71(3):390 408
9. Macovski A (1983) Physical problems of computer tomography. Proc IEEE 71(3):373 378
10. Peters TM, Lewitt RM (1977) Computerized tomography with fan beam geometry. J Comp Assist Tomogr 1:429 436
11. Ramachandran GN, Lakshminarayanan AV (1971) Three dimensional reconstruction from radiographs and electron micrographs: II. Application of convolutions instead of Fourier Transforms. Proc Natl Acad Sci 68:2236 2240
12. Ramachandran GN (1971) Reconstruction of substance from shadow: II. Mathematical theory with application to three dimensional radiology and electron microscopy. Proc Indian Acad Sci 74:14 24
13. Rosenfeld A, Kak AC (1982) Digital picture processing. Academic Press, New York
14. Shepp LA, Logan BF (1974) The Fourier reconstruction of a head section. IEEE Trans Nucl Sci NS 21(3):21 43
15. Slepian D (1976) On banwidth. Proc IEEE 64:292 300

Chapter 6
Reconstruction from Fan-beam Projections

The limitations of CT scanner projection systems that used parallel beams of radiation had become a major obstacle to the development of computed tomography. In order to overcome these growing technical barriers, engineers searched for solutions that used a single X-ray tube in which the radiation was collimated into a narrow beam in the shape of a fan (a fan-beam). This increased the speed with which each projection was carried out, as it eliminated unnecessary lateral movement of the tube-detector system. At the same time, it made more efficient use of the power emitted by the tube; the beam angle of the radiation was significantly increased compared to previous designs resulting in a shorter radiation exposure time for the patient and the distortions due to patient movement were minimised. This solution represents essentially a compromise between the simplicity of the projection system and an increase in the speed of the scanner.

The change to the shape of the radiation beam made it necessary to adapt the reconstruction algorithms to the new projection geometry. This chapter will introduce two basic types of reconstruction algorithm [2, 3, 4, 5, 6, 9] that were devised for fan-beam projections. However, we will not cover other popular solutions, descriptions of which can be found in the literature of the subject [1, 7, 8].

6.1 Geometry of the Fan-beam Scanner

A diagram of a projection system that uses X-rays collimated into the shape of a fan is shown in Fig. 6.1, together with key geometrical relationships [6].

As can be seen from Fig. 6.1, the moving fan-beam system consists of an X-ray tube and a screen in the shape of the arc, on which a matrix of detectors is placed. The axis of rotation of the system and the axis of symmetry of the radiation beam both play an important role in determining the geometric relationships in the system. The axis of rotation is directed along a line perpendicular to the cross-section of the test object, and its point of intersection with this cross-section is

R. Cierniak, *X Ray Computed Tomography in Biomedical Engineering*,
DOI: 10.1007/978 0 85729 027 4 6, © Springer Verlag London Limited 2011

Fig. 6.1 A fan beam scanner **a** a 3D view of the system, **b** basic geometrical relationships

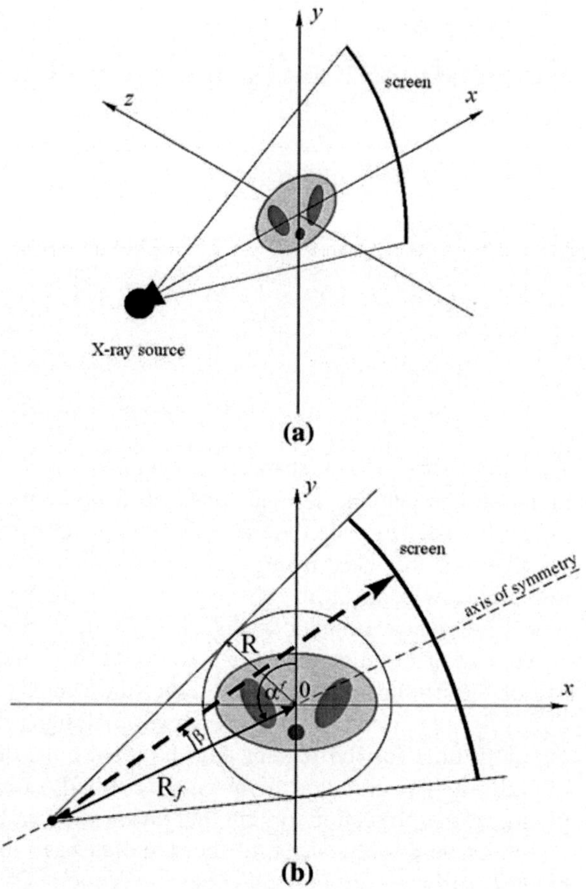

indicated on the diagram by 0. The system rotates about this axis when making projections. The distance of the X-ray tube from the axis of rotation is represented by R_f. The whole of the cross-section of the test object must lie within the fan of X-rays produced by the tube, regardless of the angle at which the projection is made. We can identify a ray emitted by the tube at a given angle of rotation and reaching a particular radiation detector, by the pair of parameters (β, α^f) where:

β the angle that the ray makes with the principal axis of the radiation beam;
α^f the angle of rotation of the fan-beam system.

In contrast to the parallel-beam system, the projections in this system are carried out during one complete revolution. Thus, the angle α^f, at which a projection is made, will be in the range $[0,2\pi)$. The angle varies within the range $[\beta_{\min}, \beta_{\max}]$, where:

$$\beta_{\max} = -\beta_{\min} = \arcsin\left(\frac{R}{R_f}\right), \tag{6.1}$$

where: R is the radius of the circle defining the space in which the examination is made; R_f is the radius of the circle described by the focus of the tube.

If we also assume that:

$$R_f = 2R, \tag{6.2}$$

then possible values for the angle β lie within the range $[-\pi/6, \pi/6]$.

We will represent the projection function acquired in a fan-beam system by the expression $p^f(\beta, \alpha^f)$. All of the procedures described below will use these projections $p^f(\beta, \alpha^f)$; $[\beta_{min}, \beta_{max}]$; $[0, 2\pi)$ to reconstruct the image using solutions obtained for parallel-beam systems. There are two dominant solutions to this problem. The first of these relies on inspecting the rays in the fan-beam for rays that correspond to those in a parallel beam, a process known as rebinning. The second solution makes direct use of the convolution and back-projection reconstruction method.

6.2 Geometry of the Discrete Projection System

Fan-beam scanners can be divided into two systems: those that have an even distribution of useful rays in the fan (*equiangular sampling*), and those that have an even distribution of detectors on the screen (*equispaced sampling*). We can combine the features of both these systems by using a screen curved in an arc in which the focus of the radiation source is situated. Each of these two systems will require a different approach to the reconstruction algorithm. For technical reasons, in medical tomography we use a fan-beam system with equiangular sampling.

In fan-beam scanners, we must also take into account the discrete nature of the projection function. Individual projections are obtained at predetermined angles α_γ^f, using radiation detectors placed on a screen in the shape of an arc. The angular distance β_η is determined by the location of the detectors. The angular distances between the detectors have a constant value Δ_β. We can therefore state that only the projection values $\hat{p}^f(\eta, \gamma)$, obtained at specific projection angles and only for the angles β, determined by the position of the detectors on the screen, are used by the reconstruction algorithm. Details of this fan-beam system are shown in Fig. 6.2.

In practical fan-beam scanners, the individual projections are evenly spaced throughout a complete revolution. Thus, the discrete angles at which the projections are made can be written as:

$$\alpha_\gamma^f = \gamma \cdot \Delta_\alpha^f, \tag{6.3}$$

where: Δ_α^f is the angle through which the tube-screen system is rotated after each projection; $\gamma = 0, 1, \ldots, \Gamma - 1$ is the sample index of each projection; $\Gamma = 2\pi \; div \; \Delta_\alpha^f$ is the maximum number of projections.

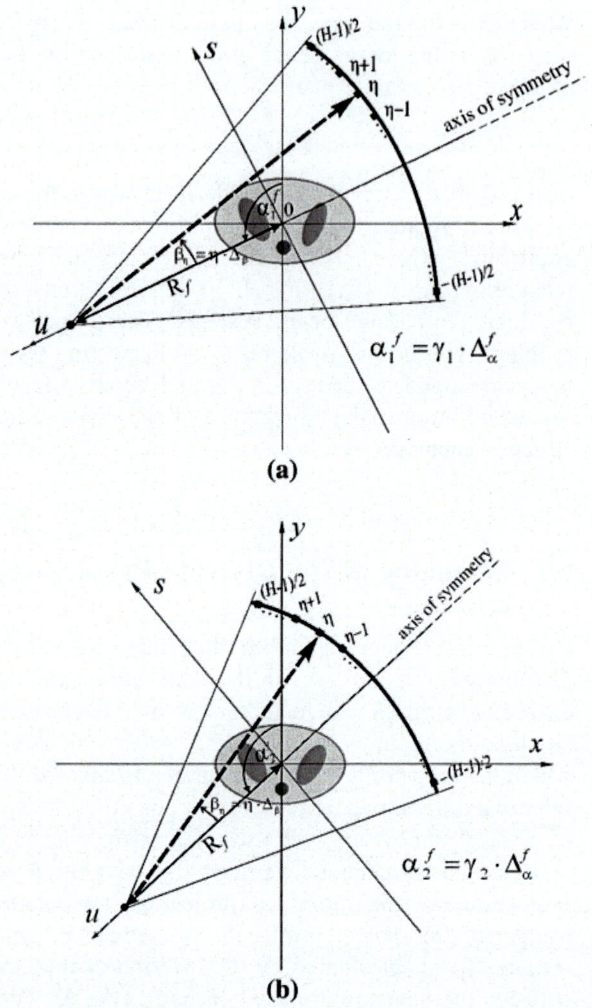

Fig. 6.2 Discrete fan beam system: **a** a projection at an angle $\alpha^f{}_1$, **b** a projection at an angle $\alpha^f{}_2$

If we assume that the total number of detectors is odd and that they are arranged on the screen so that the angles between the rays reaching them are equal, then a particular location on the arc can be defined by the angle:

$$\beta_\eta = \eta \cdot \Delta_\beta, \tag{6.4}$$

where: Δ_β is the angular distance between the radiation detectors; $\eta = -(\mathrm{H}-1)/2, \ldots, 0, \ldots, (\mathrm{H}-1)/2$ is the index of the detectors in the matrix; $\mathrm{H} = 2(\arcsin\frac{\mathrm{R}}{\mathrm{R}_f}\ div\ \Delta_\beta) + 3$ is the maximum number of detectors on the screen.

At this point, we will ignore concerns about the transfer functions of the various radiation detectors and we will make an assumption similar to that in (5.23).

This means that for a fan-beam system, the projection values available are as follows:

$$\hat{p}^f(\eta, \gamma) = p^f\left(\eta\Delta_\beta, \gamma\Delta_\alpha^f\right), \tag{6.5}$$

where: γ is the number of the projection; η is the number of the detector in the matrix.

Frequency issues concerning the projections have been discussed extensively in Chap. 5, so we will now move on to look at some reconstruction methods for this type of scanner.

6.3 Reconstruction Method with Rebinning

This method uses rebinning (sometimes referred to as re-sorting) [2, 3, 4, 9] to reconstruct images from fan-beam projections. In the first stage of the method we inspect all of the projections $p^f(\beta, \alpha^f)$; $\beta \in [\beta_{min}, \beta_{max}]$; $0 \leq \alpha^f < 2\pi$ for rays whose paths would correspond to those of the hypothetical parallel rays $p^p(s,\alpha^p)$; $-\mathrm{R} \leq s \leq \mathrm{R}$; $0 \leq \alpha^p < 2\pi$. This process is based on the premise that, in one of the fan-beams emitted in the course of making all of the projections, there will always be a ray, which would be equivalent to a ray in the virtual parallel-beam, directed towards the radiation detectors at an angle α^p and at a distance s from the centre of rotation. We can use this collection of parallel projections to reconstruct the image using well-known methods devised for actual parallel-beam systems. A flowchart outlining this method is shown in Fig. 6.3.

Using the geometric relationships between the parameters of a ray in one system with those of the corresponding ray in the other system, as shown in Fig. 6.4, we can derive the following:

$$p^f(\beta, \alpha^f) = p^p(s, \alpha^p) = p^p\left(\mathrm{R}_f \sin\beta, \alpha^f + \beta\right), \tag{6.6}$$

which is equivalent to:

$$p^p(s, \alpha^p) = p^f(\beta, \alpha^f) = p^f\left(\arcsin\left(\frac{s}{\mathrm{R}_f}\right), \alpha^p - \arcsin\left(\frac{s}{\mathrm{R}_f}\right)\right). \tag{6.7}$$

From (6.7), we can easily find the ray in the fan-beam system equivalent to a ray in the parallel-beam system, for which:

$$\alpha^f = \alpha^p - \arcsin\frac{s}{\mathrm{R}_f}, \tag{6.8}$$

and

$$\beta = \arcsin\frac{s}{\mathrm{R}_f}. \tag{6.9}$$

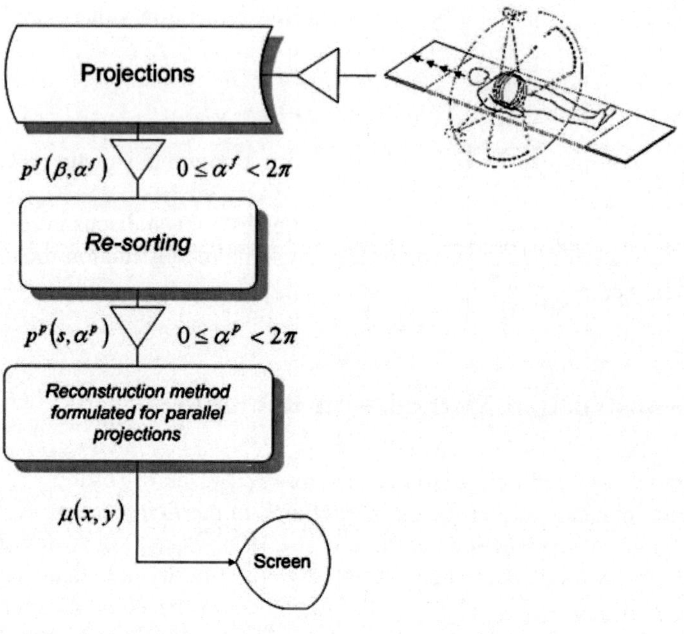

Fig. 6.3 The image reconstruction method with rebinning, for a fan beam system

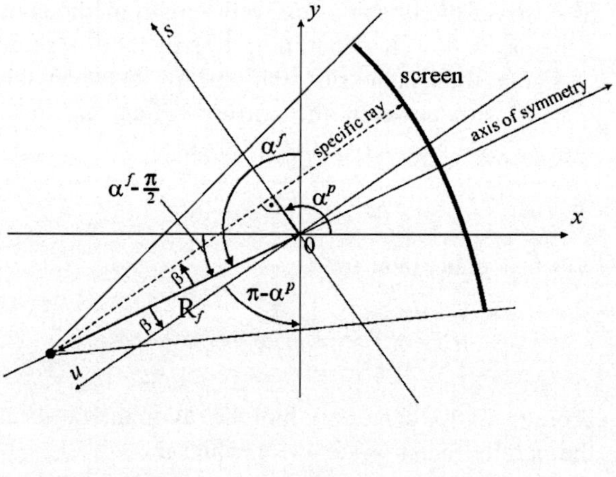

Fig. 6.4 Geometrical relationships between a fan beam and a parallel beam projection system

All of the parallel projection values obtained in this way then become inputs for the reconstruction procedures developed for actual parallel-beam systems.

In practice however, we need to adapt the rebinning method described above to the discrete nature of the projections obtained by the scanner with respect to both the angle α^f at which the projections are carried out, and to the angle β at which the radiation intensities are measured by the detectors on the screen.

6.4 Discrete Implementation of the Reconstruction Method with Rebinning

In implementing the discrete version of the reconstruction method with rebinning [3] we will first of all consider how the fan-beam projection values specified by the parameters $(\beta_\eta, \alpha^f{}_\gamma)$ are related to the parallel-beam raster determined by the pair $(s_l, \alpha^p{}_\psi)$, where:

$$s_l = l \cdot \Delta_s^p, \tag{6.10}$$

where: $l = -(\mathrm{L} - 1)/2, \ldots, 0, \ldots, (\mathrm{L} - 1)/2$ is the sample index of the detectors in the parallel-beam system; $\mathrm{L} = 2(\mathrm{R}\ \mathit{div}\ \Delta_s^p) + 1$ is the maximum number of detectors on the screen in the parallel-beam system; Δ_s^p is the distance between detectors in the parallel-beam system, and

$$\alpha_\psi^p = \psi \cdot \Delta_\psi^p, \tag{6.11}$$

where: $\psi = 0, \ldots, \Psi - 1$ is the index of the individual projections in the parallel-beam system; $\Psi = 2\pi\ \mathit{div}\ \Delta_\alpha^p$ is the maximum number of projections; Δ_α^p is the angular distance between projections.

The next step will be to reconstruct the image using one of the methods devised for the parallel-beam system.

A detailed discussion of both these basic phases of the algorithm is given below as consecutive steps in the processing of the projection values $\hat{p}^f(\eta, \gamma) = p^f(\eta\Delta_\beta, \gamma\Delta_\alpha^f)$; $\eta = -(\mathrm{H} - 1)/2, \ldots, 0, \ldots, (\mathrm{H} - 1)/2$; $\gamma = 0, 1, \ldots, \Gamma - 1$, obtained using the discrete fan-beam scanner.

Step I In order to convert the projection values from one system to the other we use the relationships:

$$\beta_{l\psi} = \arcsin \frac{s_l}{\mathrm{R}_f}; \tag{6.12}$$

$$\alpha_{l\psi}^f = \alpha_\psi^p - \arcsin \frac{s_l}{\mathrm{R}_f}. \tag{6.13}$$

This means that we more or less know the projection value in the fan-beam system, which is equivalent to the projection value in the hypothetical parallel-beam system at a given point on the screen and a given angle of projection. Unfortunately, more often than not, the ray with these particular calculated parameters is missing from the set of rays emitted in the fan-beam. As a result, the parameters must be interpolated based on projection values from the immediate neighbourhood of the calculated pair $(\beta_{l\psi}, \alpha^f{}_{l\psi})$. With this in mind, we first determine the relative values of the parameters of the interpolated ray:

$$\eta_{l\psi} = \frac{\beta_{l\psi}}{\Delta_\beta^f}; \tag{6.14}$$

$$\gamma_{l\psi} = \frac{\alpha_{l\psi}^f}{\Delta_\alpha^f}, \tag{6.15}$$

and then define the neighbourhood mentioned above as a group of four projection values:

$$\hat{p}^f\left(\eta_{l\psi}^{\uparrow}, \gamma_{l\psi}^{\uparrow}\right);\ \hat{p}^f\left(\eta_{l\psi}^{\downarrow}, \gamma_{l\psi}^{\uparrow}\right);\ \hat{p}^f\left(\eta_{l\psi}^{\uparrow}, \gamma_{l\psi}^{\downarrow}\right);\ \hat{p}^f\left(\eta_{l\psi}^{\downarrow}, \gamma_{l\psi}^{\downarrow}\right), \tag{6.16}$$

where: $\eta_{l\psi}^{\downarrow} = Trunc(\eta_{l\psi}, 1); \eta_{l\psi}^{\uparrow} = \eta_{l\psi}^{\downarrow} + 1; \gamma_{l\psi}^{\downarrow} = Trunc(\gamma_{l\psi}, 1); \gamma_{l\psi}^{\uparrow} = \gamma_{l\psi}^{\downarrow} + 1$.

There then only remains for us to make use of this selection of projection values to interpolate the values $\hat{p}^p(l,\psi) = p^p\left(s_l, \alpha_\psi^p\right)$. We could use bilinear interpolation, for instance, to estimate the projection value of the hypothetical ray:

$$\begin{aligned}\hat{\hat{p}}^p(l,\psi) = {} & \left(\gamma_{l\psi}^{\uparrow} - \gamma_{l\psi}\right)\left[\left(\eta_{l\psi}^{\uparrow} - \eta_{l\psi}\right)\hat{p}^f\left(\eta_{l\psi}^{\downarrow}, \gamma_{l\psi}^{\downarrow}\right) + \left(\eta_{l\psi} - \eta_{l\psi}^{\downarrow}\right)\hat{p}^f\left(\eta_{l\psi}^{\uparrow}, \gamma_{l\psi}^{\downarrow}\right)\right] \\ & + \left(\gamma_{l\psi} - \gamma_{l\psi}^{\downarrow}\right)\left[\left(\eta_{l\psi}^{\uparrow} - \eta_{l\psi}\right)\hat{p}^f\left(\eta_{l\psi}^{\downarrow}, \gamma_{l\psi}^{\uparrow}\right) + \left(\eta_{l\psi} - \eta_{l\psi}^{\downarrow}\right)\hat{p}^f\left(\eta_{l\psi}^{\uparrow}, \gamma_{l\psi}^{\uparrow}\right)\right]\end{aligned} \tag{6.17}$$

The process of obtaining these virtual parallel projections is repeated for all projection angles $\psi = 0, 1, \ldots, \Psi - 1$ (in this case, it is best to assume that $\Delta_\alpha^f = \Delta_\alpha^p$) and for all the hypothetical radiation detectors situated at locations identified by the index $l = -(L - 1)/2, \ldots, 0, \ldots, (L - 1)/2$, where it can be assumed that:

$$\Delta_s^p = R_f \sin \Delta_\beta. \tag{6.18}$$

Step II These approximate values of the virtual parallel-beam projections $\hat{\hat{p}}^p(l,\psi); l = -(L-1)/2, \ldots, 0, \ldots, (L-1)/2; \psi = 0, 1, \ldots, \Psi - 1$ can be used with any of the reconstruction methods developed for parallel-beam systems. Because it is easy to implement, this could be the convolution and back projection method discussed in Sect. 5.4. As the projection angles in our virtual parallel-beam system can vary within the range $0 \le \alpha^p < 2\pi$, the result of the reconstruction procedure needs to be divided by 2.

The flowchart in Fig. 6.5 shows the stages in the signal processing for the discrete version of the method with rebinning.

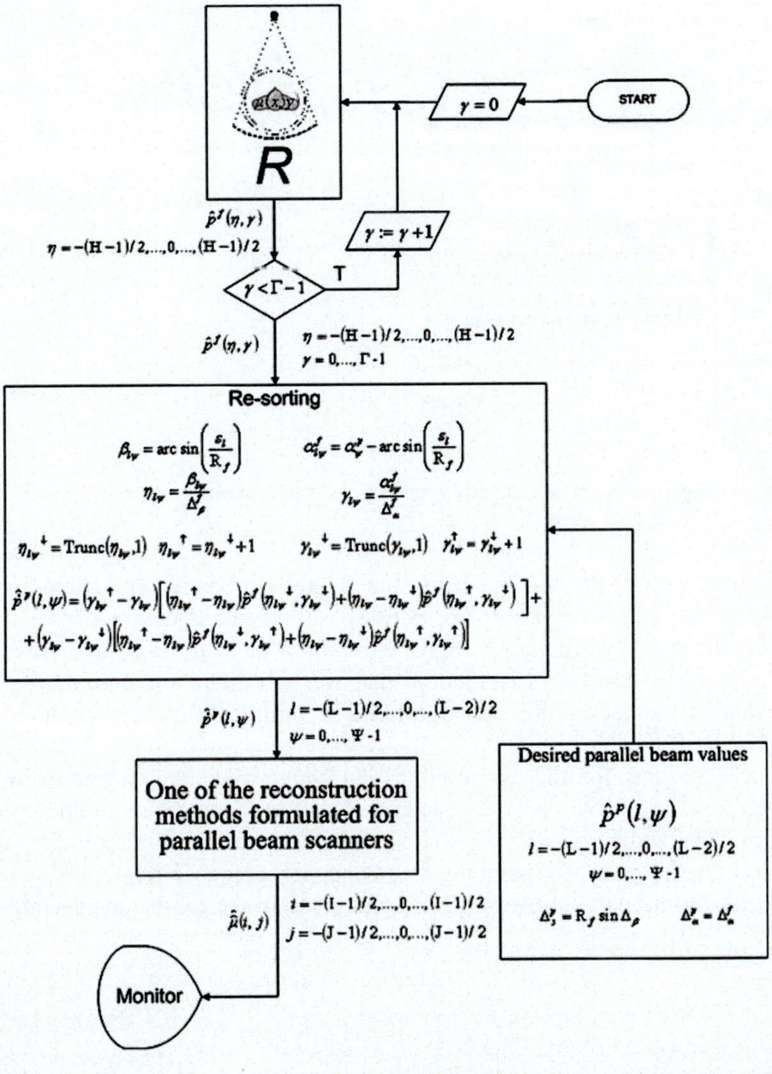

Fig. 6.5 A flowchart of the discrete version of the image reconstruction method with rebinning, for fan beam projections

6.5 Direct Fan-beam Reconstruction Method

An alternative to the previous approach to the problem of image reconstruction from fan-beam projections is a method that involves the direct use of the fan-beam projections in an algorithm designed originally for the parallel-beam system [4, 5, 6]. This method deals with the same problem as the rebinning algorithm: the

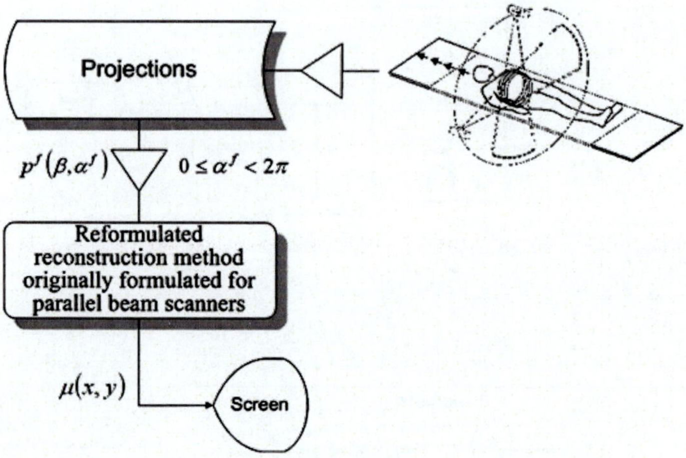

Fig. 6.6 Image reconstruction directly from fan beam projections

reconstruction of the image from the same fan-beam projections $p^f(\beta, \alpha^f)$; $\beta \in [\beta_{min}, \beta_{max}]$; $0 \leq \alpha^f < 2\pi$. The purpose of this technique however is to find a parallel-beam reconstruction formula into which the fan-beam projection values can be entered directly. The method that we will adapt for this purpose is the convolution and back-projection algorithm. A simplified flowchart of the approach adopted in this section is given in Fig. 6.6.

Key equations for the convolution and back-projection reconstruction algorithm, (5.50) and (5.51), will be adapted here to handle fan-beam projections. For a better understanding of how this can be done, it is worth returning to Fig. 6.4. We can use this diagram to derive the following trigonometric relationships between quantities in the parallel-beam system and those in the fan-beam system:

$$s = R_f \cdot \sin \beta \tag{6.19}$$

and

$$\alpha^p = \alpha^f + \beta. \tag{6.20}$$

However, in further discussions of the fan-beam system, we need to be able to express the trigonometric relationships in polar coordinates, as shown in Fig. 6.7. This diagram shows how to determine the parameters of points inside the test cross-section during a fan-beam projection. The following equations show relationships between selected parameters of a point during the projection $p^p(s, \alpha^p)$:

$$r \cos(\alpha^p - \phi) - s = \dot{u} \sin(\dot{\beta} - \beta), \tag{6.21}$$

Fig. 6.7 Determination of the polar coordinates of a point in the plane of a fan beam projection: **a** derivation of (6.21), **b** derivation of (6.22) and (6.23)

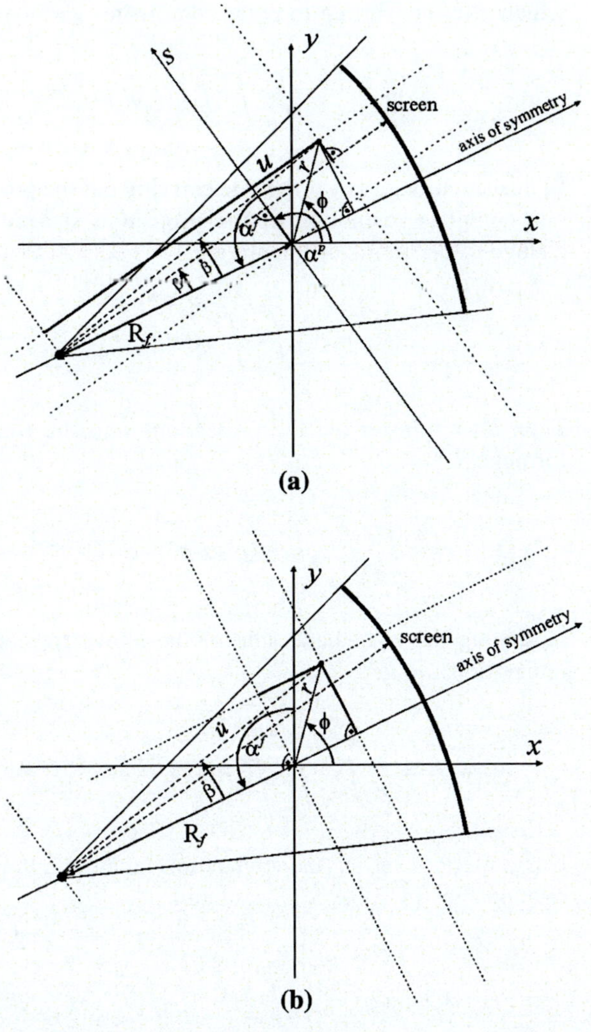

$$\dot{\beta} = \arctan\left(\frac{\alpha^f - \phi}{R_f + r\sin(\alpha^p - \phi)}\right), \tag{6.22}$$

$$\dot{u}^2 = [r\cos(\alpha^p - \phi)]^2 + [R_f + r\sin(\alpha^p - \phi)]^2. \tag{6.23}$$

The following sequence of equations is based on relationships described in earlier chapters and if we begin by taking into consideration the definition of the two-dimensional inverse Fourier transform, we obtain:

$$\mu(x, y) = \int_{\infty}^{\infty}\int_{\infty}^{\infty} M(f_1, f_2)\cdot e^{j2\pi(f_1x+f_2y)}\mathrm{d}f_1\mathrm{d}f_2, \tag{6.24}$$

which after converting to polar coordinates and using (5.34) takes the form:

$$\mu(x,y) = \int_{0}^{\pi} \int_{\infty}^{\infty} |f| P(f,\alpha^p) \cdot \mathrm{e}^{j2\pi f(x\cos\alpha^p + y\sin\alpha^p)} \mathrm{d}f\,\mathrm{d}\alpha^p. \tag{6.25}$$

In this situation, it is worthwhile carrying out the process of back projection during one complete revolution of the projection system. This leads to the following change to the limits of integration:

$$\mu(x,y) = \frac{1}{2} \int_{0}^{2\pi} \int_{\infty}^{\infty} |f| P(f,\alpha^p) \cdot \mathrm{e}^{j2\pi f(x\cos\alpha^p + y\sin\alpha^p)} \mathrm{d}f\,\mathrm{d}\alpha^p. \tag{6.26}$$

Then after transferring the projections into the frequency domain, we have the formula:

$$\mu(x,y) = \frac{1}{2} \int_{0}^{2\pi} \int_{\infty}^{\infty} \int_{\infty}^{\infty} |f| p^p(s,\alpha^p) \cdot \mathrm{e}^{j2\pi f(x\cos\alpha^p + y\sin\alpha^p)} \cdot \mathrm{e}^{\ j2\pi fs} \mathrm{d}s\mathrm{d}f\,\mathrm{d}\alpha^p. \tag{6.27}$$

Arranging the right hand side of the above formula and changing the order of integration, we get:

$$\mu(x,y) = \frac{1}{2} \int_{\infty}^{\infty} \int_{\infty}^{\infty} \int_{0}^{2\pi} |f| p^p(s,\alpha^p) \cdot \mathrm{e}^{j2\pi f(x\cos\alpha^p + y\sin\alpha^p\ \ s)} \mathrm{d}\alpha^p \mathrm{d}s\mathrm{d}f. \tag{6.28}$$

Next, after converting the attenuation function into polar coordinates by using the relationships in Table 5.1 we obtain:

$$\mu(r\cos\phi, r\sin\phi) = \frac{1}{2} \int_{\infty}^{\infty} \int_{\infty}^{\infty} \int_{0}^{2\pi} |f| p^p(s,\alpha^p) \cdot \mathrm{e}^{j2\pi f[r\cos(\alpha^p\ \ \phi)\ \ s]} \mathrm{d}\alpha^p \mathrm{d}s\mathrm{d}f. \tag{6.29}$$

Note here that the substitution $x\cos\alpha^p + y\sin\alpha^p = \dot{s} = r\cos(\alpha^p - \phi)$ refers to the point (r, ϕ), to which the reconstruction process applies, and the variable s specifies the location on the screen. Of course, we should also take into account the application of the window function, which, according to Sect. 5.4 and (5.45), should be placed appropriately in the formula above to finally obtain:

$$\breve{\mu}(r\cos\phi, r\sin\phi) = \frac{1}{2} \int_{\infty}^{\infty} \int_{\infty}^{\infty} \int_{0}^{2\pi} |f| \cdot W(f) p^p(s,\alpha^p) \cdot \mathrm{e}^{j2\pi f[r\cos(\alpha^p\ \ \phi)\ \ s]} \mathrm{d}\alpha^p \mathrm{d}s\mathrm{d}f. \tag{6.30}$$

By using Eqs. (6.21) (6.23) in the above equation and at the same time changing the limits of integration we obtain a relationship, which is fundamental for the fan-beam image reconstruction method:

$$\breve{\mu}(r\cos\phi, r\sin\phi) = \frac{R_f}{2}\int\limits_{\infty}^{\infty}\int\limits_{\beta_{\min}}^{\beta_{\max}}\int\limits_{\beta}^{2\pi\ \beta}|f|\cdot W(f)\cdot p^f(\beta,\alpha^f)\cdot\cos\beta \cdot e^{j2\pi f\dot{u}\sin(\dot{\beta}\ \beta)}\mathrm{d}\alpha^f\,\mathrm{d}\beta\mathrm{d}f. \tag{6.31}$$

The angle α^f has a periodicity of 2π, which means that we can change the limits of integration to the range: 0 to 2π. This would give us the following equation:

$$\breve{\mu}(r\cos\phi, r\sin\phi) = \frac{R_f}{2}\int\limits_{\infty}^{\infty}\int\limits_{\beta_{\min}}^{\beta_{\max}}\int\limits_{0}^{2\pi}|f|\cdot W(f)\cdot p^f(\beta,\alpha^f)\cdot\cos\beta \cdot e^{j2\pi f\dot{u}\sin(\dot{\beta}\ \beta)}\mathrm{d}\alpha^f\,\mathrm{d}\beta\mathrm{d}f. \tag{6.32}$$

We are now ready to begin adapting the equation above to the convolution and back projection method, which we met during our discussion of the parallel-beam system. To do this, we will rework (6.32) to resemble (5.78) as much as possible, that is to say, to the form:

$$\breve{\mu}(r\cos\phi, r\sin\phi) = \int\limits_{0}^{2\pi} p^f(\dot{\beta},\alpha^f)\mathrm{d}\alpha^f, \tag{6.33}$$

where

$$p^f(\dot{\beta},\alpha^f) = \int\limits_{\beta_{\min}}^{\beta_{\max}} p^f(\beta,\alpha^f)\cdot\frac{R_f}{2}\cos\beta\cdot h(\dot{u}\cdot\sin(\dot{\beta}-\beta))\mathrm{d}\beta, \tag{6.34}$$

and the convolving function has the following interpretation:

$$h(\dot{u}\cdot\sin(\dot{\beta}-\beta)) = \int\limits_{\infty}^{\infty}|f|\cdot W(f)\cdot e^{j2\pi f\dot{u}\sin(\dot{\beta}\ \beta)}\mathrm{d}f. \tag{6.35}$$

Unfortunately, there is a serious drawback associated with the use of the fan-beam reconstruction method formulated like this. It stems from the dependence of (6.35) on the parameter $\dot{u}$, which poses certain practical problems when carrying out the calculations during the reconstruction process. Instead of a simple formula for the convolution kernel, as we had in the case of the parallel-beam system, it now becomes necessary to determine a different form of the kernel for every point of the object's cross-section. This is because $\dot{u}$ represents the distance of the point (r, ϕ) from the radiation source at coordinates $(\mathrm{R}_f, \alpha^f + \frac{\pi}{2})$. Therefore, by changing the angle α^f, we also change $\dot{u}$ and consequently we need to adjust the value of the convolution kernel. We will take action later to eliminate this undesirable situation. With this in mind, we will reverse our strategy for this method; we will make the relationship defining the convolving function, introduced for the convolution and back-projection method in the parallel-beam system, resemble (6.34), formulated for the fan-beam system. This adjustment is based on a term in (5.79), which is reproduced here in a suitably amended form:

$$h(s) = \int_{f_0}^{f_0} |f| \cdot W(f) \cdot e^{j2\pi fs} df. \tag{6.36}$$

In this equation, the integration is carried out with respect to the frequency f. The next step will be to make a substitution for f, using the following expression:

$$f^f = \frac{f \cdot \dot{u} \cdot \sin\beta}{\mathrm{R}_f \cdot \beta}. \tag{6.37}$$

If at the same time we change the limits of integration, the convolving function will be modified to:

$$h(\dot{u}\sin\beta) = \left(\frac{\mathrm{R}_f \cdot \beta}{\dot{u} \cdot \sin\beta}\right)^2 \cdot h^f(\mathrm{R}_f \cdot \beta), \tag{6.38}$$

where

$$h^f(\mathrm{R}_f \cdot \beta) = \int_{f_0^f}^{f_0^f} |f| \cdot \mathrm{W}\left(\frac{f \cdot f_0}{f_0^f}\right) \cdot e^{j2\pi f \mathrm{R}_f \beta} df \tag{6.39}$$

and

$$f_0^f = \frac{f_0 \cdot \dot{u} \cdot \sin\beta}{\mathrm{R}_f \cdot \beta}. \tag{6.40}$$

This substitution now allows us to use the convolution kernel $h^f(\mathrm{R}_f \cdot \beta)$, which we already know from its use in the parallel-beam system (see Table 5.3). Unfortunately, even here we encounter problems caused by the dependence of the cut-off frequency f_0^f on the parameter $\dot{u}$. On the other hand, if we were to establish a constant value for f_0^f it would mean that the reconstruction process for the point (r, ϕ) would have a different resolution (determined by the value of the cut-off frequency f_0) for every angle α^f. However, if we put aside the assumption of uniform resolution for the resulting reconstructed image, then, by manipulating the values $\dot{u}$ and f_0, the varying value of f_0^f can be fixed as f_0^f. Assuming a constant cut-off frequency $f_0^f = \mathrm{f}_0^f$, (6.38) can be written as:

$$\tilde{h}(\dot{u}\sin\beta) = \left(\frac{\mathrm{R}_f \cdot \beta}{\dot{u} \cdot \sin\beta}\right)^2 \cdot \tilde{h}^f(\beta), \tag{6.41}$$

where:

$$\tilde{h}^f(\beta) = \int_{\mathrm{f}_0^f}^{\mathrm{f}_0^f} |f| \cdot W\left(\frac{f \cdot f_0}{f_0^f}\right) \cdot \mathrm{e}^{j2\pi f \mathrm{R}_f \beta} \mathrm{d}f. \tag{6.42}$$

This compromise allows us to put (6.38) into a more convenient form for carrying out the calculation:

$$\tilde{h}(\dot{u}\sin\beta) = h'(f_0, \dot{u}) \cdot h''(\beta). \tag{6.43}$$

After obtaining this form of the convolution kernel, the equation describing the filtering of the projections becomes:

$$p^f(\dot{\beta}, \alpha^f) = h'(f_0, \dot{u}) \cdot \int_{\beta_{\min}}^{\beta_{\max}} p^f(\beta, \alpha^f) \cdot \frac{\mathrm{R}_f}{2} \cos\beta \cdot h''(\dot{\beta} - \beta) \mathrm{d}\beta, \tag{6.44}$$

which automatically reduces the computational inputs necessary for this method.

At this point, we now have the theoretical framework for deriving the discrete algorithm for the convolution and back-projection reconstruction method for fan-beam systems.

6.6 Discrete Implementation of the Direct Fan-beam Reconstruction Method

The process of implementing the discrete version of the convolution and back-projection reconstruction algorithm for the fan-beam system is similar to the solution for the parallel-beam system. Once again, there are geometric factors introduced by the limited number of projections made during one revolution of the tube and by the limited resolution at which the radiation intensities are measured during each projection. These elements of the algorithm, discrete at the design level, were introduced by (6.3) and (6.4).

Possible practical reconstruction procedures for this method are aimed at implementing (6.33) and (6.44). The various stages in this process are given below [4].

Step I We need to begin our discussion of the discrete version of the convolution and back-projection reconstruction algorithm by making corrections for the geometry of the fan-beam projections: $\hat{p}^f(\eta,\gamma); \eta = -(\mathrm{H}-1)/2,\ldots, 0,\ldots,(\mathrm{H}-1)/2; \gamma = 0,1,\ldots,\Gamma-1$. To do this, each projection value $\hat{p}^f(\eta,\gamma)$ is processed for every projection angle using the following formula:

$$\hat{p}^f_{\mathrm{cor}}(\eta,\gamma) = \hat{p}^f(\eta,\gamma)\cdot\cos(\eta\Delta_\beta). \tag{6.45}$$

Step II At this stage, the geometrically corrected functions $\hat{p}^f_{\mathrm{cor}}(\eta,\gamma)$ are filtered using an appropriate convolution kernel, as we did with the convolution and back-projection method for the parallel-beam system. By carrying out the convolution operation given in (6.44) and using the modified and conditioned convolving function we obtain:

$$\hat{p}^f(\dot{\eta},\gamma) \cong \Delta_\beta \cdot \sum_{\eta=\;(\mathrm{H}\;\;1)/2}^{(\mathrm{H}\;\;1)/2} \hat{p}^f_{\mathrm{cor}}(\eta,\gamma)\cdot\hat{\hat{h}}^{XX}(\dot{u}\cdot\sin(\dot{\eta}-\eta)\Delta_\beta), \tag{6.46}$$

where: $\hat{\hat{h}}^{XX}(\dot{u}\cdot\sin(\eta\Delta_\beta))$ is one of the discrete convolution kernels whose argument is related to that of its continuous form given in (6.41); *XX* is a symbol representing the selected convolution kernel (e.g. "*RL*" or "*SL*").

As a result of this operation, we obtain "prophylactic" cleared projections, free from geometrical distortions. At this point, the definition of the convolution kernel $\hat{\hat{h}}^{XX}(l)$ becomes extremely important. Consequently, we will select the window function:

$$W\left(\frac{f\cdot f_0}{f_0^f}\right) = \begin{cases} 1-\dfrac{\varepsilon\left|\frac{f\cdot f_0}{f_0^f}\right|}{f_0} & \text{for } \left|\frac{f\cdot f_0}{f_0^f}\right| \le f_0^f \\ 0 & \text{for } \left|\frac{f\cdot f_0}{f_0^f}\right| > f_0^f \end{cases}, \tag{6.47}$$

where: f_0^f is the cut-off frequency of the filter; ε is a value in the range [0,1], which will then be substituted into (6.35). At the same time, we will take into account the assumption made in the previous section concerning the constant value of the cut-off frequency:

$$f_0^f = \mathrm{f}_0^f = \frac{1}{2\mathrm{R_f}\cdot\Delta_\beta}, \tag{6.48}$$

in order to obtain the following family of convolution kernels, based on (5.59) and (6.47):

$$\hat{\hat{h}}^{XX}(\dot{u}\cdot\sin(\eta\Delta_\beta)) = \begin{cases} \frac{1}{\dot{u}^2}\frac{3\ \ 2\varepsilon}{12(\Delta_\beta)^2} & \text{for} \quad \eta = 0 \\ -\frac{1}{\dot{u}^2}\frac{\varepsilon}{\pi^2\sin^2(\eta\Delta_\beta)} & \text{for} \quad \eta \text{ even and } \eta \neq 0\,. \\ -\frac{1}{\dot{u}^2}\frac{1\ \ \varepsilon}{\pi^2\sin^2(\eta\Delta_\beta)} & \text{for} \quad \eta \text{ odd} \end{cases} \tag{6.49}$$

If, in addition, we assume that $\varepsilon = 0$, this equation then represents the Ram-Lak convolution kernel for the fan-beam system:

$$\hat{\hat{h}}^{RL}(\dot{u}\cdot\sin(\eta\cdot\Delta_\beta)) = \begin{cases} \frac{1}{\dot{u}^2}\frac{1}{4\left(\Delta_\beta\right)^2} & \text{for} \quad \eta = 0 \\ 0 & \text{for} \quad \eta \text{ even and } \eta \neq 0\,. \\ -\frac{1}{\dot{u}^2}\frac{1}{\pi^2\sin^2\left(\eta\cdot\Delta_\beta\right)} & \text{for} \quad \eta \text{ odd} \end{cases} \tag{6.50}$$

By applying this to (6.46), we obtain an equation for removing geometrical distortions from the projections. It is important to note that (6.50) describing the convolving function also satisfies the condition established in (6.43), because in the elements of the Ram-Lak convolution kernel, we can isolate the components:

$$\hat{\hat{h}}^{RL'}(f_0, \dot{u}) = \frac{1}{(\dot{u})^2} \tag{6.51}$$

and

$$\hat{\hat{h}}^{RL''}(\eta\cdot\Delta_\beta) = \begin{cases} \frac{1}{4\left(\Delta_\beta\right)^2} & \text{for} \quad \eta = 0 \\ 0 & \text{for} \quad \eta \text{ even and } \eta \neq 0\,. \\ -\frac{1}{\pi^2\sin^2\left(\eta\Delta_\beta\right)} & \text{for} \quad \eta \text{ odd} \end{cases} \tag{6.52}$$

Therefore, we can now take the opportunity to rewrite (6.46) in a form that allows for easier calculation:

$$\hat{p}^f(\dot{\eta}, \gamma) \cong \Delta_\beta \cdot \sum_{\eta = \ (H\ \ 1)/2}^{(H\ \ 1)/2} \hat{p}^f_{\text{cor}}(\eta, \gamma)\cdot \hat{\hat{h}}^{RL''}((\dot{\eta} - \eta)\Delta_\beta), \tag{6.53}$$

where the factor $\frac{1}{\dot{u}^2}$ is taken into account at a later stage.

Step III Unfortunately, these projection values most often relate to rays which do not pass through the raster points (i, j) of the reconstructed image. Because of this, we need to introduce one more stage in the processing of these projections: linear interpolation based on the projection values $\hat{p}^f(\dot{\eta}, \gamma)$ of the two rays passing nearest to the point (*i*, *j*). The interpolation problem for the fan-beam system is illustrated in Fig. 6.8.

The interpolation stage for the projection $\hat{p}^f(\dot{\eta}, \gamma)$ can be written as follows:

$$\dot{p}^f\left(\dot{\beta}_{ij}, \gamma \cdot \Delta_\alpha^f\right) \cong \Delta_\beta \cdot \sum_{\dot{\eta}} \hat{p}^f(\dot{\eta}, \gamma) \cdot I(\dot{\beta}_{ij} - \dot{\eta} \cdot \Delta_\beta), \tag{6.54}$$

where: $I(\dot{\beta}_{ij} - \dot{\eta} \cdot \Delta_\beta)$ is the interpolation function, defining the dependence of the value of $\dot{p}^f(\dot{\beta}_{ij}, \gamma \cdot \Delta_\alpha^f)$ at any point on the screen, on the value $\hat{p}^f(\dot{\eta}, \gamma)$ at a measured point, as a function of the distance between the two points.

If we use the linear interpolation function defined by the formula:

$$I^L(\Delta\dot{\beta}) = \begin{cases} \frac{1}{\Delta_\beta^2} \cdot \left(1 - \frac{|\Delta\dot{\beta}|}{\Delta_\beta}\right) & \text{for } |\Delta\dot{\beta}| \le \Delta_\beta \\ 0 & \text{for } |\Delta\dot{\beta}| > \Delta_\beta \end{cases}, \tag{6.55}$$

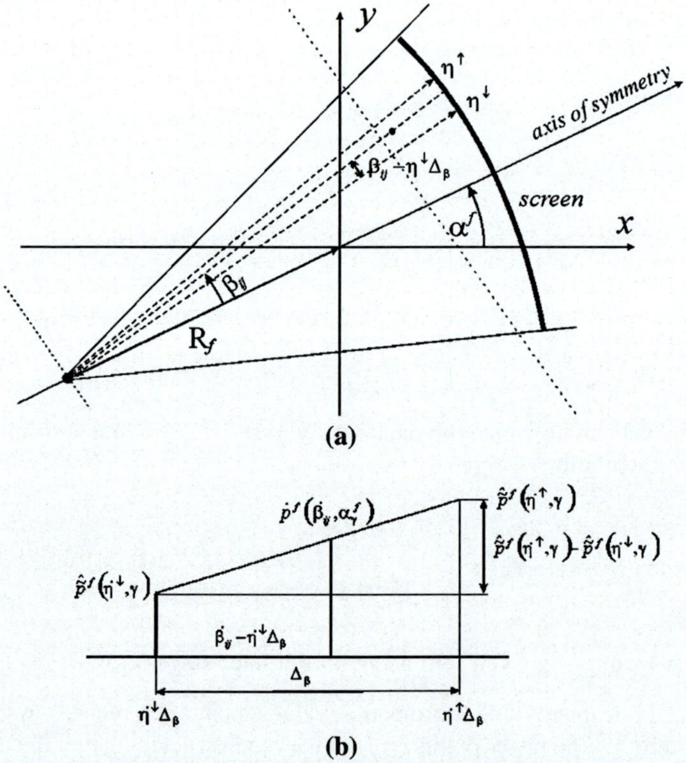

Fig. 6.8 Interpolation of projection values in a fan beam system: **a** selection of the rays to use for the interpolation, **b** trigonometric analysis of linear interpolation

where:

$$\Delta\dot{\beta} = \dot{\beta}_{ij} - \dot{\eta} \cdot \Delta_\beta \tag{6.56}$$

and

$$\dot{\beta}_{ij} = \arctan \frac{i\Delta_x \cdot \cos\gamma\Delta^f_\alpha + j\Delta_y \cdot \sin\gamma\Delta^f_\alpha}{\mathrm{R}_f + i\Delta_x \cdot \sin\gamma\Delta^f_\alpha - j\Delta_y \cdot \cos\gamma\Delta^f_\alpha}, \tag{6.57}$$

then the projection values at discrete points of the image are expressed as follows:

$$\dot{p}^f\left(\dot{\beta}_{ij}, \alpha^f_\gamma\right) \cong \hat{\dot{p}}^f\left(\dot{\eta}^\downarrow, \gamma\right) + \left(\frac{\dot{\beta}_{ij}}{\Delta_\beta} - \dot{\eta}^\downarrow\right)\left(\hat{\dot{p}}^f\left(\dot{\eta}^\uparrow, \psi\right) - \hat{\dot{p}}^f\left(\dot{\eta}^\downarrow, \psi\right)\right), \tag{6.58}$$

where, $\dot{\beta}_{ij}$ is the parameter defining the position of the point (i, j) on the screen, for a projection angle $\alpha^f_\gamma = \gamma\Delta^f_\alpha; \dot{\eta}^\downarrow = Trunc\left(\dot{\beta}_{ij}, \Delta_\beta\right)$ is the position of the first of the rays passing in the neighbourhood of the point $(i, j); \dot{\eta}^\uparrow = \dot{\eta}^\downarrow + 1$ is the position of the second of the rays passing near the point (i, j).

In this way, we can calculate the approximate projection values $\dot{p}^f(\dot{\beta}_{ij}, \alpha^f_\gamma)$ for all points of the discrete image with raster $i = -(\mathrm{I} - 1)/2, \ldots, 0, \ldots, (\mathrm{I} - 1)/2$; $j = -(\mathrm{J} - 1)/2, \ldots, 0, \ldots, (\mathrm{J} - 1)/2$, for each projection angle $0 \leq \alpha^f_\gamma < 2\pi$.

Step IV Equation (6.33), describing the fundamental relationship for the convolution and back-projection reconstruction method, says that we can reconstruct the image of an object using suitably pre-prepared projections. Of course, the original projections must be processed in such a way that the inversibility principle of the Radon transform is maintained (see Sect. 5.4). In the discrete case, we can replace the integral in (6.33) with the trapezoidal rule (which approximates to the integral), according to the formula:

$$\hat{\mu}(i,j) \cong \Delta^f_\alpha \cdot \frac{\mathrm{R}_f}{2} \cdot \sum_{\gamma=0}^{\Gamma-1} \frac{1}{\dot{u}^2(i,j,\gamma)} \dot{p}^f\left(\dot{\beta}_{ij}, \gamma\Delta^f_\alpha\right). \tag{6.59}$$

It is also important to take into account (6.23), which defines the value of the variable $\dot{u}$, representing the distance of the point in the (x, y) space from the radiation source. In order to make this variable dependent on the discrete parameters (i, j, γ), we can convert (6.23) using the equations for converting polar coordinates into rectangular coordinates given in Table 5.1. This gives us the following relationship:

$$\dot{u}(i,j,\gamma) = \left(i\Delta_x \cdot \cos\gamma\Delta^f_\alpha + j\Delta_y \cdot \sin\gamma\Delta^f_\alpha\right)^2 + \left(\mathrm{R}_f + i\Delta_x \cdot \sin\gamma\Delta^f_\alpha - j\Delta_y \cdot \cos\gamma\Delta^f_\alpha\right)^2. \tag{6.60}$$

In the context of the whole procedure for implementing the convolution and back-projection method, this is essentially the last step in the reconstruction of the image. The implementation of the discrete version of this algorithm is illustrated in Fig. 6.9.

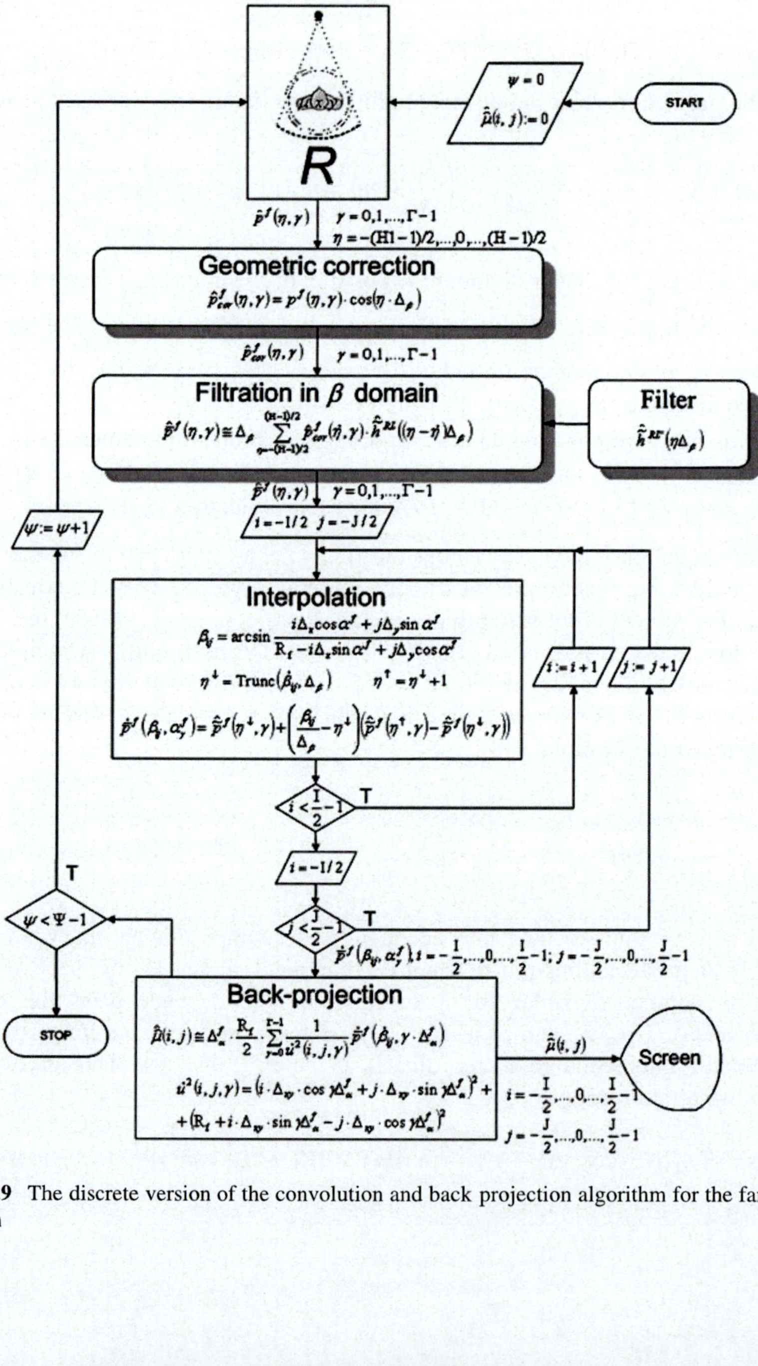

Fig. 6.9 The discrete version of the convolution and back projection algorithm for the fan beam system

References

1. Herman GT, Lakshminarayanan AV, Naparstek A (1976) Convolution reconstruction techniques for divergent beams. Comput Biol Med 6:259 271
2. Herman GT, Lung H P (1980) Reconstruction from divergent beams: a comparison of algorithms with and without rebinning. Comput Biol Med 10:131 139
3. Jain AK (1989) Fundamentals of digitals image processing. Prentice Hall, Englewood Cliffs
4. Kak AC, Slanley M (1988) Principles of computerized tomographic imaging. IEEE Press, New York
5. Lakshminarayanan AV (1975) Reconstruction from divergent ray data. Tech Rep TR 92, Department of Computer Science. State University New York, Buffalo, New York
6. Lewitt RM (1983) Reconstruction algorithms: transform methods. Proc IEEE 71(3):390 408
7. Naparstek A (1980) Short scan fan beam algorithms for CT. IEEE Trans Nucl Sci NS 27:1112 1120
8. Parker DL (1982) Optimal short scan convolution reconstruction for fan beam CT. Med Phys 9:254 257
9. Peters TM, Lewitt RM (1977) Computerized tomography with fan beam geometry. J Comp Assist Tomogr 1:429 436

Chapter 7
Spiral Tomography

Since the beginning of the 1990s, the use of *spiral tomography* scanners has been increasingly widespread [7, 35, 44, 54]. The name comes from the shape of the path that the X-ray tube and its associated detector array follow with respect to the patient. In the English-language literature, there is still some debate concerning the choice of name for this type of device: *helical* or *spiral tomography* scanner. The spiral path of the projection system as it rotates around the patient is the result of a combination of two types of movement: a longitudinal translation of the table with the patient on it and a rotary movement of the projection system around the longitudinal axis of the patient. This type of path could not have been achieved if it had not been for the development of slip rings in 1985. These rings enabled the supply of high voltage electricity to the X-ray tube through special brushes that allowed the continuous rotation of the projection system around the patient [12, 14].

Spiral tomography scanners are distinguished from their predecessors by an increased scan rate and improved high- and low-contrast resolution [35, 65, 67]. For this type of scanner, we can identify three main groups of design solution, three consecutive stages in the development of spiral tomography:

- *single-slice computed tomography* (SSCT),
- *multi-slice computed tomography* (MSCT),
- *cone-beam computed tomography* (CBCT).

In all these designs, the same procedure for carrying out a tomographic examination is appropriate, as shown in Fig. 7.1a [7].

In earlier designs of spiral CT scanners, because of the limited power of the tube and its limited rate of rotation around the test object, the projection parameters were essentially a compromise between scan resolution (i.e. the image density along the axis of the test object), the level of noise, as well as the time to acquire the images and adapt the radiation power to the type of material being examined. The use of spiral tomography was to eliminate the barriers that had prevented the further development of the older techniques. By using a projection

R. Cierniak, *X Ray Computed Tomography in Biomedical Engineering*,
DOI: 10.1007/978 0 85729 027 4 7, © Springer Verlag London Limited 2011

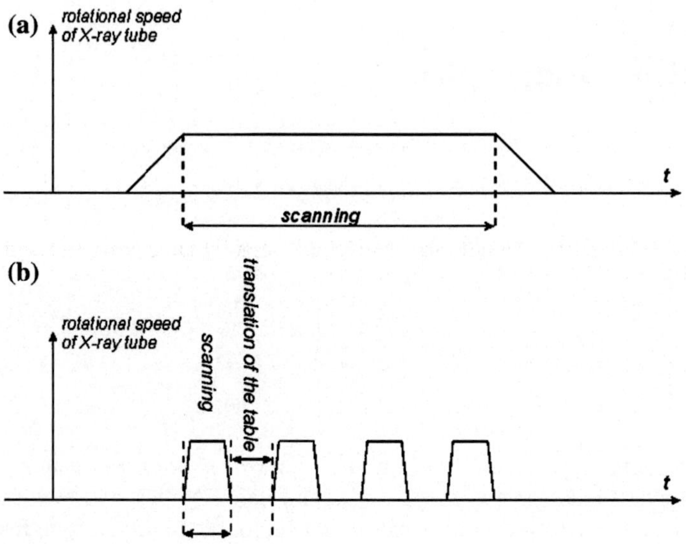

Fig. 7.1 The procedure for carrying out a CT examination: **a** using spiral tomography; **b** using previous generations of scanners

system that moved in a spiral path, it was possible to increase the scanning resolution and reduce the time needed for the whole examination as well as the time for each individual scan. During a spiral scan, X-rays are emitted continuously throughout the whole examination, until all necessary projections have been obtained. Note that, unfortunately, this also increases the demands made on the thermal durability of the X-ray tube.

With the introduction of CBCT technology and the use of a *cone-beam* of radiation in conjunction with a matrix of radiation detectors instead of a single row of detectors came other significant improvements. In addition to a considerable improvement in the scan rate and an increase in the resolution of the scanner along the axis of the patient, there was also a reduction in both the level of noise in the reproduced image and the amount of heat emitted by X-ray tube.

With all these advantages, spiral scanners have become the currently prevailing standard in the market for medical devices, superseding scanners in which the table was stationary during the scan.

7.1 Single Slice Computed Tomography—SSCT

The very first design of spiral tomography device, the *single slice computed tomography* scanner (SSCT), used an array of X-ray detectors arranged in a single row. As with fan-beam scanners, these detectors were placed on an arc-shaped screen in a plane perpendicular to the axis of the patient. The main distinguishing feature of the new design, however, was the combination of the rotary motion of the projection system with a steady forward displacement of the patient during the scan. This resulted in the elimination of the time interval between each individual scan and so significantly reduced the time taken for the entire CT examination.

There are many algorithms that use the projections obtained from spiral projection systems having a single row of detectors. These methods include 360° *linear interpolation* (360° LI) [35, 44], 80° *linear interpolation* (180° LI) [22], 180° *linear extrapolation* (180° LE) [7], *non-linear interpolation* [3] and others. However, we will only discuss the first two of these in this chapter, due mostly to their popularity amongst the manufacturers of CT scanners.

7.1.1 The Geometry of the Scanner

The geometry of a spiral projection system with a single row of detectors is illustrated in Figs. 7.2 and 7.3.

The moving projection system consists of an X-ray tube rigidly connected to a detector matrix on an arc-shaped screen. The matrix consists of a single row of detectors. The tube together with the detectors rotates around the z-axis, the principal axis of the system. At the same time as the projection system rotates, the patient table steadily moves forward. This means that the rotating projection system moves around the z-axis along a spiral path. A fan-beam of radiation emitted by the tube passes through the test object and finally reaches the detector matrix on the screen. Figure 7.3a shows the projection geometry in the

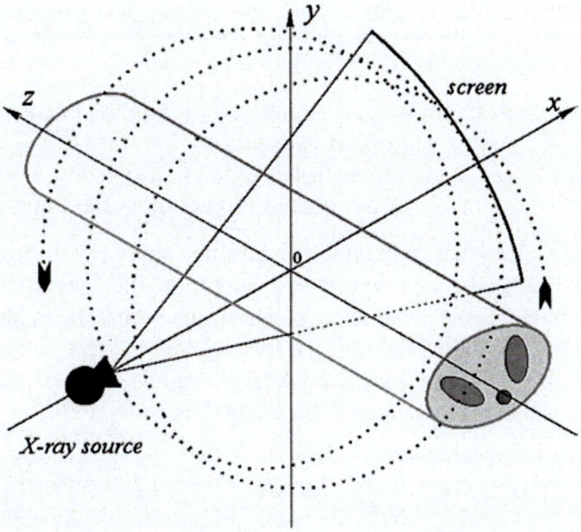

Fig. 7.2 The projection system of a single slice spiral scanner: a three dimensional perspective view

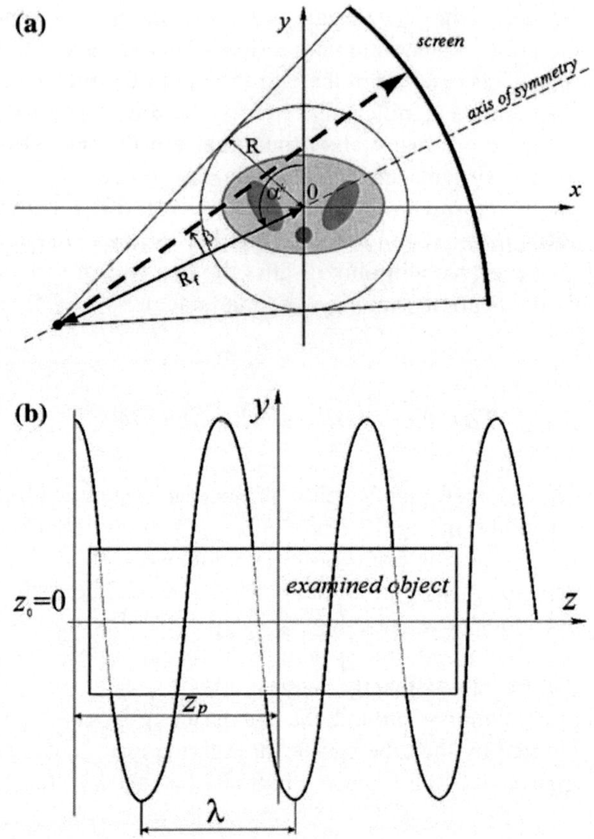

Fig. 7.3 The projection system of a single slice spiral scanner: **a** the geometry of the fan beam projection system in the plane perpendicular to the axis of rotation; **b** the path traced by projection system relative to the test object in the plane along the axis of rotation

(x, y) plane, i.e. the plane of the reconstructed slices. In this system, the rays that are emitted by the tube and that reach the screen are identified by:

β the angle between a particular ray in the beam and the axis of symmetry of the moving projection system;

α^h the angle at which the projection is made, i.e. the angle between the axis of symmetry of the rotated projection system and the y-axis.

This pair of parameters specifies every ray during the whole projection process. The projection values measured on the screen in a fan-beam system can be represented by $p^h(\beta, \alpha^h)$. The projections are made throughout the entire multi-rotation movement of the tube around the test object. Thus, the angles α^h at which the radiation measurements are made will be within the range $0 \leq \alpha^h \leq 2\pi$ whereas the range of the angle β is $[-\beta_{\max}, \beta_{\max}]$, where $\beta_{\max}$ is defined as:

$$\beta_{\max} = -\beta_{\min} = \arcsin\left(\frac{\mathrm{R}}{\mathrm{R}_f}\right), \tag{7.1}$$

where R is the radius of the circle defining the space in which the scan is carried out; R_f is the radius of the circle described by the focus of the tube.

If we assume that the patient table moves forward continuously and that the system starts at the point $z_0 = 0$ when $\alpha^h = 0$, we can use the following linear function to determine the location of the centre of the projection system z_0:

$$z_0 = \lambda \cdot \frac{\alpha^h}{2\pi}, \tag{7.2}$$

where λ is the translation of the table during one complete rotation of the tube around the patient, i.e. the relative travel of the spiral path traced by the tube, measured in $\left[\frac{\text{m}}{\text{rad}}\right]$.

The array of detectors placed in an arc on the screen is designed to measure the intensity of the X-rays passing through the test object. As with fan-beam scanners, this is done by placing the screen in a plane perpendicular to the z-axis. The main difference between spiral tomography and previous solutions is the continuous change of position of the projection system during successive projections.

7.1.2 The Geometry of the Discrete Scanner

The design of the single slice spiral scanner has to take into account the discrete nature of the projections. A general view of the design of a discrete spiral fan-beam projection system is given in Fig. 7.4.

In this system, the acquisition of the measurements of the projection function $p^h(\beta, \alpha^h)$ only takes place at certain angles of rotation α^h, determined by the relationship:

$$\alpha^h_\theta = \theta \cdot \Delta^h_\alpha, \tag{7.3}$$

where $\Delta^h_\alpha = \frac{2\pi}{\Theta^{2\pi}}$ is the angle through which the tube-screen system is rotated following each projection; $\Theta^{2\pi}$ is the number of projections made during one full rotation of the projection system; $\theta = 0, \ldots, \Theta - 1$ is the global projection index; $\Theta = number\_of\_rotations \cdot \Theta^{2\pi}$ is the total number of projections.

The position of the detector in the matrix is determined by the index η. In practice, in view of the fact that the detector array consists of a finite number of detectors, the value of the projection function $p^h(\beta, \alpha^h)$ is only obtained at certain angles β, determined by the relationship:

$$\beta_\eta = \eta \cdot \Delta^f_\beta, \tag{7.4}$$

where Δ^f_β is the angular distance between the individual radiation detectors placed on the screen; $\eta = -(\text{H}-1)/2, \ldots, 0, \ldots, (\text{H}-1)/2$; H is an odd number of detectors in the array.

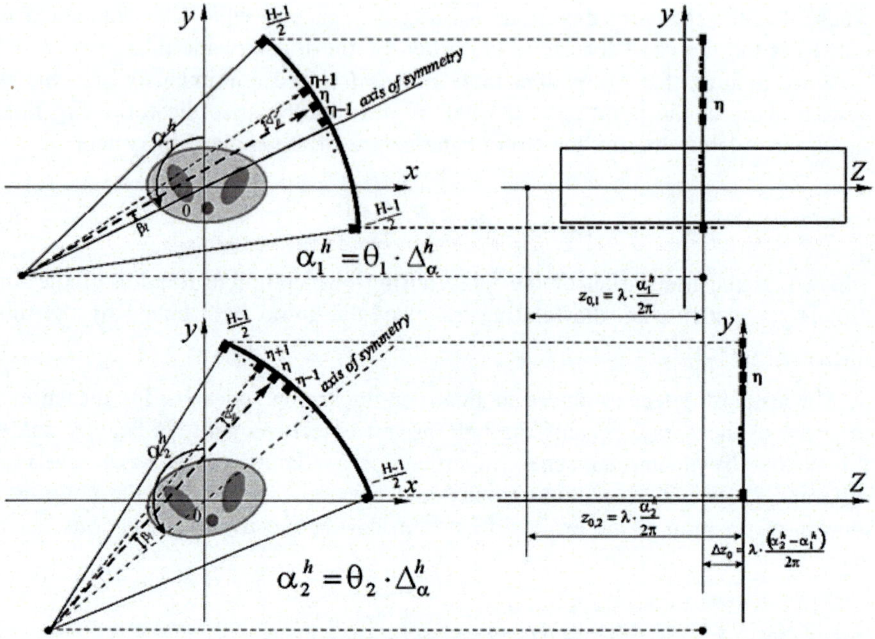

Fig. 7.4 A sequence of two projections in the discrete version of the SSCT spiral scanner

Therefore, in summary, we can say that in the discrete projection system of the SSCT spiral scanner we only obtain projection values $\hat{p}^h(\eta, \theta) = p^h(\beta_\eta, \alpha_\theta^h)$, for $\eta = -(\mathrm{H}-1)/2, \ldots, 0, \ldots, (\mathrm{H}-1)/2$ and $\theta = 0, \ldots, \Theta - 1$.

Bearing in mind the reconstruction algorithms used in SSCT spiral scanners, we might pause for a moment to consider the problem of determining the thickness of the slices, represented in the literature by the abbreviation SW (*slice width*). As in spiral tomography a projection is only made once for any given angle α^h, the rest of the data needed for the reconstruction process have to be obtained from projections made at other angles. The faster the forward movement of the patient table, the greater the errors involved in recovering the missing projections and the poorer the quality of the reconstructed image of the slice. The following parameter specifies the rate of translation of the table in relation to the width of the slice:

$$pitch = \frac{\lambda}{\mathrm{SW}}, \tag{7.5}$$

where SW is the nominal width of the slice whose image is to be reconstructed (related to the width of the collimated X-ray beam).

Figure 7.5 shows the geometry of three commonly used pitch values:

- *pitch* > 1.0 the consecutive loops of the path traced by the radiation beam around the patient's body are separate from each other (similar to an extended spring);

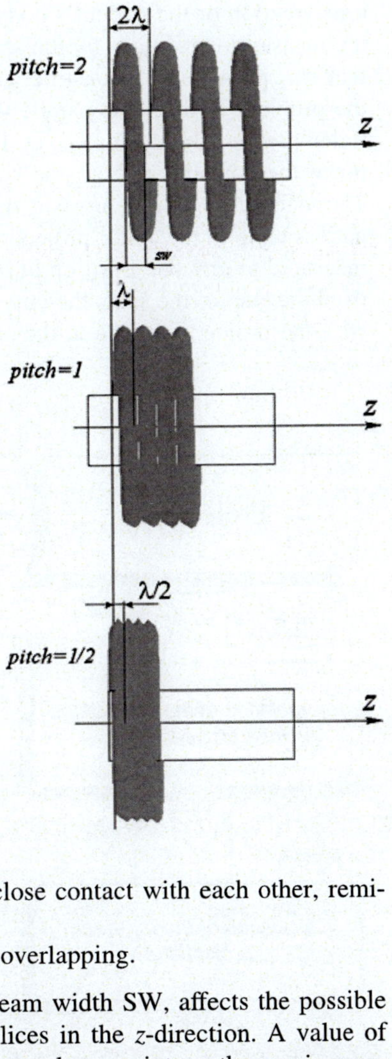

Fig. 7.5 A spiral projection system with various values of pitch

- *pitch* $= 1.0$ the consecutive loops are in close contact with each other, reminiscent of a compressed spring;
- *pitch* > 1.0 the consecutive loops exhibit overlapping.

The choice of the value of λ, for a fixed beam width SW, affects the possible levels of resolution RI of the reconstructed slices in the z-direction. A value of pitch ≥ 1.0 means that the radiation passes through no point on the z-axis more than once. For all values of pitch less than one, the radiation passes through the same point on the z-axis several times. It is worth mentioning that projections are usually carried out at a pitch setting of 1.5.

7.1.3 The 360° LI Reconstruction Algorithm

The 360° LI (360° *linear interpolation*) reconstruction algorithm [7, 35, 44] uses projections $p^h(\beta, \alpha^h)$ obtained from a spiral projection system. We can obtain the fan-beam projections $p^f(\beta, \alpha^f); \beta \in [-\beta_{\max}, \beta_{\max}]$ needed for reconstructing a cross-section of the patient's body by applying a suitable interpolation formula to the measurements made by the scanner. However, we already know from Chap. 6 that it is possible to reconstruct an image from fan-beam projections by reducing the problem to that of a parallel-beam system. The full 360° LI method is illustrated graphically in Fig. 7.6. In the first stage of this reconstruction algorithm, we make the conversion from the spiral projection system to the fan-beam system. The main problem that arises is that, because of the translational movement of the patient table in the spiral projection system, only one projection value $p^h(\beta, \alpha^h)$ is measured at any one position of the table. If the slice lies in a plane a distance z_p from the start of the scan, the only beam of radiation in this plane is that associated with the projection made at the angle:

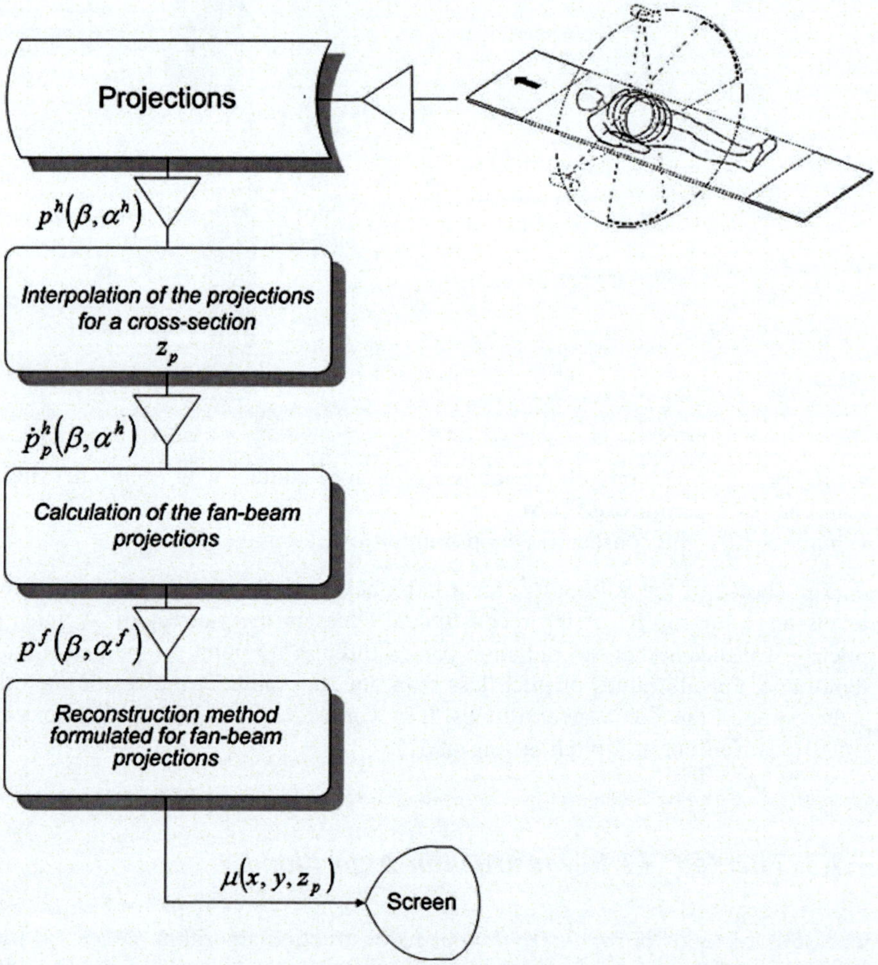

Fig. 7.6 Stages in the 360° LI reconstruction algorithm (applicable also to the 180° LI method)

$$\alpha_p^h = \frac{2\pi \cdot z_p}{\lambda}. \tag{7.6}$$

One projection is not enough, however, to complete the reconstruction process for the whole slice. Therefore, we have to find other ways to make up for this deficiency.

The 360° LI reconstruction algorithm relies on the linear interpolation (LI) of the missing fan-beam projections to reconstruct a slice from the measurements made in the spiral system. In this algorithm, the missing values for the angles $\alpha^f \in [0, 2\pi) - \left\{\alpha_p^h \; mod \; 2\pi\right\}$ are made up for by projections at angles in the range $\left(\alpha_p^h - 2\pi, \alpha_p^h + 2\pi\right)$ using linear interpolation, as follows:

$$\dot{p}_p^h(\beta, \alpha_1^h) = w_1 \cdot p_p^h(\beta, \alpha_1^h) + w_2 \cdot p_p^h(\beta, \alpha_2^h), \tag{7.7}$$

where

$$w_1 = \frac{\alpha_p^h - \alpha_2^h}{\alpha_1^h - \alpha_2^h} \tag{7.8}$$

and

$$w_2 = \frac{\alpha_1^h - \alpha_p^h}{\alpha_1^h - \alpha_2^h}, \tag{7.9}$$

for $\alpha_2^h = \alpha_1^h - 2\pi; \alpha_1^h \in \left(\alpha_p^h, \alpha_p^h + 2\pi\right)$.

Figure 7.7 illustrates the method of carrying out linear interpolation using the 360° LI algorithm.

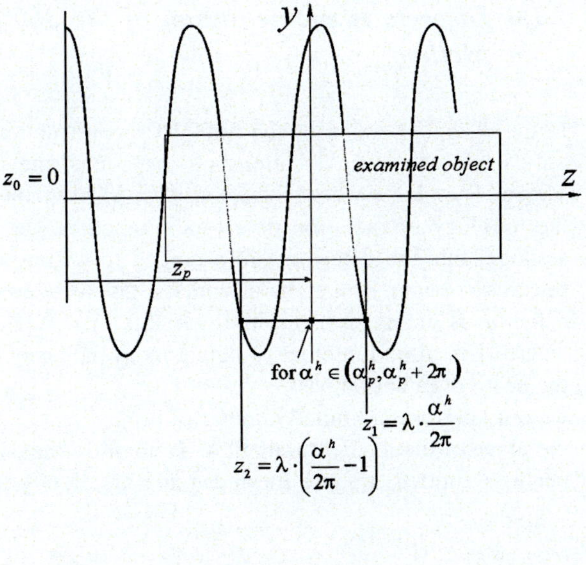

Fig. 7.7 Linear interpolation using the 360° LI reconstruction algorithm

Using Eq. 7.7 it is possible to acquire all the projections $\dot{p}_p^h(\beta, \alpha^h)$; $\alpha^h \in \left[\alpha_p^h, \alpha_p^h + 2\pi\right)$ lying in the plane of the slice, independently of the variable z. Therefore, for any $z = z_p$, we can describe the conversion from the spiral to the fan-beam projection system as follows:

$$p^f(\beta, \alpha^f) \equiv \dot{p}_p^h(\beta, \alpha^h), \tag{7.10}$$

where

$$p^f(\beta, \alpha^f) = \begin{cases} \dot{p}_p^h(\beta, \alpha^h - \alpha_0^h) & \text{for} \quad \alpha^h \in \left[\alpha_0^h, \alpha_p^h + 2\pi\right) \wedge \beta \in [-\beta_{\max}, \beta_{\max}] \\ \dot{p}_p^h(\beta, \alpha^h - \alpha_0^h + 2\pi) & \text{for} \quad \alpha^h \in \left[\alpha_p^h, \alpha_0^h\right) \wedge \beta \in [-\beta_{\max}, \beta_{\max}] \end{cases}, \tag{7.11}$$

and α_0^h is calculated using:

$$\alpha_0^h = 2\pi\left(Trunc\left(\frac{\alpha_p^h}{2\pi}, 1\right) + 1\right). \tag{7.12}$$

The assignment described using Eqs. 7.10 7.12 allows us to obtain the projections $p^f(\beta, \alpha^f); \beta \in [-\beta_{\max}, \beta_{\max}]$ in the hypothetical fan-beam projection system in the range $\alpha^f \in [0, 2\pi)$.

These projections $p^f(\beta, \alpha^f); \beta \in (-\beta_{\max}, \beta_{\max}]; \alpha^f \in [0, 2\pi)$ are further processed using the methods developed for the fan-beam projection system discussed in Chap. 6.

7.1.4 Discrete Implementation of the 360° LI Reconstruction Method

In the discrete version of the 360° LI reconstruction method, the projections are only made at certain locations on the z-axis and only at certain points on the screen. The places where the intensity measurements are made are determined by the topology of radiation detectors situated on the arc-shaped screen. It is also assumed that the detectors are arranged to ensure an even distribution of useful rays in the beam. The angle at which a given ray in the fan-beam falls on a given detector is indexed using the variable $\eta = -(\mathrm{H}-1)/2, \ldots, 0, \ldots, (\mathrm{H}-1)/2$, where H is an odd number of detectors in the array. During a scan, the middle of the beam of radiation passes through a particular point on the z-axis only once. As we only perform a limited number of projections, not all places on the z-axis lie in the plane of the incident radiation. To identify the angles α_θ^h at which the radiation beam is emitted, we use the index $\theta = 0, \ldots, \Theta - 1$; where Θ is the number of projections made during the scan. It is also convenient to assume that the value Δ_α^h is a complete divisor of the angle 2π.

We can summarise this by saying that only those discrete projection values defined for $\hat{p}^h(\eta,\theta); \eta = -(\mathrm{H}-1)/2,\ldots,0,\ldots,(\mathrm{H}-1)/2; \theta = 0,\ldots,\Theta-1$, are available to the reconstruction algorithm.

Before beginning the scan, we need to decide on the positions on the z-axis of the slices to be reconstructed. The projections to be considered in later stages of the process are chosen relative to one of the slices; let us say the slice at z_p. If the first projection takes place at an angle $\alpha^h = 0$, the hypothetical beam will pass through the point z_p at the angle described by (7.6).

The projections that will take part in the reconstruction of the slice at z_p are represented by $\hat{p}^h(\eta,\theta); \eta = -(\mathrm{H}-1)/2,\ldots,0,\ldots,(\mathrm{H}-1)/2; \theta = 0,\ldots,\Theta-1$, for which $\frac{(\alpha_p^h\ 2\pi)}{\Delta_\alpha^h} \le \theta \le \frac{(\alpha_p^h+2\pi)}{\Delta_\alpha^h}$. The following procedure leads to the reconstruction of the image based on these projections.

Step I Instead of using Eq. 7.7, we can start by establishing the weightings for each of the projections $\hat{p}^h(\eta,\theta)$ performed at angles in the range $\frac{(\alpha_p^h\ 2\pi)}{\Delta_\alpha^h} \le \theta \le \frac{(\alpha_p^h+2\pi)}{\Delta_\alpha^h}$ using the following weighting function (a graph of the function $w(\theta)$ is shown in Fig. 7.8):

$$w(\theta) = \begin{cases} \frac{2\pi+\alpha_p^h\ \theta\cdot\Delta_\alpha^h}{2\pi} & \text{for} \quad \alpha_p^h < \theta\cdot\Delta_\alpha^h \le \alpha_p^h + 2\pi \\ 1 & \text{for} \quad \theta\cdot\Delta_\alpha^h = \alpha_p^h \\ \frac{2\pi+\theta\cdot\Delta_\alpha^h\ \alpha_p^h}{2\pi} & \text{for} \quad \alpha_p^h - 2\pi \le \theta\cdot\Delta_\alpha^h < \alpha_p^h \\ 0 & \text{for} \quad \theta\cdot\Delta_\alpha^h > \alpha_p^h + 2\pi \vee \theta\cdot\Delta_\alpha^h < \alpha_p^h - 2\pi \end{cases} . \tag{7.13}$$

Each projection value $\hat{p}^h(\eta,\theta)$ is then multiplied by the appropriate weighting:

$$\dot{\hat{p}}_p^h(\eta,\theta) = w(\theta)\cdot\hat{p}^h(\eta,\theta). \tag{7.14}$$

As filtration and back-projection is a linear transformation, we can interpret it as an interpolation carried out at later stages of the process.

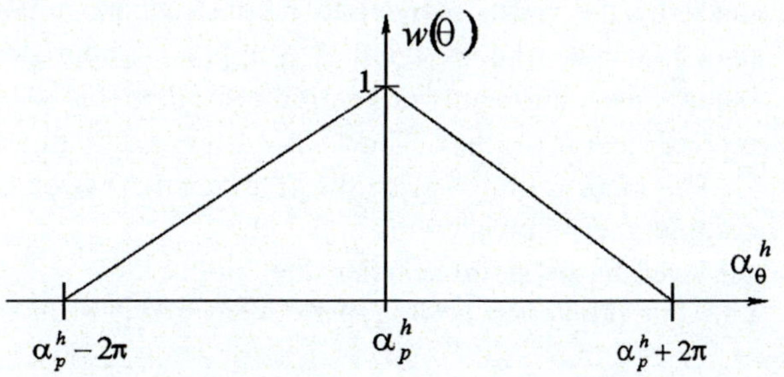

Fig. 7.8 A graph of the function $w(\theta)$ defining the weightings given to each projection $\hat{p}^h(\eta,\theta)$ in the 360° LI method

Step II In order to reconstruct the image, we use one of the methods devised for fan-beam projection systems and make the following assignment:

$$p^f(\eta, \gamma) \equiv \dot{\hat{p}}_p^h(\eta, \theta), \tag{7.15}$$

substituting:

$$\gamma = \begin{cases} \theta - \theta_0 & \text{if} \quad \theta \geq \theta_0 \\ \theta - \theta_0 + \Theta^{2\pi} & \text{if} \quad \theta < \theta_0 \end{cases} \tag{7.16}$$

and calculating θ_0 using:

$$\theta_0 = \left(\alpha_p^h \; div \; 2\pi\right) \cdot \Theta^{2\pi}. \tag{7.17}$$

We also assume that all the calculations are carried out with indices in the ranges: $\frac{(\alpha_p^h \; 2\pi)}{\Delta_\alpha^h} \leq \theta \leq \frac{(\alpha_p^h + 2\pi)}{\Delta_\alpha^h}$; $-(\mathrm{H} - 1)/2 \leq \eta \leq (\mathrm{H} - 1)/2$.

Step III The projections $p^f(\eta, \gamma); \eta = -(\mathrm{H} - 1)/2, \ldots, 0, \ldots, (\mathrm{H} - 1)/2; \gamma = 0, \ldots, \Gamma - 1$, obtained from the previous stage of the processing can then be subjected to any of the reconstruction procedures originally intended for fan-beam projection systems. At the same time, the number of fan-beam projections taken into account by the algorithm is set at:

$$\Gamma = 2 \cdot \Theta^{2\pi}. \tag{7.18}$$

The flowchart shown in Fig. 7.9 illustrates all the steps and signals for the discrete version of the 360° LI algorithm used in the SSCT scanner.

7.1.5 The 180° LI Reconstruction Algorithm

The 180° LI (*linear interpolation*) algorithm [7, 47] uses the projections $p^h(\beta, \alpha^h)$ made by the spiral scanner to reconstruct the image of individual slices of the patient's body. Once again, we apply an appropriate interpolation formula to obtain the fan-beam projections $p^f(\beta, \alpha^f); \beta \in [-\beta_{max}, \beta_{max}]$ needed for the reconstruction process. The 180° LI method is illustrated by Fig. 7.6.

The main problem with the implementation of this algorithm is the lack of a complete set of projections in the plane of the slice at a distance z_p from the start of the scan. In the spiral scanner, the patient table moves, and therefore the values of only one projection $p^h(\beta, \alpha^h)$ are measured at each angle of rotation α^h of the tube.

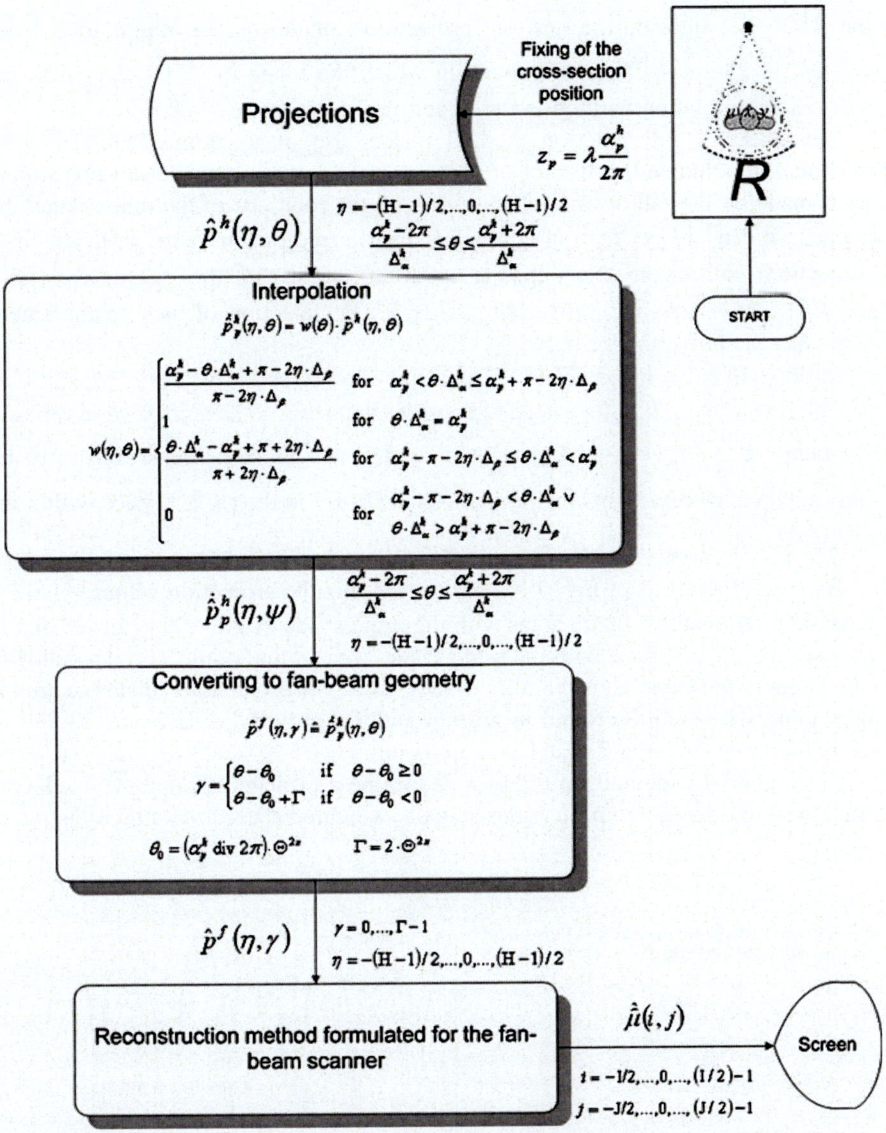

Fig. 7.9 A flowchart of the 360° LI algorithm used in the SSCT scanner

In order to obtain the missing projections, the 360° LI method uses linear interpolation based on projections made when $z \neq z_p$.

When the beam of radiation passes through the point $z = z_p$, the angle at which the projection is performed α_p^h can be determined using Eq. 7.6.

The main difference between the 180° LI and 360° LI algorithms is the method of selecting the projections to be interpolated. In contrast to the previous method, the 180° LI algorithm relies on projections made in the range $\alpha^h \in \left[\alpha_p^h - \pi - 2\beta_{\max}, \alpha_p^h + \pi + 2\beta_{\max}\right]$. The way in which the range of α^h is selected in the 180° LI interpolation method is illustrated in Fig. 7.10.

The 180° LI interpolation method makes use of a certain redundancy of information contained in the set of projections. So, if we consider all the projections made by the fan-beam system during all the rotations of the tube around the z-axis, we can always find an equivalent for the projection value $p^f\left(\beta, \dot{\alpha}^f\right)$ from projection values on the opposite side, at angles in the range $\alpha^f \in \left[\dot{\alpha}^f - \pi - 2\beta_{\max}, \dot{\alpha}^f - \pi + \beta_{\max}\right]; \beta \in [-\beta_{\max}, \beta_{\max}]$. The selection of these complementary pairs is shown in Fig. 7.11.

In order to solve the problem of acquiring the projection values $p^f\left(\beta, \dot{\alpha}^f\right); \dot{\alpha}^f \in [0, 2\pi]; \beta \in [-\beta_{\max}, \beta_{\max}]$ we need to consider that $p^h(\beta,\ \alpha^h)$ occurs several times in the range $\alpha^h \in \left[\alpha_p^h - \pi - 2\beta_{\max}, \alpha_p^h + \pi + 2\beta_{\max}\right]$. This situation is illustrated by Fig. 7.12, which represents the projections $p^h\left(\beta, \dot{\alpha}^h\right)$ in the $(\beta,\ \alpha^h)$ space within the ranges: $\beta \in [-\beta_{\max}, \beta_{\max}], \alpha^h \in \left[\alpha_p^h - \pi - 2\beta_{\max}, \alpha_p^h + \pi + 2\beta_{\max}\right]$.

By careful analysis of Fig. 7.12, we can see that the projection values $p^h\left(\beta, \dot{\alpha}^h\right)$ have their equivalents in the areas with the same shade of grey. This means that in areas in the $(\beta,\ \alpha^h)$ space with the same shade, we can find points corresponding to rays lying in the same plane parallel to the z-axis. For projections related to area 1, their equivalents can be found in areas 4 and 7. Similarly, area 2 corresponds to areas 5 and 8, and area 3 matches area 6.

In the 360° LI method, in order to determine a projection value for a selected slice, we considered two projections suitably weighted according to their degree of

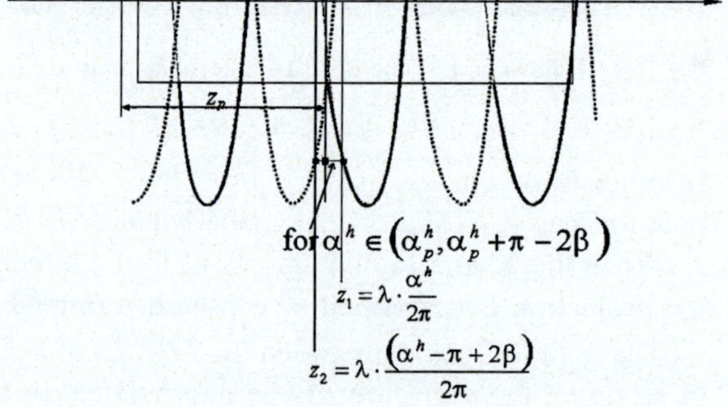

Fig. 7.10 Linear interpolation in the reconstruction algorithm

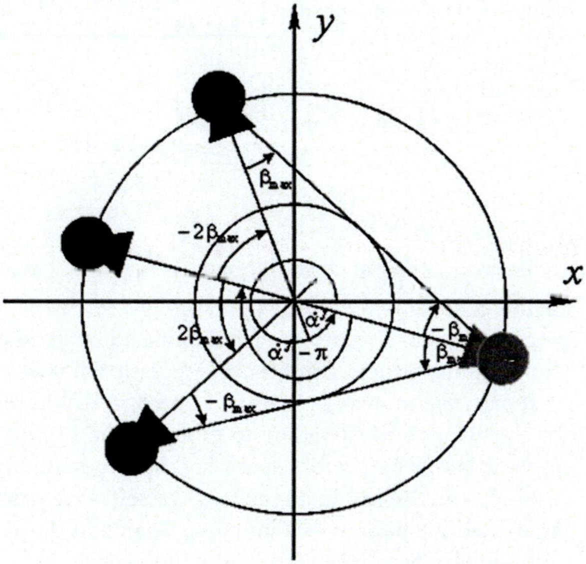

Fig. 7.11 Selecting complementary projection values

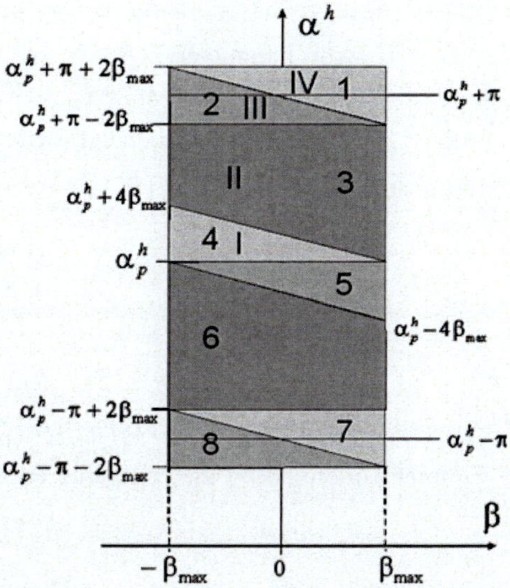

Fig. 7.12 The projections $p^h(\beta, \dot{\alpha}^h)$ in the (β, α^h) space

influence on the outcome of the interpolation. In the 180° LI method, the weighting is determined in a much more complex way. This is because when obtaining some of the projection values $p^f(\beta, \dot{\alpha}^f)$ we have two and in some cases three suitable projections $p^h(\beta, \alpha^h)$ to choose from. These can be seen as identical shaded areas in Fig. 7.12. These areas can be formed into pairs as shown in Table 7.1, each pair assigned to one of four groups of interpolated projection values.

Table 7.1 The assignment of pairs of areas from Fig. 7.12 to groups of interpolated projection values

Group number	Pairs of areas from Fig. 7.12
I	$4 \leftrightarrow 7; 4 \leftrightarrow 1$; (extrapolation);
II	$3 \leftrightarrow 6$
III	$2 \leftrightarrow 5; 2 \leftrightarrow 8$;
IV	$1 \leftrightarrow 7; 1 \leftrightarrow 4$; (extrapolation);

To avoid having to extrapolate projection values, we need to choose corresponding areas that are on opposite sides of the $\alpha^h = \alpha_p^h$ axis. There are two such pairs of areas in Table 7.1, each duplicated by another pair, which therefore allows us to eliminate them from the interpolation process.

If we were to disregard areas 1 and 8, it would result only in the elimination of the duplicates corresponding to groups I and IV. As we can see, areas 1 and 8 are on the edge of the (β, α^h) space and have a negligible effect on the interpolation.

So, having looked at all the ways of selecting pairs of areas for groups I-IV, and eliminated the pairs $1 \leftrightarrow 7$ and $2 \leftrightarrow 8$, and all those involving extrapolation, there only remain three suitable combinations of areas in groups I-III.

After careful analysis of these choices, based on Fig. 7.12, we can deduce a general rule for interpolating the value $\dot{p}^h\left(\dot{\beta}, \dot{\alpha}^h\right); \alpha_p^h \leq \dot{\alpha}^h \leq \alpha_p^h + \pi + 2\beta$ from $p^h(\beta, \alpha^h)$, with parameters (β, α^h) within the ranges $-\beta_{\max} \leq \beta \leq \beta_{\max}$ and $\dot{\alpha}^f - \pi - 2\beta_{\max} \leq \alpha^h \leq \dot{\alpha}^f + 2\pi + \beta_{\max}$. The rule says that in order to obtain any projection value $\dot{p}_p^h\left(\dot{\beta}, \dot{\alpha}^h\right)$ needed for reconstructing the slice at $z = z_p$, we must find a suitable projection $p_1^h(\beta_1, \alpha_1^h)$, where

$$\alpha_1^h = \dot{\alpha}^h \tag{7.19}$$

and

$$\beta_1 = \dot{\beta}. \tag{7.20}$$

The other projection value $p_2^h(\beta_2, \alpha_2^h)$ needed to perform the interpolation has parameters defined by the following equations:

$$\beta_2 = -\beta_1 \tag{7.21}$$

and

$$\alpha_2^h = \alpha_1^h - \pi + 2\beta_1. \tag{7.22}$$

Linear interpolation of the value $\dot{p}_p^h\left(\dot{\beta}, \dot{\alpha}^h\right)$ from the values $p_1^h(\beta_1, \alpha_1^h)$ and $p_2^h(\beta_2, \alpha_2^h)$ is performed using the equation:

$$\dot{p}_p^h\left(\dot{\beta}, \dot{\alpha}^h\right) = w_1 \cdot p_1^h(\beta_1, \alpha_1^h) + w_2 \cdot p_2^h(\beta_2, \alpha_2^h), \tag{7.23}$$

where the weights in the above relationship are calculated as follows:

$$w_1 = \frac{\alpha_p^h - \alpha_2^h}{\alpha_1^h - \alpha_2^h}, \tag{7.24}$$

and

$$w_2 = \frac{\alpha_1^h - \alpha_p^h}{\alpha_1^h - \alpha_2^h}. \tag{7.25}$$

After calculating all $\dot{p}_p^h\left(\dot{\beta}, \dot{\alpha}^h\right); -\beta_{\max} \leq \dot{\beta} \leq \beta_{\max}; \alpha_p^f < \dot{\alpha}^h \leq \alpha_p^h + \pi + 2\dot{\beta}$, we can then transpose them to the hypothetical fan-beam system and obtain the values $p^f(\beta, \alpha^f)$. To do this, we simply make the appropriate assignment:

$$p^f\left(\beta, \alpha^f\right) \equiv \dot{p}_p^h\left(\dot{\beta}, \dot{\alpha}^h\right). \tag{7.26}$$

To adapt the values of the function $p^f(\beta, \alpha^f)$ obtained from (7.26) to the reconstruction methods described in Chap. 6, we need to take care to preserve the usual ranges for these projections, namely: $\beta \in [-\beta_{\max}, \beta_{\max}]$ and $\alpha^f \in [0, 2\pi)$. We can do this by giving parts of the projection values from areas 5 to 7 in Fig. 7.12 appropriate values from areas 2 to 4, using the equation:

$$\dot{p}_p^h\left(\dot{\beta}, \dot{\alpha}^h\right) = \dot{p}_p^h\left(-\dot{\beta}, \dot{\alpha}^h + \pi + 2\dot{\beta}\right), \tag{7.27}$$

for $\dot{\beta} \in [-\beta_{\max}, \beta_{\max}] \wedge \dot{\alpha}^h \in \left(\alpha_p^h - \pi - 2\dot{\beta}, \alpha_p^h\right)$.

After extending the range of the interpolated projections $\dot{p}_p^h\left(\dot{\beta}, \dot{\alpha}^h\right)$ as described above, we still need to fill the gaps in relation to parts of areas 1 and 8, which we can write as follows:

$$\dot{p}_p^h\left(\dot{\beta}, \dot{\alpha}^h\right) = \begin{cases} \dot{p}_p^h\left(\dot{\beta}, \dot{\alpha}^h\right) & \text{for} \quad \dot{\beta} \in [0, \beta_{\max}] \wedge \dot{\alpha}^h \in \left[\alpha_p^h + \pi - 2\dot{\beta}, \alpha_p^h + \pi\right] \\ \dot{p}_p^h\left(\dot{\beta}, \dot{\alpha}^h + 2\pi\right) & \text{for} \quad \dot{\beta} \in [-\beta_{\max}, 0] \wedge \dot{\alpha}^h \in \left[\alpha_p^h - \pi, \alpha_p^h - \pi - 2\dot{\beta}\right] \end{cases}. \tag{7.28}$$

After increasing the ranges of $\dot{p}_p^h\left(\dot{\beta}, \dot{\alpha}^h\right)$ we are now able to implement assignment (7.26) using the following formula:

$$p^f\left(\beta, \alpha^f\right) = \begin{cases} \dot{p}_p^h\left(\dot{\beta}, \dot{\alpha}^h - \dot{\alpha}_0^h\right) & \text{if} \quad \dot{\alpha}^h \geq \dot{\alpha}_0^h \\ \dot{p}_p^h\left(\dot{\beta}, \dot{\alpha}^h - \dot{\alpha}_0^h + 2\pi\right) & \text{if} \quad \dot{\alpha}^h < \dot{\alpha}_0^h \end{cases}, \tag{7.29}$$

where $\dot{\alpha}_0^h$ is calculated from:

$$\dot{\alpha}_0^h = 2\pi\left(\dot{\alpha}^h \; div \; 2\pi\right). \tag{7.30}$$

With the set of fan-beam projections $p^f(\beta, \alpha^f)$ calculated for the angle of rotation $\alpha^f \in [0, 2\pi)$ and for $\beta \in [-\beta_{\max}, \beta_{\max}]$, we can then start the reconstruction of the image of the slice at $z_p = \lambda \frac{\alpha_p^h}{2\pi}$.

7.1.6 Discrete Implementation of the 180° LI Reconstruction Method

The implementation of the discrete 180° LI reconstruction method relies on measurements made only at particular projection angles and only at particular points on the screen. The places where the radiation intensities are measured are determined by the location of the detectors in the array on the arc-shaped screen. If the useful rays are evenly distributed in the fan-beam, the angle at which a ray strikes a detector is represented by the variable $\eta = -(\mathrm{H}-1)/2, \ldots, 0, \ldots, (\mathrm{H}-1)/2$, where H is an odd number of detectors in the array. During a scan, only a limited number of projections are made, so only certain places on the z-axis will lie in the plane of the incident radiation. The indices $\theta = 0, \ldots, \Theta - 1$ are used to identify the angles α_θ^h at which the beam of radiation is emitted, where Θ is the number of projections made during the scan. We can therefore say that only those discrete projection values $\hat{p}^h(\eta, \theta)$ defined for $\eta = -(\mathrm{H}-1)/2, \ldots, 0, \ldots, (\mathrm{H}-1)/2; \theta = 0, \ldots, \Theta - 1$, are available to the reconstruction algorithm.

Before beginning the actual scan, we need to decide on the positions on the z-axis of the slices to be reconstructed. Let us say for argument's sake that a particular slice is located at z_p. If the first projection is made at an angle $\alpha^h = 0$, then the angle at which the hypothetical beam passes through the point z_p is determined by Eq. 7.6.

In reconstructing the image of the slice at z_p, the projections that are involved are represented by $\hat{p}^h(\eta, \theta)$, where $\frac{\left(\alpha_p^h \;\; \pi \;\; 2\beta_{\max}\right)}{\Delta_\alpha^h} \leq \theta \leq \frac{\left(\alpha_p^h + \pi + 2\beta_{\max}\right)}{\Delta_\alpha^h}$.

The following steps are designed to lead to the reconstruction of the image, based on these projections.

Step I Due to the linearity of the filtration and back-projection process, Eqs. 7.24 and 7.25, defining the weightings assigned to individual projection values, can be replaced by the function $w(\eta, \theta)$ defined by the following formula:

$$
w(\eta,\theta)=\begin{cases}\frac{\alpha_p^h\quad\theta\cdot\Delta_\alpha^h+\pi\quad 2\eta\cdot\Delta_\beta}{\pi\quad 2\eta\cdot\Delta_\beta} & \text{for } \alpha_p^h<\theta\cdot\Delta_\alpha^h\leq\alpha_p^h+\pi-2\eta\cdot\Delta_\beta\\ 1 & \text{for } \theta\cdot\Delta_\alpha^h=\alpha_p^h\\ \frac{\theta\cdot\Delta_\alpha^h\quad\alpha_p^h+\pi+2\eta\cdot\Delta_\beta}{\pi+2\eta\cdot\Delta_\beta} & \text{for } \alpha_p^h-\pi-2\eta\cdot\Delta_\beta\leq\theta\cdot\Delta_\alpha^h<\alpha_p^h\\ 0 & \text{for } \theta\cdot\Delta_\alpha^h<\alpha_p^h-\pi-2\eta\cdot\Delta_\beta\vee\theta\cdot\Delta_\alpha^h>\alpha_p^h+\pi-2\eta\cdot\Delta_\beta\end{cases}.
\tag{7.31}
$$

A graph of the function $w(\beta_\eta, \alpha_\theta^h)$, which is the continuous equivalent of the discrete weighting function $w(\eta, \theta)$ from Eq. 7.31, is shown in Fig. 7.13.

It is easy to show that the sum of two weights on opposite sides of the $w(\beta_\eta, \alpha_\theta^h)$ axis, a distance $\pi - 2\beta_1$ away from each other on the α_θ^h axis and satisfying the relationship $\beta_2 = -\beta_1$ is equal to 1, i.e. that:

$$
w(\beta_1, \alpha_1^h) + w(-\beta_1, \alpha_1^h - \pi + 2\beta_1) = 1. \tag{7.32}
$$

The individual projection values $\hat{p}^h(\eta, \theta)$ within the ranges $-(\mathrm{H}-1)/2 \leq \eta \leq (\mathrm{H}-1)/2; \frac{(\alpha_p^h\quad\pi\quad 2\eta\cdot\Delta_\beta)}{\Delta_\alpha^h} \leq \theta \leq \frac{(\alpha_p^h+\pi\quad 2\eta\cdot\Delta_\beta)}{\Delta_\alpha^h}$, obtained from the detectors, can be transformed using these weightings. This is a form of interpolation performed in later stages of the procedure. The linear transformation of the entire set of projection functions needed for the reconstruction of the image of the slice at z_p is implemented using:

$$
\dot{\hat{p}}_p^h(\eta, \theta) = w(\eta, \theta)\hat{p}^h(\eta, \theta). \tag{7.33}
$$

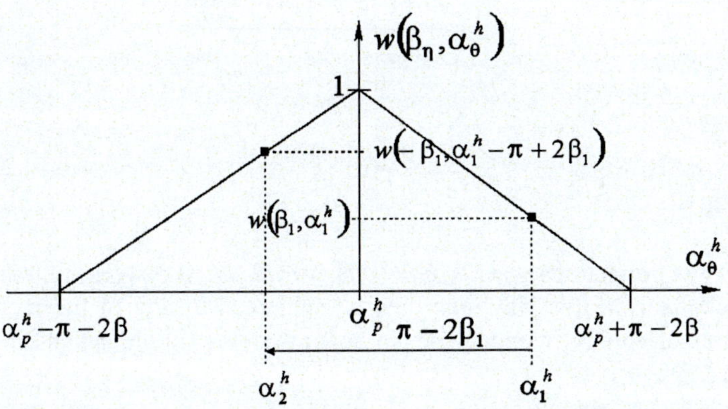

Fig. 7.13 A graph of the weighting function $w(\beta_\eta, \alpha_\theta^h)$ determining the weight assigned to each projection $\hat{p}^h(\eta, \theta)$ in the 180° LI method

Step II In order to reconstruct the image of the cross-section at $z = z_p$, we use one of the methods designed for fan-beam projection systems and in order to obtain the hypothetical fan-beam projection we use the following:

$$p^f(\eta,\gamma) \equiv \dot{\hat{p}}_p^h(\eta,\theta), \tag{7.34}$$

for the ranges $-(\mathrm{H}-1)/2 \leq \eta \leq (\mathrm{H}-1)/2; \frac{(\alpha_p^h\ \ \pi\ \ 2\beta)}{\Delta_\alpha^h} \leq \theta \leq \frac{(\alpha_p^h+\pi\ \ 2\beta)}{\Delta_\alpha^h}$.

The projection values $p^f(\eta, \gamma)$ obtained from (7.34) can be used directly in any of the reconstruction methods originally devised for fan-beam systems, as considered in Chap. 6. But first, we need to adapt the projections $\dot{\hat{p}}_p^h(\eta,\theta)$ so that the indexing and the range are suitable for fan-beam reconstruction algorithms:

$$\dot{\hat{p}}_p^h(\eta,\theta) = \begin{cases} \hat{p}_p^h\left(\eta, \theta - \frac{2\pi}{\Delta_\alpha^h}\right) & \text{for} \quad \eta \in \left[0, \frac{\mathrm{H}\ \ 1}{2}\right] \wedge \theta \in \left(\frac{\alpha_p^h+\pi\ \ 2\eta\Delta_\beta}{\Delta_\alpha^h}, \frac{\alpha_p^h+\pi}{\Delta_\alpha^h}\right] \\ \hat{p}_p^h\left(\eta, \theta + \frac{2\pi}{\Delta_\alpha^h}\right) & \text{for} \quad \eta \in \left[-\frac{\mathrm{H}\ \ 1}{2}, 0\right] \wedge \theta \in \left(\frac{\alpha_p^h\ \ \pi}{\Delta_\alpha^h}, \frac{\alpha_p^h\ \ \pi\ \ 2\eta\Delta_\beta}{\Delta_\alpha^h}\right] \\ \dot{\hat{p}}_p^h(\eta,\theta) & \text{for} \qquad\qquad \text{the remaining} \end{cases}. \tag{7.35}$$

It remains only to convert the indices of the two projection systems:

$$\gamma = \begin{cases} \theta - \theta_0 & \text{if} \quad \theta \geq \theta_0 \\ \theta - \theta_0 + \Gamma & \text{if} \quad \theta < \theta_0 \end{cases}, \tag{7.36}$$

for $-\frac{\beta_{\max}}{\Delta_\beta} \leq \eta \leq \frac{\beta_{\max}}{\Delta_\beta}; \frac{\alpha_p^h\ \ \pi}{\Delta_\alpha^h} \leq \theta \leq \frac{\alpha_p^h+\pi}{\Delta_\alpha^h}$, calculating θ_0 using:

$$\theta_0 = \frac{2\pi\left(\left(\alpha_p^h + \pi\right) \mathit{div}\ 2\pi\right)}{\Delta_\alpha^h}, \tag{7.37}$$

where

$$\Gamma = \frac{2\pi}{\Delta_\alpha^h}. \tag{7.38}$$

Step III The projections $p^f(\eta,\gamma); \eta = -(\mathrm{H}-1)/2, \ldots, 0, \ldots, (\mathrm{H}-1)/2; \gamma = 0, \ldots, \Gamma - 1$, obtained in this way, can then be subjected to any of the reconstruction procedures originally intended for fan-beam systems (implementation details are given in Chap. 6).

The flowchart shown in Fig. 7.14 illustrates all the steps and signals for the discrete version of the 180° LI algorithm used in SSCT scanners.

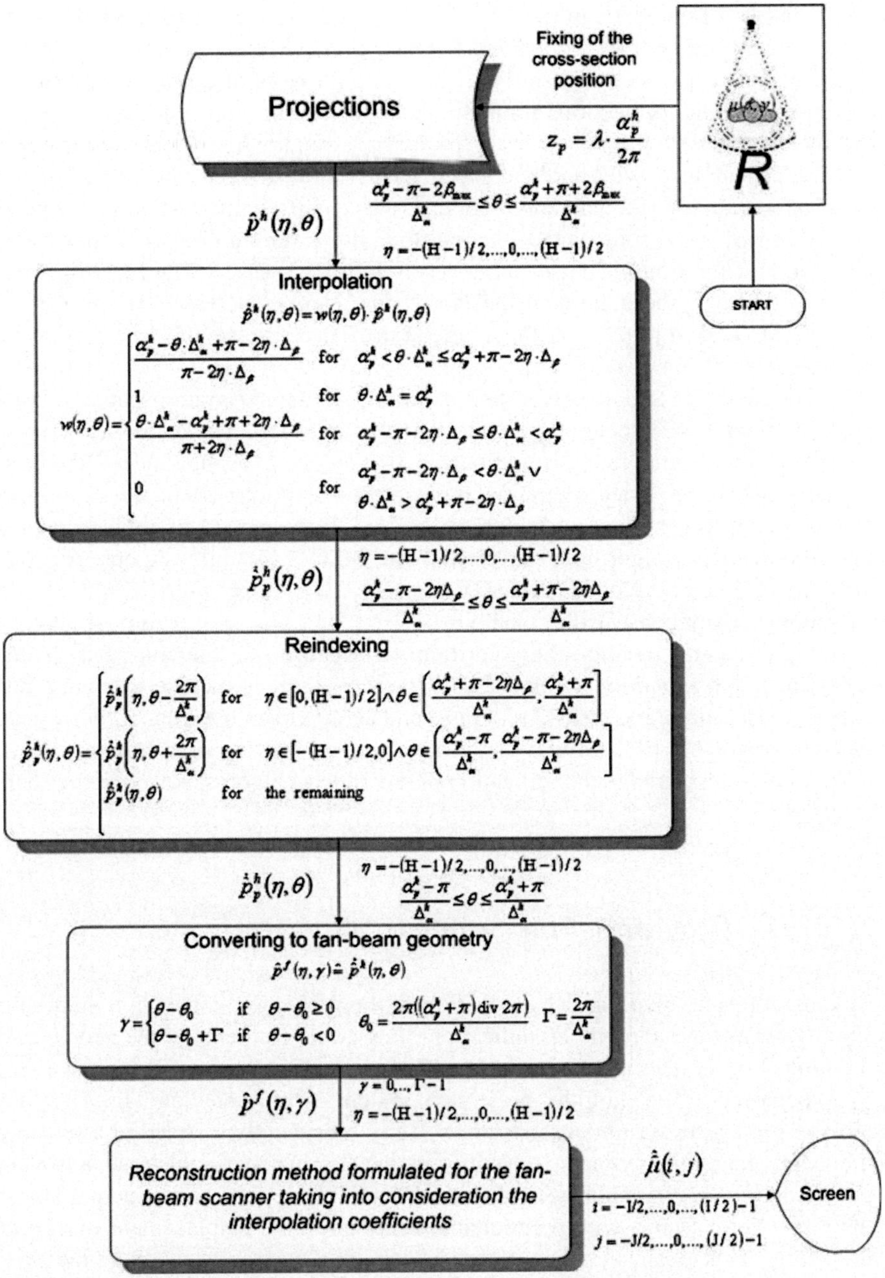

Fig. 7.14 A flowchart of the 180° LI algorithm used in SSCT scanners

7.2 Multi-Slice Computed Tomography—MSCT

The previous design of spiral scanner, the single-slice CT scanner (SSCT), had only one row of detectors in the array. Adding additional rows of detectors to the array created the *multi-slice computed tomography* (MSCT) scanner [2, 22, 43]. Practical MSCT devices contain between 8 and 34 rows of detectors and so it is possible to acquire projections simultaneously for the subsequent reconstruction of up to four slices [52].

MSCT scanners have improved specifications compared to spiral scanners that have only one row of detectors. There is an eightfold increase in the rate of acquisition of the reconstructed images (four times the number of reconstructed slices in half the time). The scanning resolution is increased. The level of image noise is reduced (the current in the X-ray tube can be increased because of the reduced time taken to perform the whole scan). There is also a more effective use of the power of X-ray tube [15].

It should be stressed, however, that in large part the procedure for acquiring the projections in MSCT technology is the same as in SSCT. The similarity between the two types of tomography is particularly marked as far as the shape of the beam of radiation is concerned; there are the same assumptions about the fan-shaped beams reaching each row of detectors in the MSCT scanner. As might be expected, the reconstruction algorithms developed for MSCT are only slightly modified versions of those developed for SSCT.

Amongst the reconstruction methods devised for use in MSCT tomography, we should particularly mention the algorithm described in the literature as *extended 360° linear interpolation* (ex-360° LI). Other approaches include extended 180° *linear interpolation* (ex-180° LI) [34, 60] and an approach using an *adaptive axial interpolator* (AAI) [52]. In this book, however, we will consider the *ex-180° LI algorithm*, as it is simply a modification of the 180° LI algorithm used in the SSCT technique.

7.2.1 The Geometry of the Scanner

Key quantities involved in the acquisition of the projection values in a multi-slice spiral scanner together with an indication of essential elements of the geometry of the projection system are given in Figs. 7.15 and 7.16.

A perspective view of the projection system is presented in Fig. 7.15. The moving projection system consists of an X-ray tube rigidly coupled to a screen in the shape of a partial cylinder. A multi-row detector matrix (in this case, 4 rows) is placed on the screen. This system rotates around the z-axis (the principal axis of the projection system) with a simultaneous longitudinal displacement during the projection. This means that the rotating projection system moves around the z-axis along a spiral path. A cone-beam of radiation emitted by the tube travels through

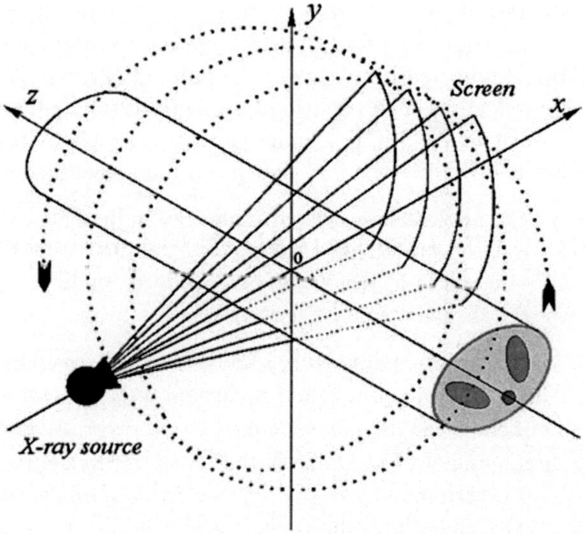

Fig. 7.15 The projection system of a multi slice spiral scanner a three dimensional perspective view

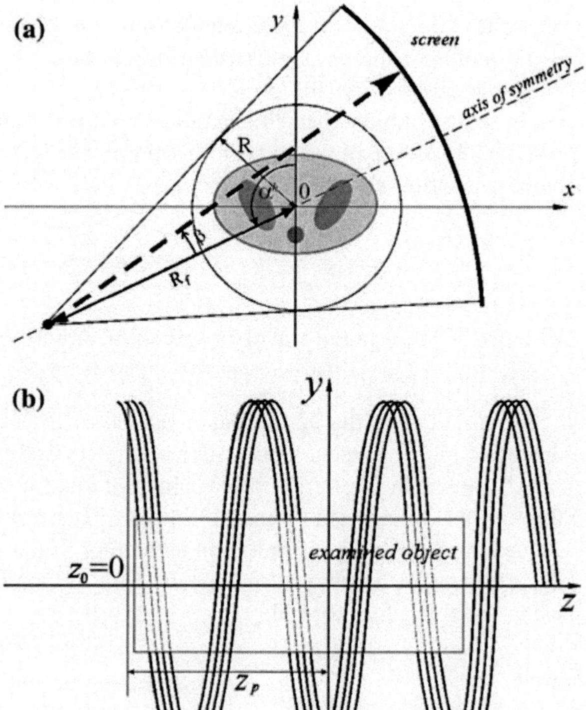

Fig. 7.16 The projection system of a multi slice spiral scanner: **a** the geometry of the fan beam projection system in the plane perpendicular to the axis of rotation; **b** the location of the test object in the plane containing the axis of rotation

the test object and finally reaches the detector matrix on the screen. Owing to the limited number of rows in the matrix and the small distance between them, the projections reaching each of the individual rows are essentially fan-beams and can be treated as such [52]. Figure 7.16b illustrates the projection geometry, identical to that in an SSCT scanner, in the $x\ y$ plane. In this system, the rays that are emitted by the tube and that reach the screen are identified by:

β the angle between a particular ray in the beam and the axis of symmetry of the moving projection system;
α^h the angle at which the projection is made;
$\dot{z}$ the displacement of the ray relative to the start of the z-axis.

These three parameters specify every ray during the whole projection process. Thus, the projection values measured on the screen in a system made up of a set of fan-beams can be represented by $p^h(\beta, \alpha^h, \dot{z})$. As the projections are made during a large number of rotations of the projection system around the test object, the angle α^h is determined by $0 \leq \alpha^h \leq 2\ \pi \cdot number\ \ of\ \ rotations$. The values of the angle β are situated within the range $[-\beta_{\max}, \beta_{\max}]$, in which:

$$\beta_{\max} = \arcsin\left(\frac{\mathrm{R}}{\mathrm{R}_f}\right), \tag{7.39}$$

where R is the radius of the circle defining the space in which the scan is made; R_f is the radius of the circle described by the tube.

The location z_0 of the projection system along the z-axis is a function of the angle α^h. Assuming the patient table moves forward uniformly and that $z_0 = 0$ when $\alpha^h = 0$ we can write the following linear relationship, which determines the current location z_0:

$$z_0 = \lambda \cdot \frac{\alpha^h}{2\pi}, \tag{7.40}$$

where λ is the relative travel of the spiral described by the tube around the test object, measured in $\left[\frac{\mathrm{m}}{\mathrm{rad}}\right]$.

In this design, the X-ray beam falls on a much broader, multi-row array of detectors on the screen. This is demonstrated by Fig. 7.17.

As shown in Fig. 7.17, the beam of radiation emitted by the source passes through the narrow slit of the collimator. This results in a cone-beam. As a consequence of the beam of radiation spreading in the plane parallel to the z-axis we need to convert the distances appearing on the screen into distances on the z-axis using the following formula:

$$\dot{z} = z_0 + z_d \frac{\mathrm{R}_d}{\mathrm{R}_d + \mathrm{R}_f}, \tag{7.41}$$

where R_d is the radius of the circle described by the screen.

Fig. 7.17 The geometry of the spiral projection system of the MSCT

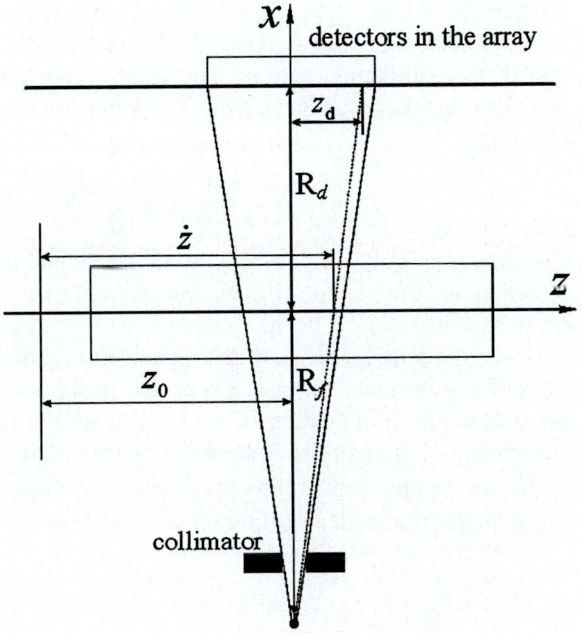

The array of detectors placed on the cylindrical screen is designed to measure the intensity of the X-rays passing through the test object. The detectors in the array are arranged in rows encompassing the z-axis. Further details of the construction of the detector array will be given when we discuss the discrete version of this projection system.

A further problem that needs to be considered by reconstruction algorithms is the inclination of the gantry during a scan. The solution to this problem, for projection systems with up to four rows of detectors, can be found in the articles [23, 24].

7.2.2 The Geometry of the Discrete Scanner

The projection system presented above with its multi-row detector array found its practical application in spiral scanners. As with all previous designs, the MSCT spiral scanner also had to take into account the discrete nature of the projections obtained.

Figure 7.18 shows orthogonal views of the projection system at two different projection angles. As we can see from the diagram, the quantities R_d and R_f are many times greater than the width of the detectors d_w. In addition, the gaps between the individual rows of detectors are very small. We can therefore regard the beams travelling from tube to detector as being approximately parallel. This allows us to assume that the radiation beam is made up of fans with a total thickness BW (the *beam width*). Since each detector has a width d_w, the intensity measurements are made only within this restricted area. This arrangement forms a part of the collimation system. The width of the cross-section, SW (*slice width*), can therefore be calculated from the value of d_w in the z-direction, using the equation:

$$\mathrm{SW} = \mathrm{d}_w \frac{\mathrm{R}_d}{\mathrm{R}_d + \mathrm{R}_f}. \tag{7.42}$$

The individual rows of detectors in the array, and therefore the individual fans of radiation, are numbered using the index $k = 1, 2, \ldots$, K. In the case of the detector array shown in Fig. 7.18, K = 4.

The remaining elements of the quantisation process of the projection values do not differ from those discussed for other designs of fan-beam scanner. However, because of the introduction of a new convention for representing the projection parameters in this approach, they are described again below.

In this system, acquisition of the projection values $p^h\left(\beta, \alpha^h, \dot{z}\left(\alpha^h, k\right)\right)$ only takes place at specific angles of rotation α^h, determined by the relationship:

$$\alpha_\theta^h = \theta \cdot \Delta_\alpha^h, \tag{7.43}$$

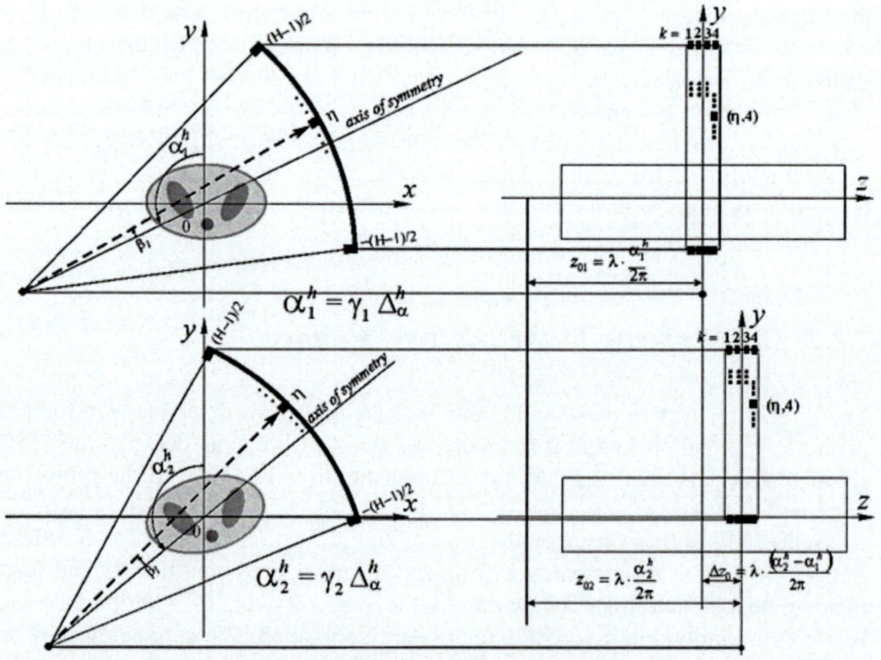

Fig. 7.18 The discrete version of the MSCT scanner

where $\Delta_{\alpha}^{h} = \frac{2\pi}{\Theta^{2\pi}}$ is the angle through which the tube-screen system is rotated following each projection; $\Theta^{2\pi}$ is the number of projections made during one full rotation of the projection system; $\theta = 0, \ldots, \Theta - 1$ is the global projection index; $\Theta = \textit{number of rotations} \cdot \Theta^{2\pi}$ is the total number of projections.

The position of the detector in the matrix is determined by the pair (η, k), where $\eta = -(\mathrm{H}-1)/2, \ldots, 0, \ldots, (\mathrm{H}-1)/2$ is number of the detector in the row and $k = 1, 2, \ldots, \mathrm{K}$ is the number of the row in which the detector is located. L and K represent, respectively, the total number of detectors in each row and the total number of rows. It is convenient to assume that K is an even number.

With this design of detector array, we obtain projection values $p^h\left(\beta, \alpha^h, \dot{z}\right)$ only for the selected projection angle β, determined by the relationship:

$$\beta_\eta = \eta \cdot \Delta_\beta^f, \tag{7.44}$$

where Δ_β^f is the angular distance between the individual radiation detectors placed on the cylindrical screen.

Therefore, we can summarise by saying that in the discrete projection system of the MSCT spiral scanner we can only obtain the projection values $\hat{p}^h(\eta, \theta, k) = p^h\left(\beta_\eta, \alpha_\theta^h, k\right)$ for $\eta = -(\mathrm{H}-1)/2, \ldots, 0, \ldots, (\mathrm{H}-1)/2; \theta = 0, \ldots, \Theta - 1; k = 1, 2, \ldots, \mathrm{K}$.

Looking back to the discussion summarised by Eq. 7.42, it is advisable, for discrete projections, to reformulate the relationship describing the displacement of the detectors with respect to the z-axis. As the detector array has multiple rows, it is necessary to consider the position of each of the rows of detectors individually. In addition, it is convenient to establish the point $z_0 = 0$ as a point of reference in the z direction. Finally, we can conclude that the position of a given row of detectors with respect to the z-axis is given by:

$$\dot{z}\left(\alpha^h, k\right) = \lambda \frac{\alpha^h}{2\pi} + \left(k - \frac{\mathrm{K}+1}{2}\right) \cdot \mathrm{SW}. \tag{7.45}$$

Another very important scan parameter in a spiral scanner is the pitch. Unlike the definition of the similar quantity given in Eq. 7.5, the definition in the MSCT projection system must take into account the number of rows of detectors in the array:

$$\mathrm{pitch}_d = \frac{\lambda}{\mathrm{K} \cdot \mathrm{SW}}. \tag{7.46}$$

Figure 7.19 shows a graphical interpretation of the parameter pitch_d defined by Eq. 7.46, relative to the parameter pitch. It is clear from this that the faster the forward movement of the patient table (i.e. higher values of pitch and pitch_d), the greater the errors involved in recovering the missing projections and the poorer the quality of the resulting reconstructed image.

Fig. 7.19 A graphical interpretation of the parameter $pitch_d$ in the MSCT scanner

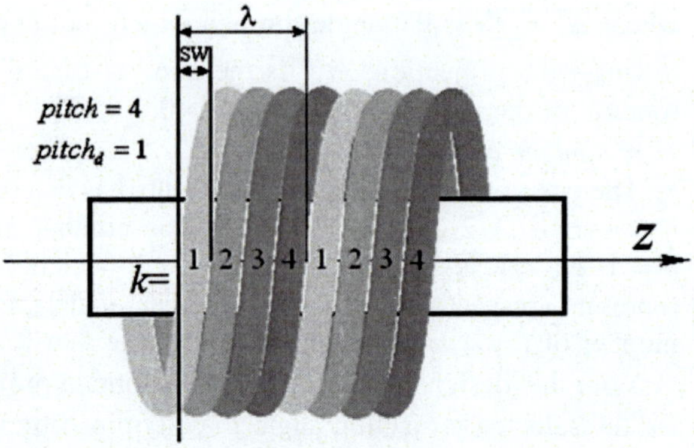

The choice of the value for λ (for a fixed beam width SW) affects the z-axis resolution attainable for the reconstructed images. For a standard detector array with 4 rows, the $pitch_d$ is four times smaller than the pitch.

7.2.3 The z-Filtering Reconstruction Algorithm

The z-filtering reconstruction algorithm is based on linear interpolation methods used for SSCT scanners (360° LI and 180° LI). In this case, however, we use projections $p^h(\beta, \alpha^h, \dot{z})$ obtained from a spiral projection system with a multi-row detector array to reconstruct the image of the selected cross-section. In the z-filtering algorithm, the function $p^h(\beta, \alpha^h, \dot{z})$ is used to calculate the hypothetical fan-beam projections $p^f(\beta, \alpha^f)$; $[-\beta_{\max}, \beta_{\max}]$; $\alpha^h \in [0, 2\pi)$, which are then used to reconstruct the image of the slice at location $z = z_p$.

Before proceeding to a discussion of the z-filtering algorithm, we should first examine the circumstances in which the projections $p^h(\beta, \alpha^h, \dot{z})$ are performed in an MSCT scanner [26, 27, 58]. What is important here is the pitch parameter that determines the relative positions of the projections $p^h(\beta, \alpha^h, \dot{z}(\alpha^h, k))$ along the z-axis. Figure 7.20a illustrates a situation where $pitch_d = 2$ (for simplicity, only rays corresponding to $\beta = 0$ for each projection are indicated in the diagram). The different lines in this diagram represent the rays assigned to specific rows of detectors, more specifically to one of the detectors in each row. The dotted lines represent the rays corresponding to projection values $p^h(0, \alpha^h + \pi, \dot{z})$ made after half a rotation. As can be seen from the diagram, the rays of the two adjacent projections $p^h(0, \alpha^h, \dot{z})$ and $p^h(0, \alpha^h + 2\pi, \dot{z})$ coincide in two instances. In addition, all the rays of the complementary projection $p^h(0, \alpha^h + \pi, \dot{z})$ are duplicated by rays coming from $p^h(0, \alpha^h, \dot{z})$ or $p^h(0, \alpha^h + 2\pi, \dot{z})$. This duplication of the radiation measurements is not helpful, as it means that in spite of an expanded array of detectors, there is no increase in the measurement resolution. The situation can be

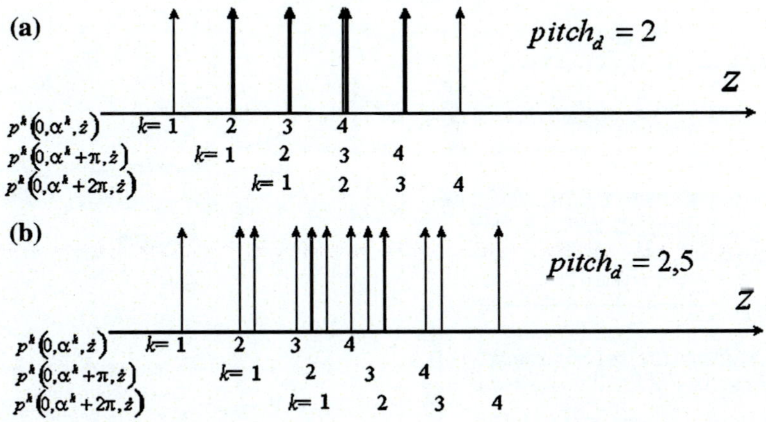

Fig. 7.20 Selecting values of pitch_d: **a** the overlap of the rays when pitch_d 2; **b** the increase in the density of the rays when pitch_d 2.5

avoided, however, by using non-integer values for pitch_d [27, 66], for example: $\text{pitch}_d = 0.5; 1.5$. Figure 7.20b shows the advantage of this, in terms of the spread of the rays from the projections $p^h(0, \alpha^h, \dot{z}), p^h(0, \alpha^h + \pi, \dot{z})$ and $p^h(0, \alpha^h + 2\pi, \dot{z})$. If we were also to draw the extra rays associated with the complementary projection $p^h(0, \alpha^h - \pi, \dot{z})$, we would see an evenly spaced, four-fold increase in the density of the rays for $\beta = 0$. In general, this means an increase in the density of the projections for all angles β and consequently a potential increase in the z-axis resolution of the reconstructed slice images.

However, the direct transfer of any of the SSCT spiral scanner reconstruction methods (such as 360° LI or 180° LI) to a scanner with a multi-row detector array would not result in any benefit from the increased z-axis sampling resolution. Therefore, a new method designed for MSCT scanners has been proposed: z-filtering [27, 58]. A diagram of this method is shown in Fig. 7.21.

The z-filtering reconstruction algorithm makes use of projection values from every detector row to obtain the hypothetical projections made in the plane of the slice. The interpolation process in this method uses a filter of width *FW* (*filter width*). The main elements of the interpolation are shown located on the z-axis in Fig. 7.22 [58].

As shown in Fig. 7.22, the range used to interpolate the projections $\dot{p}^h(\beta, \alpha^h, z_p)$ is restricted to $\dot{z} \in \left[z_p - \frac{\text{FW}}{2}, z_p + \frac{\text{FW}}{2}\right]$. But we also take into account two additional projections: the projection on the z-axis just before $\dot{z} = z_p - \frac{\text{FW}}{2}$ and the one just after $\dot{z} = z_p + \frac{\text{FW}}{2}$. It should be stressed that in this arrangement, as well as using measurements from all the detector rows, we also use the projections made after complete rotations and the complementary projections, i.e. those obtained after half-rotations (or more specifically, when the angle of rotation of the projection system is $\alpha^h + integer\_value \cdot \pi - 2\beta$ and the angle of the ray in the fan is $-\beta$). All of the projections in the set are arranged temporarily in order of their

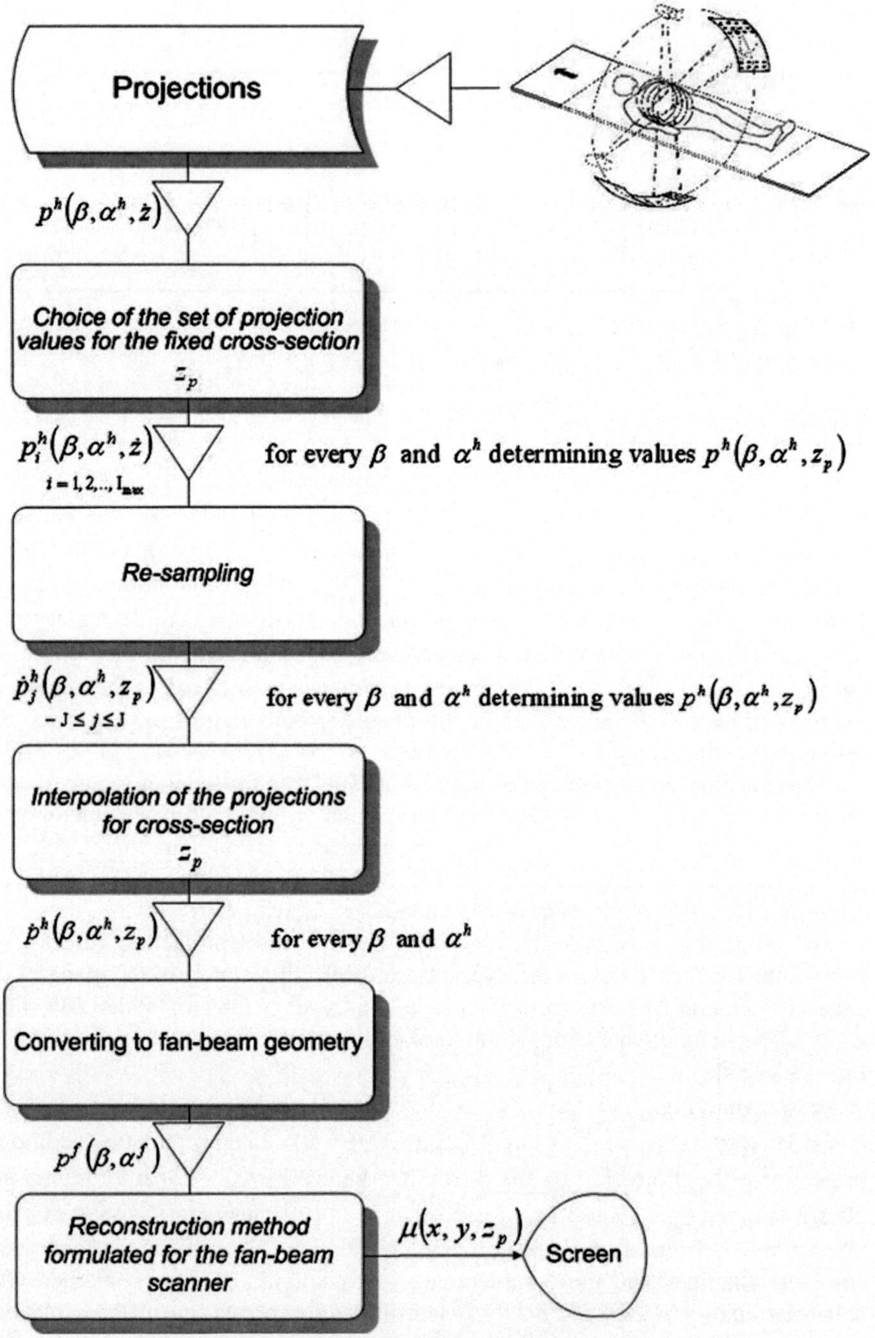

Fig. 7.21 The z filtering algorithm used in MSCT tomography

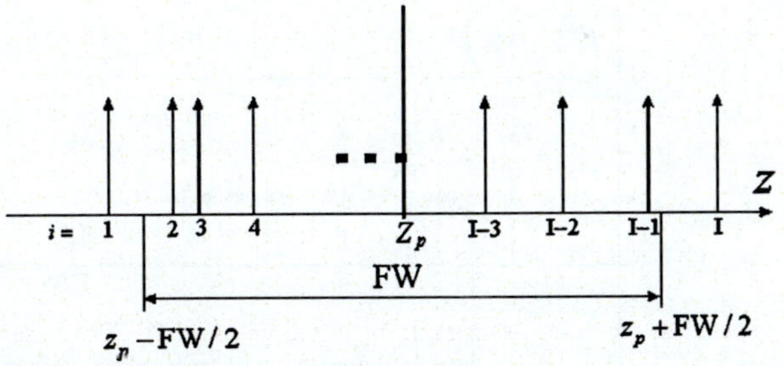

Fig. 7.22 Determining the neighbourhood of a slice using a filter of width FW

occurrence on the z-axis and are indexed using the index $i = 1, 2, \ldots, \mathrm{I}_{\max}$. The projection value $p_1^h(\beta, \alpha^h, \dot{z})$ represents the additional projection lying just before $\dot{z} = z_p - \frac{\mathrm{FW}}{2}$ and the projection value $p_{\mathrm{I}_{\max}}^h(\beta, \alpha^h, \dot{z})$ the one just after $\dot{z} = z_p + \frac{\mathrm{FW}}{2}$.

The interpolation procedure used in the z-filtering algorithm then proceeds as described below [58].

The first stage in the processing of the projection values $p^h(\beta, \alpha^h, \dot{z})$ involves *re-sampling* within the range $\left[z_p - \frac{\mathrm{FW}}{2}, z_p + \frac{\mathrm{FW}}{2}\right]$ with a resolution:

$$\Delta_z = \frac{\mathrm{FW}}{2\mathrm{J} + 1}, \tag{7.47}$$

where J is the number of re-sampling points.

The individual positions where re-sampling occurs are arranged in the order:

$$\dot{z}_j = z_p + j \cdot \Delta_z, \tag{7.48}$$

where $-\mathrm{J} \le j \le \mathrm{J}$.

The re-sampled values $\dot{p}_j^h(\beta, \alpha^h, z_p)$ are determined from two adjacent projections $p_i^h(\beta, \alpha^h, \dot{z})$ on the z-axis, using an interpolation formula, for example:

$$\begin{aligned} \dot{p}_j^h(\beta, \alpha^h, z_p) = {} & \left(1 - w(\beta, \alpha^h, i(j))\right) \cdot p_{i(j)}^h(\beta, \alpha^h, \dot{z}) + w(\beta, \alpha^h, i(j)) \\ & \cdot p_{i(j)+1}^h(\beta, \alpha^h, \dot{z}), \end{aligned} \tag{7.49}$$

in which:

$$w(\beta, \alpha^h, i(j)) = \left| \frac{\dot{z}_j - \dot{z}_1}{\dot{z}_2 - \dot{z}_1} \right|, \tag{7.50}$$

where $i(j)$ is the index of the last in the series of projections $p_i^h(\beta, \alpha^h, \dot{z})$, where $\dot{z} \le \dot{z}_j$; $\dot{z}_1$ is the $\dot{z}$-coordinate of the projection $p_{i(j)}^h(\beta, \alpha^h, \dot{z})$; $\dot{z}_2$ is the $\dot{z}$-coordinate of the projection $p_{i(j)+1}^h(\beta, \alpha^h, \dot{z})$.

The next step of the process is to filter the re-sampled projections $\dot{p}_j^h(\beta, \alpha^h, z_p)$. Examples of different shapes of filter are shown in Fig. 7.23 [58].

In each case, the equation defining the filtering process can be written as follows:

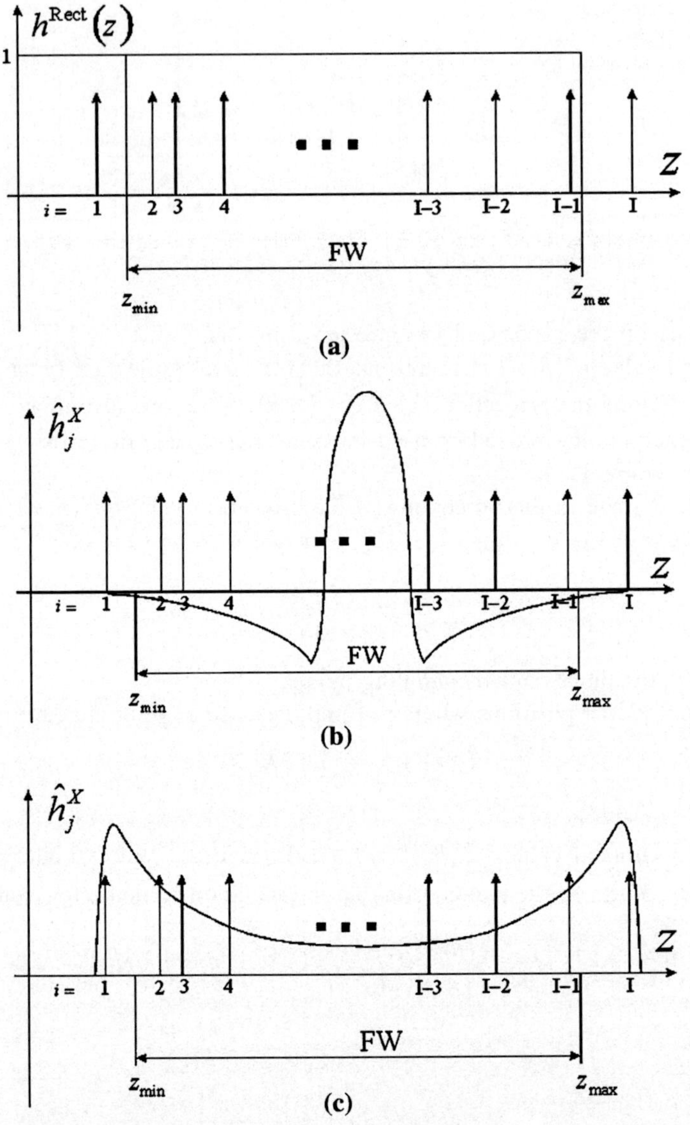

Fig. 7.23 Filter function shapes: **a** rectangular function (smoothing filter); **b** edge enhancement function; **c** modified function

$$\dot{p}^h\left(\beta, \alpha^h, z_p\right) = \frac{\sum_{j=-J}^{J} \hat{h}_j^X \cdot \dot{p}_j^h\left(\beta, \alpha^h, z_p\right)}{\sum_{j=-J}^{J} \hat{h}_j^X}, \tag{7.51}$$

where $\hat{h}_j^X$ is the discrete form of the convolving function.

Using this two-stage interpolation formula, we obtain the projection values $\dot{p}^h(\beta, \alpha^h, z_p)$, in the reconstruction plane z_p. In this way, the problem of the multi-row detector matrix system has been reduced to that of the SSCT scanner.

Use of the procedure described by Eqs. 7.10 7.12 then allows us to define the projections $p^f(\beta, \alpha^f)$ made in the hypothetical fan-beam projection system in the $z = z_p$ plane. After this operation, we can begin to reconstruct the image using a method designed for fan-beams.

7.2.4 Discrete Implementation of the z-filtering Reconstruction Method

The discrete version of the z-filtering reconstruction algorithm operates only on certain projections carried out at particular locations on the z-axis and for X-ray intensity measurements made only at particular places on the screen. The points on the screen where the measurements are made are determined by the location of the detectors on the partial drum-shaped array.

During the whole scan, the middle of the radiation beam only passes through each point on the z-axis once and as only a limited number of projections are carried out, only certain locations on the z-axis lie in the plane of the incident radiation. These places are referenced using the index $\theta = 0, \ldots, \Theta - 1$, where Θ is the number of projections made during the entire scan.

The angle at which a particular ray in the beam falls on a suitable detector will be indexed using the variable $\eta = -(\mathrm{H} - 1)/2, \ldots, 0, \ldots, (\mathrm{H} - 1)/2$, where H is an odd number of detectors in each row of the array. The number of the row in which a specific detector is situated is determined by the variable $k = 1, 2, \ldots, \mathrm{K}$, where K is the total number of rows of detectors in the array (this is usually an even number).

Therefore, we can summarise by saying that only the discrete projection values $\hat{p}^h(\eta, \theta, k)$ for $\eta = -(\mathrm{H} - 1)/2, \ldots, 0, \ldots, (\mathrm{H} - 1)/2; \theta = 0, \ldots, \Theta - 1$; $k = 1, 2, \ldots, \mathrm{K}$ are available to the reconstruction algorithm.

In order to carry out the z-filtration reconstruction process, we reduce the problem to that of a hypothetical fan-beam projection system and then use any of the methods devised for the fan-beam system to obtain an image of the slice at z_p. To do this, we need to calculate all the necessary projections $\hat{p}^f(\eta^f, \gamma); \eta^f = -(\mathrm{H} - 1)/2, \ldots, 0, \ldots, (\mathrm{H} - 1)/2; \gamma = 0, \ldots, \Gamma - 1$, where $\Gamma = \frac{2\pi}{\Delta_\alpha^f}$.

It is also important to pay attention to the relationships between the parameters of the spiral projection system and those of the fan-beam system, for rays lying in the same plane parallel to the z-axis. These relationships can be determined by the following systems of equations:

$$\theta = \begin{cases} \gamma + \theta_0 + n\pi & \text{if} \quad \gamma\Delta_\beta < \alpha_p^h + \pi - \theta_0 \\ \gamma + \theta_0 - \Gamma + n\pi & \text{if} \quad \gamma\Delta_\beta \geq \alpha_p^h + \pi - \theta_0 \end{cases} \tag{7.52}$$

and

$$\eta = \eta^f \tag{7.53}$$

for $n = 0, \pm 2, \pm 4, \pm 6, \ldots$; and for the complementary rays, i.e. those projected from the opposite side:

$$\theta = \begin{cases} \gamma + \theta_0 + n\pi - 2\eta^f & \text{if} \quad \gamma\Delta_\beta < \alpha_p^h + \pi - \theta_0 \\ \gamma + \theta_0 - \Gamma + n\pi - 2\eta^f & \text{if} \quad \gamma\Delta_\beta \geq \alpha_p^h + \pi - \theta_0 \end{cases} \tag{7.54}$$

and

$$\eta = -\eta^f \tag{7.55}$$

for $n = \pm 1, \pm 3, \pm 5, \ldots$; where in all instances θ_0 is calculated using:

$$\theta_0 = \frac{2\pi\left(\left(\alpha_p^h + \pi\right) \, div \, 2\pi\right)}{\Delta_\alpha^h}. \tag{7.56}$$

Consecutive stages in the determination of the projection values $\hat{p}^f\left(\eta^f, \gamma\right)$; $\eta^f = -(\mathrm{H}-1)/2, \ldots, 0, \ldots, (\mathrm{H}-1)/2; \gamma = 0, \ldots, \Gamma - 1$ are presented below.

Step I During the preliminary phase, when the parameters for the scan are established, the radiologist determines the position $z = z_p$ of the reconstruction plane. If the projections start at angle $\alpha_0^h = 0$, then the angle of the principal axis of the hypothetical beam, at the moment it passes through the point z_p, can be determined from Eq. 7.6. Knowing this, and parameters such as the distance d_w between the rows of detectors, the resolution Δ_α^h at which the projections are made, and λ, we can use Eqs. 7.52 7.56 to establish which of the projection values $\hat{p}^h(\eta, \theta, k)$ (the direct and the complementary projections) will cross the z-axis through the section $\left[z_p - \frac{\mathrm{FW}}{2}, z_p + \frac{\mathrm{FW}}{2}\right]$, i.e. which of them satisfy the condition:

$$z_p - \frac{\mathrm{FW}}{2} \leq \lambda\frac{\theta \cdot \Delta_\alpha^h}{2\pi} + \left(k + \frac{\mathrm{K}+1}{2}\right) \cdot \mathrm{d}_w \leq z_p + \frac{\mathrm{FW}}{2}, \tag{7.57}$$

where FW is the width of the filter; d_w is the distance between the detectors along the z-axis.

The projections satisfying these conditions are arranged in the order in which they occur along the z-axis, starting from the point $z = z_p - \frac{\mathrm{FW}}{2}$, and given an index $i = 2, 3, \ldots, \mathrm{I} - 1$. The value $\mathrm{I} - 2$ represents the number of projection values situated within the range specified by (7.57).

The projection value $\hat{p}_1^h(\eta, \theta, k)$ situated just before this range is given the index $i = 1$; the next sample to be selected is the first projection value $\hat{p}_I^h(\eta, \theta, k)$ just after the range. So the sequence of projections $\hat{p}_i^h(\eta, \theta, k)$ finally taken into account in subsequent stages of the process is indexed $i = 1, 2, 3, \ldots, \mathrm{I}$.

Step II All of the projections $\hat{p}_i^h(\eta, \theta, k); \quad i = 1, 2, 3, \ldots, I$, obtained from the first stage of the process, are filtered as follows:

$$p^f\left(\beta^f, \alpha^f\right) = \frac{\sum_{i=1}^{\mathrm{I}} \hat{p}_i^h(\eta, \theta, k) \cdot \hat{h}_i^{\mathrm{Rect}}}{\sum_{i=1}^{\mathrm{I}} \hat{h}_i^{\mathrm{Rect}}}, \tag{7.58}$$

where $\hat{h}_i^{\mathrm{Rect}}$ are the weightings for the rectangular filter.

The weighting factors $\hat{h}_i^{\mathrm{Rect}}$ are determined based on the premise that their values depend on the density of the sampled series $\hat{p}_i^h(\eta, \theta, k)$ at a given location on the z-axis. Figure 7.24 shows how the values of $\hat{h}_i^{\mathrm{Rect}}$ can be calculated for a rectangular filter, for selected index values $i = 2$; $i = \mathrm{I} - 2$; $i = \mathrm{I}$.

As we can see from Fig. 7.24, the value of the weighting factor $\hat{h}_i^{\mathrm{Rect}}$, assigned to a particular sample taken from the series $\hat{p}_i^h(\eta, \theta, k)$, is proportional to the sample's area of influence on the area defined by the rectangular filter function. This allows us to attempt an accurate calculation of the weightings $\hat{h}_i^{\mathrm{Rect}}$. The equations defining these values differ depending on the value of the index i. Determinations of the weights $\hat{h}_i^{\mathrm{Rect}}$ for the different categories of samples $\hat{p}_i^h(\eta, \theta, k)$ are shown below:

$$\hat{h}_1^{\mathrm{Rect}} = \frac{1}{\mathrm{FW}} \int_0^{z_2 - z_{\min}} \frac{\ddot{z}}{z_2 - z_1} d\ddot{z} = \frac{1}{\mathrm{FW}} \frac{(z_2 - z_{\min})^2}{2(z_2 - z_1)}, \tag{7.59}$$

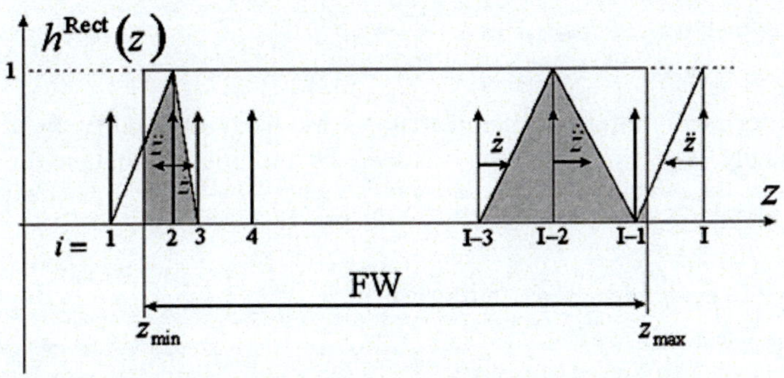

Fig. 7.24 Determining the weighting factors for a rectangular filter

$$\hat{h}_2^{\mathrm{Rect}} = \frac{1}{\mathrm{FW}}\left(\int\limits_0^{z_3\;\; z_2}\left(1-\frac{\dot{z}}{z_3-z_2}\right)d\dot{z} + \int\limits_0^{z_2\;\; z_{\min}}\left(1-\frac{\ddot{z}}{z_2-z_1}\right)d\ddot{z}\right)$$
$$= \frac{1}{\mathrm{FW}}\left(\frac{z_3-z_2}{2} + z_2 - z_{\min} - \frac{(z_2-z_{\min})^2}{2(z_2-z_1)}\right), \tag{7.60}$$

$$\hat{h}_i^{\mathrm{Rect}} = \frac{1}{\mathrm{FW}}\left(\int\limits_0^{z_i\;\; z_{i\;\;1}}\frac{\dot{z}}{z_i-z_{i\;\;1}}d\dot{z} + \int\limits_0^{z_{i+1}\;\; z_i}\left(1-\frac{\ddot{z}}{z_{i+1}-z_i}\right)d\ddot{z}\right) = \frac{1}{\mathrm{FW}}\left(\frac{z_{i+1}-z_{i\;\;1}}{2}\right), \tag{7.61}$$

for $2 < i < \mathrm{I} - 1$,

$$\hat{h}_{\mathrm{I}\;\;1}^{\mathrm{Rect}} = \frac{1}{\mathrm{FW}}\left(\int\limits_0^{z_{\max}\;\; z_{\mathrm{I}\;\;1}}\left(1-\frac{\dot{z}}{z_{\mathrm{I}}}-z_{\mathrm{I}\;\;1}\right)d\dot{z} + \int\limits_0^{z_{\mathrm{I}\;\;1}\;\; z_{\mathrm{I}\;\;2}}\left(1-\frac{\ddot{z}}{z_{\mathrm{I}\;\;1}}-z_{\mathrm{I}\;\;2}\right)dd\dot{z}\right)$$
$$= \frac{1}{\mathrm{FW}}\left(\frac{z_{\mathrm{I}\;\;1}-z_{\mathrm{I}\;\;2}}{2} + z_{\max} - z_{\mathrm{I}\;\;1} - \frac{(z_{\max}-z_{\mathrm{I}\;\;1})^2}{2(z_{\mathrm{I}}-z_{\mathrm{I}\;\;1})}\right), \tag{7.62}$$

$$\hat{h}_{\mathrm{I}}^{\mathrm{Rect}} = \frac{1}{\mathrm{FW}}\int\limits_0^{z_{\max}\;\; z_{\mathrm{I}\;\;1}}\frac{\dot{z}}{z_{\mathrm{I}}}-z_{\mathrm{I}\;\;1}d\dot{z} = \frac{1}{\mathrm{FW}}\frac{(z_{\max}-z_{\mathrm{I}\;\;1})^2}{2(z_{\mathrm{I}}-z_{\mathrm{I}\;\;1})}, \tag{7.63}$$

where z, $\dot{z}$, $\ddot{z}$ are coordinates whose ranges are indicated in Fig. 7.24; $z_{\min}$, $z_{\max}$ are, respectively, the points on the z-axis indicating the beginning and end of the area covered by the filter.

Note that the sum of all the weighting factors calculated using Eqs. 7.59 7.63 is 1, after normalisation by the filter width FW (the area determined by the shape of the filter function used). Therefore, for a rectangular filter such as that in Fig. 7.23a, Eq. 7.51 takes the form:

$$\dot{p}^f(\eta,\gamma) = \sum_{i=1} \hat{p}_i^h(\eta,\theta,k)\cdot\hat{h}_i^{\mathrm{Rect}}. \tag{7.64}$$

For a filter with different characteristics, we need to modify Eqs. 7.59 7.63 appropriately. For example, Eq. 7.61 can be modified to obtain the following equation:

$$\hat{h}_i^X = \frac{1}{\mathrm{FW}}\left(\int\limits_0^{z_i\;\; z_{i\;\;1}}\left(1-\frac{\dot{z}}{z_i-z_{i\;\;1}}\cdot\mathrm{filter}(\dot{z})\right)d\dot{z} + \int\limits_0^{z_i\;\; z_{i+1}}\left(1-\frac{\ddot{z}}{z_{i+1}-z_i}\cdot\mathrm{filter}(\ddot{z})\right)d\ddot{z}\right), \tag{7.65}$$

where filter($\dot{z}$) is the function of the filter used, such as one of those shown in Fig. 7.23b or 7.23c.

Step III Using the interpolated projection values $\dot{p}^f(\eta^f, \gamma)$ obtained from the hypothetical fan-beam projection system, we can now reconstruct the image of the slice at $z = z_p$.

A flowchart for implementing the discrete z-filtering reconstruction method is shown in Fig. 7.25.

7.3 Cone-Beam Spiral Computed Tomography—CBCT

An important factor in the design of the MSCT spiral scanner was the assumption that the individual fan-beams making up the cone-shaped beam of radiation are parallel. This assumption presented an obstacle to attempts to increase the number of rows in the detector array. With the development of *cone-beam computed tomography* (CBCT) there was a break with previous thinking, which led to a substantial increase in the width of the detector array. This in turn led to such an increase in scanning rate that it now became possible to scan organs physiologically in motion, such as the heart. Furthermore, because of the small distance between the rows of detectors it was also possible to increase the scan resolution along the z-axis significantly.

An additional advantage of the new projection geometry was the increase in the effective solid angle of the X-rays. This vastly improved the efficiency of the scanner in regard to the amount of information obtained from the radiation energy used. It reduced the amount of energy lost in the tube, which allowed the tube current to be increased, thereby reducing the level of noise in the reconstructed image.

Increasing the width of the detector array and the consequent departure from the assumption of parallel fan-beams made it necessary to develop new reconstruction algorithms that were specially designed for systems with a conical beam of radiation. Theoretical studies [36, 63] led to the conclusion that it was indeed possible to reconstruct the image using three-dimensional projections recorded by a two-dimensional detector array. A sufficient condition for the exact reconstruction of the radiation attenuation coefficient at a point in three-dimensional space from a conical projection is the existence of at least one cone-shaped source of radiation in each plane that contains the point [16, 55, 64]. This statement led to the development of a whole series of reconstruction algorithms, of which the best known are: *exact cone-beam reconstructions* based on Smith's theory [56, 71, 74], the Grangeat approach [10, 25, 37, 41, 45, 60] and the method developed by Tuy [75].

Practical medical scanners suffer from a number of technical problems, however. For example, some positions of the radiation source (the X-ray tube) are not physically possible (the problem of longitudinal irradiation of the patient's body)

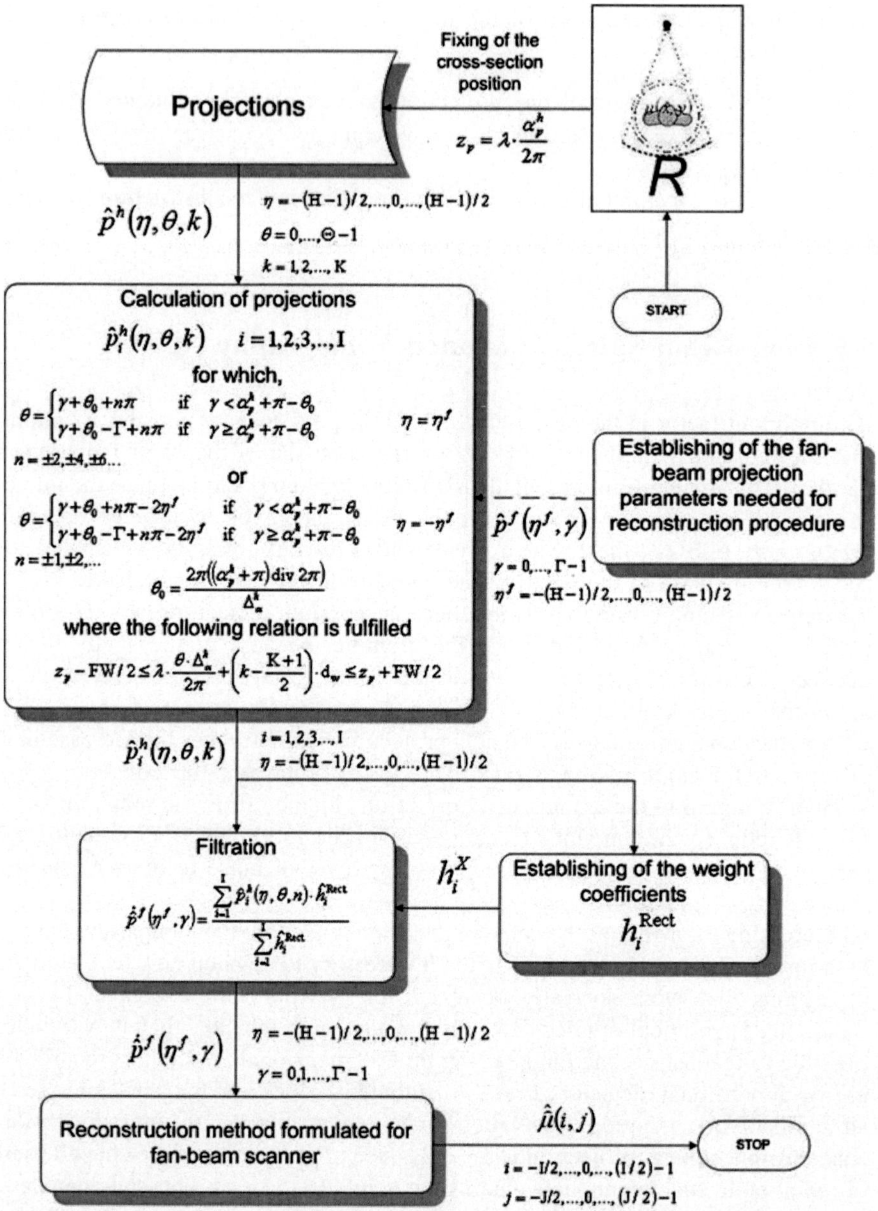

Fig. 7.25 A flowchart of the z filtering algorithm used for the MSCT scanner

and the whole body cannot be included in a simultaneous measurement of radiation intensity (the detector array has finite size). This made it necessary to develop algorithms that take these circumstances into consideration. A range of algorithms has been developed for *longitudinally truncated data* to take account of the finite number of projections of an object of theoretically infinite length (the so-called *long object*): the *local region-of-interest* (L-ROI or Local-ROI) method [50, 51, 59], *zero-boundary* (ZB) algorithms [11] and the *virtual circle* (VC) approach [38, 39].

Other approaches were also developed, which assumed an approximate solution to the problem of reconstruction from conical projections. This type of algorithm, known in the literature as *approximate cone-beam reconstruction*, includes methods such as the *PI method* (n PI) [8, 9, 48, 61, 62], *single slice reconstruction* (SSR) [46], *multi-row Fourier reconstruction* (MFR) [4, 5, 49], *adaptive multiple plane reconstruction* (AMPR) [53], *nutating slice reconstruction* (NSR) [40], *general surface reconstruction* (GSR) [6] and others [73]. These methods have a shorter calculation time than exact algorithms, as well as less noise and lower distortion in the reconstructed image.

The rest of this chapter describes two practical approximate cone-beam reconstruction methods for spiral projection systems. These are included due to their usefulness in medical applications and their commercial importance. They are the *Feldkamp algorithm* [13] and the reconstruction procedure described in the literature by its abbreviation ASSR [29 31] (*advanced single slice rebinning*).

7.3.1 The Geometry of the Cone-Beam Scanner

A diagram of the cone-beam scanner, together with key trigonometric relationships, is shown in Figs. 7.26 and 7.27 [29, 49, 68].

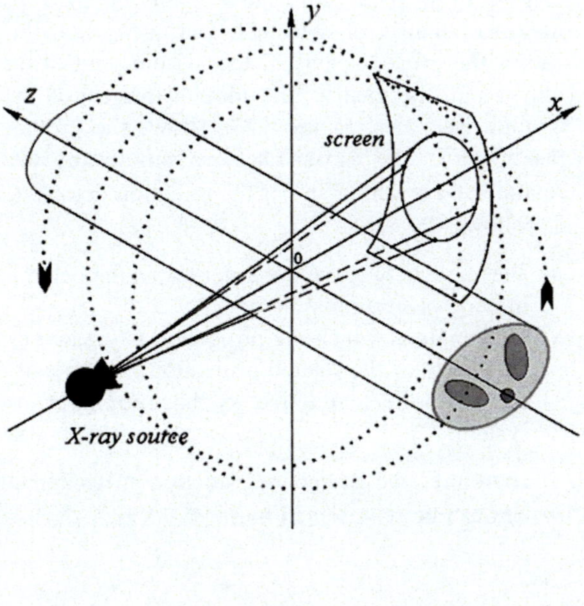

Fig. 7.26 The projection system of a cone beam scanner a three dimensional perspective view

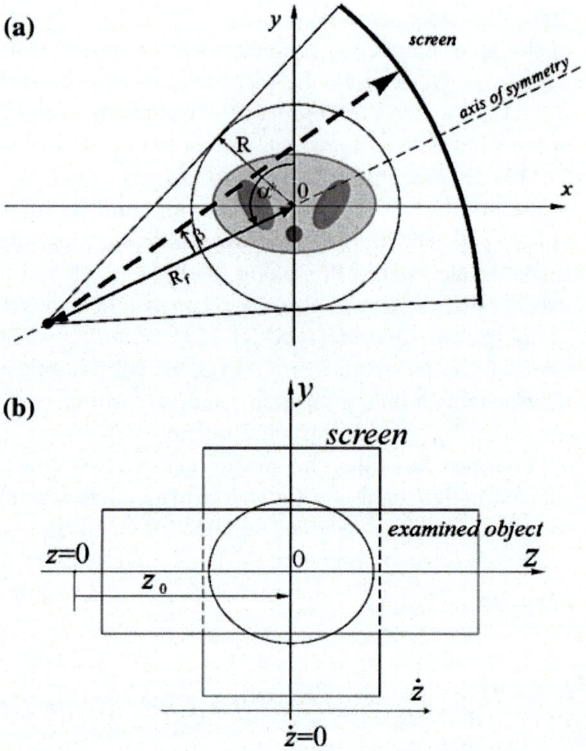

Fig. 7.27 The projection system of a cone beam scanner: **a** the geometry of the cone beam projection system in a plane perpendicular to the axis of rotation; **b** the location of the test object in the plane along the axis of rotation of the projection system

A three-dimensional view of the scanner is given in Fig. 7.26. The system consists of an X-ray tube and a rigidly coupled, partial cylindrical screen with a multi-row matrix of detectors. During a scan, this assembly rotates around the z-axis, the principal axis of the system, and at the same time, the patient table moves into the gantry. The moving projection system thus traces a spiral path around the z-axis. Figure 7.27a shows the projection geometry in a plane perpendicular to the z-axis. Each ray emitted by the tube at a particular angle of rotation and reaching any of the radiation detectors can be identified by $(\beta, \alpha^h, \dot{z})$, as follows:

β the angle between a particular ray in the beam and the axis of symmetry of the moving projection system;

α^h the angle at which the projection is made, i.e. the angle between the axis of symmetry of the rotated projection system and the y-axis;

$\dot{z}$ the z-coordinate relative to the current position of the moving projection system.

Therefore, the projection function measured at the screen in a cone-beam system can be represented by $p^h(\beta, \alpha^h, \dot{z})$.

The angle α^h at which the projections are made is determined by the double inequality $0 \leq \alpha^h \leq 2\pi \cdot number\_of\_rotations$, whilst the value of the angle β is within the range $[-\beta_{max}, \beta_{max}]$, where

$$\beta_{max} = \arcsin\left(\frac{R}{R_f}\right), \tag{7.66}$$

where R is the radius of the circle defining the space in which the scan is carried out; R_f is the radius of the circle described by the focus of the tube.

Unlike β, which is an angle, $\dot{z}$ represents a distance on the screen. It is the distance between the point where a ray strikes the screen and the vertical plane of symmetry of the projection system. For convenience, this distance is usually calculated relative to the z-axis, as shown in Fig. 7.28.

Assuming that the tube rotating around the test object starts at a projection angle $\alpha^h = 0$, the vertical plane of symmetry of the projection system (and the focus of the tube) moves along the z-axis and its current location along the axis is defined by the relationship:

$$z_0 = \lambda \cdot \frac{\alpha^h}{2\pi}, \tag{7.67}$$

where λ is the relative travel of the spiral described by the tube around the test object, measured in $\left[\frac{m}{rad}\right]$.

As with MSCT scanners, one of the basic parameters for a particular scan is the $pitch_d$ value. This is defined in Eq. 7.46 and illustrated in Fig. 7.19, but is also applicable to cone-beam tomography.

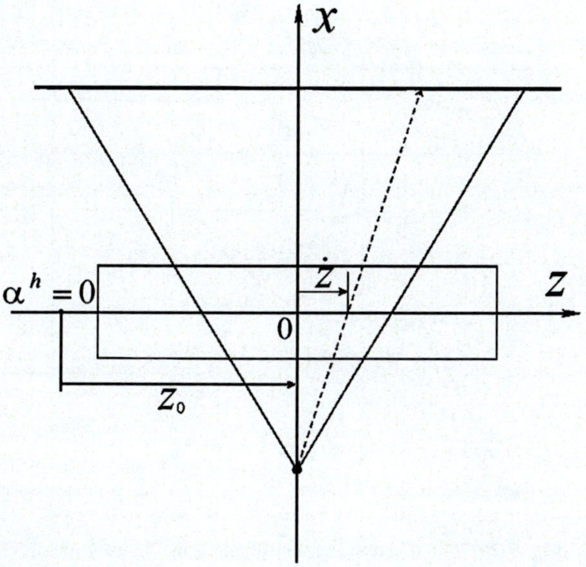

Fig. 7.28 The geometry of the scanner in the x z plane

The array of detectors on the cylindrical screen is designed to measure the intensity of the cone of X-rays. The detectors in the array are arranged in mutually perpendicular rows and columns, the rows partially encircling the z-axis. Further details of the design of the detector array will be given during discussion of the discrete version of the projection system, which is used in practice.

7.3.2 *The Geometry of the Discrete Cone-Beam Scanner*

The cone-beam projection system found application in spiral scanners. When designing this generation of device the discrete nature of the projections had to be taken into account. The stages of the discretisation process are the subject of the following discussion.

A method of measuring the X-ray intensity in a practical cone-beam scanner is shown in Fig. 7.29.

The acquisition of the projection values $p^h(\beta, \alpha^h, \dot{z})$ only takes place at specific angles of rotation α^h:

$$\alpha_\theta^h = \theta \cdot \Delta_\alpha^h, \tag{7.68}$$

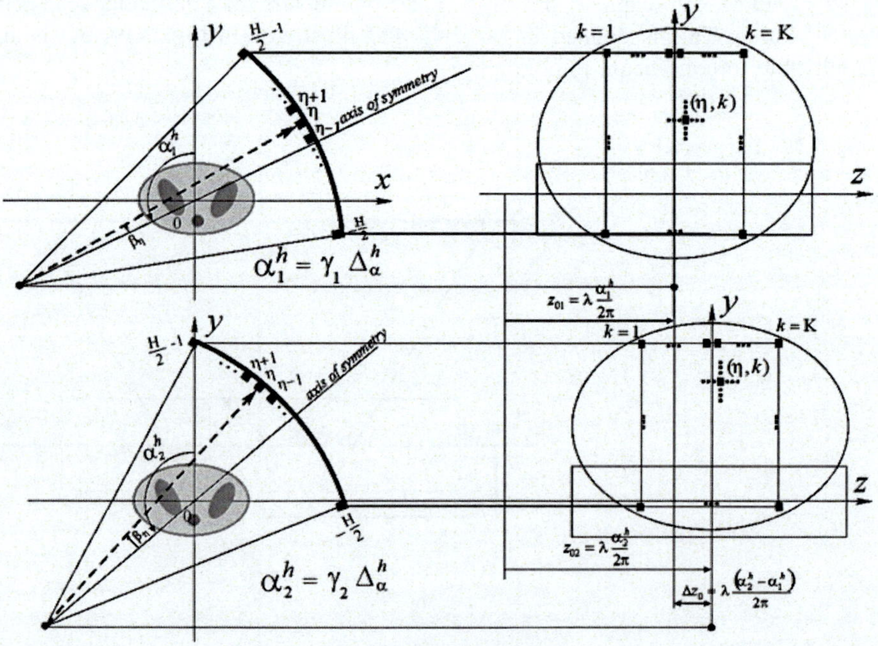

Fig. 7.29 The discrete version of the cone beam scanner

where $\Delta_{\alpha}^{h} = \frac{2\pi}{\Theta^{2\pi}}$ is the angle through which the tube-screen system is rotated following each projection; $\Theta^{2\pi}$ is the number of projections made during one full rotation of the projection system; $\theta = 0, \ldots, \Theta - 1$ is the global projection index; $\Theta = number\_of\_rotations \cdot \Theta^{2\pi}$ is the total number of projections.

The position of a detector in the matrix is determined by the pair (η, k), where $\eta = -(\mathrm{H}-1)/2, \ldots, 0, \ldots, (\mathrm{H}-1)/2$ is the number of the detector (channel) and $k = 1, 2, \ldots, \mathrm{K}$ is the number of the column (row). H and K denote the total number of detectors in the columns and the total number of columns, respectively. It is helpful to assume that the useful rays striking the detectors in the individual columns are distributed evenly, i.e. $\Delta_{\beta} = \text{const}$, and that the individual channels are equidistant from each other on the screen, i.e. $\Delta_{z}^{h} = \text{const}$. These assumptions make it easy to locate the detectors in the array on the surface of the partial cylinder, as shown in Fig. 7.30.

In practice, given this design of detector array, we obtain the projection values $p^{h}(\beta, \alpha^{h}, \dot{z})$ only at certain angles β, determined by:

$$\beta_{\eta} = \eta \cdot \Delta_{\beta}^{f}, \tag{7.69}$$

where Δ_{β}^{f} is the angular distance between the radiation detectors on the cylindrical screen.

As shown in Fig. 7.31, the angles between the individual rays, incident on the screen, vary. This means that the relative distances between the individual detectors in the z-direction also vary. However, if we assume that the number of columns is within reasonable limits, the distance between the detectors relative to the z-axis is [49]:

$$\dot{\Delta}_{z}^{h} \cong \Delta_{z}^{h} \cdot \frac{\mathrm{R}_{f}}{\mathrm{R}_{f} + \mathrm{R}_{d}}. \tag{7.70}$$

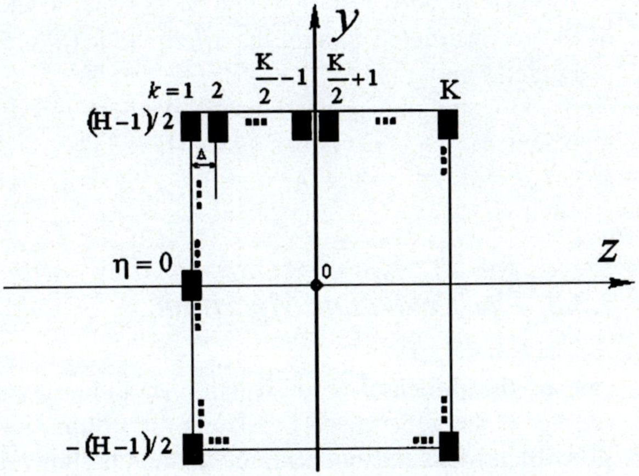

Fig. 7.30 The topology of the detectors on the screen of a multi row spiral scanner

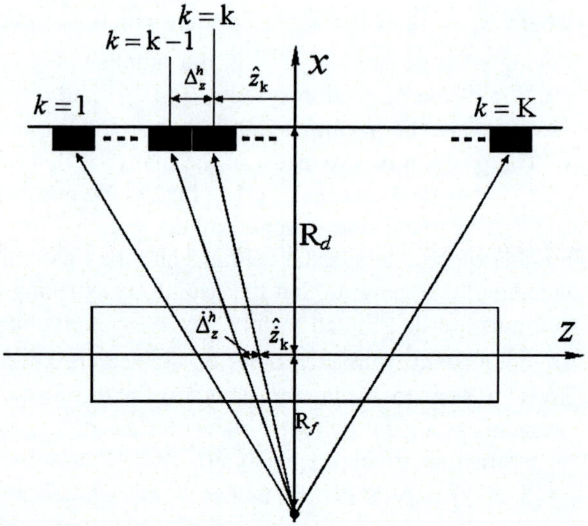

Fig. 7.31 Determining distances on the screen relative to the z axis

The further the detectors are from the y-axis, the smaller the intervals between the detectors become, relative to the z-axis. If necessary, we can compensate for this effect, during design, by increasing the size of those detectors that are more distant from the vertical plane of symmetry of the screen [29].

Using Eq. 7.70, we can calculate the distance of each detector from the x-y plane, measured along the z-axis:

$$\hat{\dot{z}}_k = \hat{z}_k \cdot \frac{\mathrm{R}_f}{\mathrm{R}_f + \mathrm{R}_d} \cong \left(k - \frac{\mathrm{K}+1}{2}\right) \cdot \Delta_z^h \cdot \frac{\mathrm{R}_f}{\mathrm{R}_f + \mathrm{R}_d}, \tag{7.71}$$

where R_f is the distance from the focus of the X-ray tube to the principal axis of the projection system; R_d is the smallest distance from the partial cylinder on which the detector matrix is placed to the principal axis of the projection system.

It is also important to note that $\dot{\Delta}_z^h$ is equal to the thickness of the cross-section of the reconstructed image, the *slice width* (SW), one of the key parameters in computed tomography.

In summary, the projections obtained in the discrete cone-beam scanner are represented by $\hat{p}(\eta, \theta, k); \eta = -(\mathrm{H}-1)/2, \ldots, 0, \ldots, (\mathrm{H}-1)/2; \quad \theta = 0, \ldots, \Theta - 1; k = 1, 2, \ldots, \mathrm{K}$.

7.3.3 The Feldkamp Algorithm

One of the principal reconstruction methods devised for the cone-beam spiral scanner is the generalised Feldkamp algorithm [13, 69]. A diagram of the reconstruction process for this heuristic method is shown in Fig. 7.32. The algorithm is a

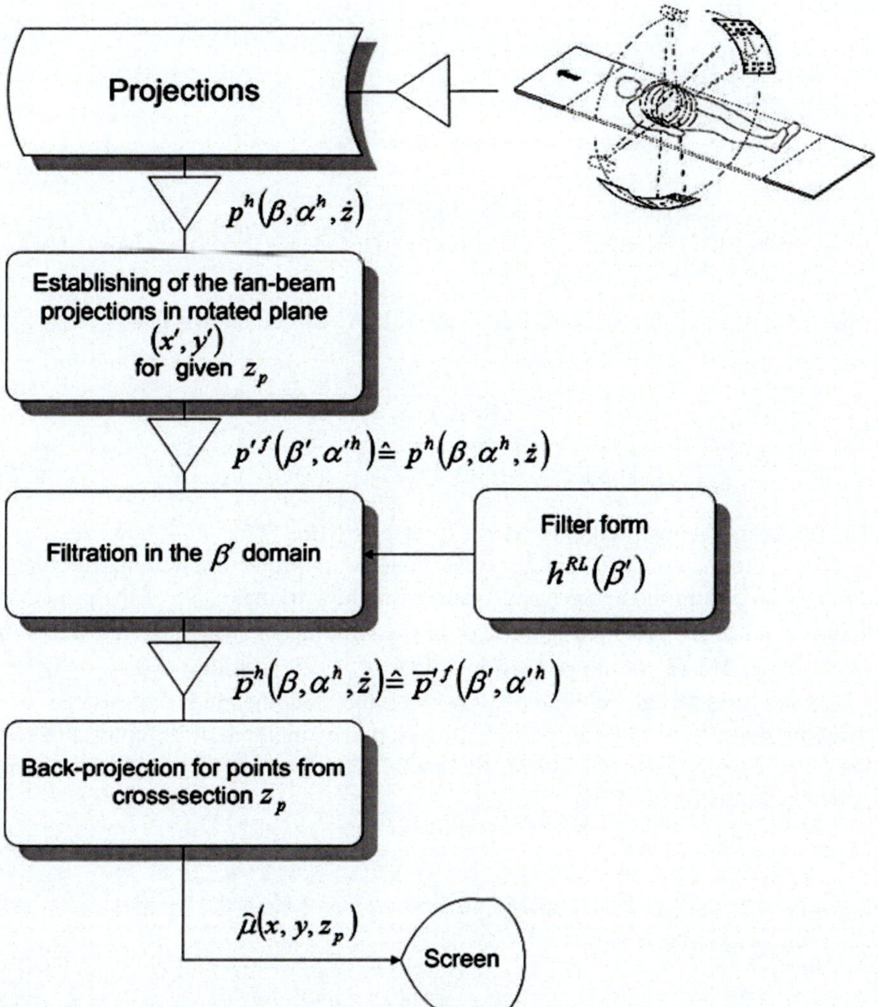

Fig. 7.32 A flowchart for the Feldkamp algorithm

development of a conventional fan-beam reconstruction approach. The fan-beam projections are filtered in two dimensions and then back-projected in three dimensions. A number of modifications to this algorithm have also been developed, such as *extended parallel back-projection* (EPBP) [28, 32] and others [17, 18, 68, 70].

Before discussing the two-dimensional filtration phase of the Feldkamp algorithm, it is worth first returning to the implementation of the direct fan-beam reconstruction method considered in Chap. 6. Accordingly, we can write a set of equations describing this reconstruction method for the Ram-Lak filter [33, 42]:

$$\breve{\mu}(x,y) = \frac{R_f}{2} \cdot \int_0^{2\pi} p^f\left(\dot{\beta}, \alpha^f\right) \mathrm{d}\alpha^f, \tag{7.72}$$

where

$$p^f\left(\dot{\beta}, \alpha^f\right) = \frac{1}{\dot{u}^2} \cdot \int_{\beta_{\min}}^{\beta_{\max}} p^f\left(\dot{\beta}, \alpha^f\right) \cdot \cos \dot{\beta}^{\mathrm{RL}}\left(\beta - \dot{\beta}\right) \mathrm{d}\dot{\beta}, \tag{7.73}$$

where, by using Table 4.3 and Eqs. 7.22 7.23, it can be shown that:

$$\dot{\beta} = \arctan\left(\frac{x \cos \alpha^f + y \sin \alpha^f}{R_f + x \sin \alpha^f - y \cos \alpha^f}\right), \tag{7.74}$$

$$\dot{u}^2 = \left(x \cos \alpha^f + y \sin \alpha^f\right)^2 + \left(R_f + x \sin \alpha^f - y \cos \alpha^f\right)^2. \tag{7.75}$$

The fan-beam reconstruction method expressed by Eqs. 7.72 7.75, however, has to be adapted to the conditions of the spiral cone-beam projection system. In order to do this, the first problem we have to address is how to make use of the projection values $p^h\left(\beta, \alpha^h, \dot{z}\right)$ obtained from rays in the cone-beam, which do not lie in the (x, y) plane. Those are the projection values $p^h\left(\beta, \alpha^h, \dot{z}\right)$ with $\dot{z} \neq 0$.

In the generalised Feldkamp algorithm, the cone-beam is considered as a combination of multiple fan-beams lying in planes inclined at different angles to the central plane perpendicular to the z-axis. The location of one of these components is illustrated in Fig. 7.33.

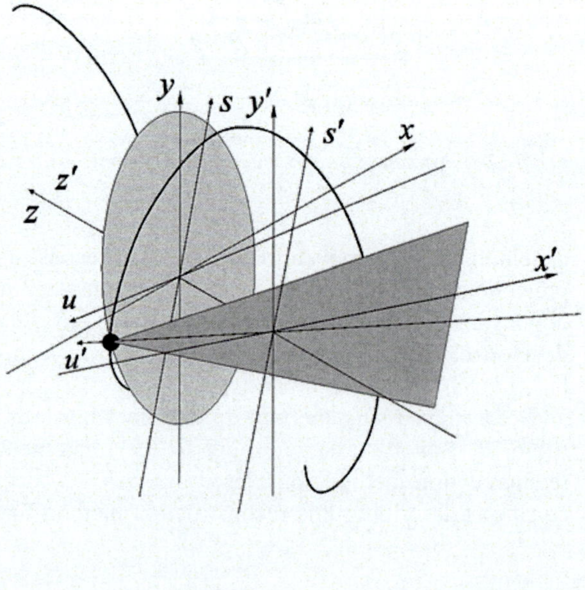

Fig. 7.33 The position of one of the components of the cone beam

If we consider this component to be lying in the plane of a new coordinate system (x', y'), then the reconstruction algorithm given by Eqs. 7.72 7.75 for the slice in this plane can be expressed as follows:

$$\breve{\mu}(x', y') = \frac{R'_f}{2} \cdot \int_0^{2\pi} p'^h\left(\dot{\beta}', \alpha'^h\right) d\alpha'^h, \tag{7.76}$$

$$p'^f\left(\dot{\beta}', \alpha'^h\right) = \frac{1}{\dot{u}'^2} \cdot \int_{\beta_{min}}^{\beta_{max}} p'^f\left(\beta', \alpha'^h\right) \cdot \cos\dot{\beta}' \cdot h^{RL}\left(\beta' - \dot{\beta}'\right) d\dot{\beta}', \tag{7.77}$$

$$\dot{\beta}' = \arctan\left(\frac{x\cos\alpha'^h + y\sin\alpha'^h}{R_f + x\sin\alpha'^h - y\cos\alpha'^h}\right), \tag{7.78}$$

$$\dot{u}'^2 = \left(x\cos\alpha'^h + y\sin\alpha'^h\right)^2 + \left(R'_f + x\sin\alpha'^h - y\cos\alpha'^h\right)^2. \tag{7.79}$$

The contribution that the filtered projection $p'^f(\beta', \alpha'^h)$ makes to the value assigned to the voxel $\breve{\mu}(x, y, z)$ of the reconstructed image is determined by the relationship:

$$d\breve{\mu}(x, y, z) = \frac{R'_f}{2 \cdot \dot{u}'^2} \cdot \int_{\beta_{min}}^{\beta_{max}} p\left(\dot{\beta}', \alpha'^h\right) \cdot \cos\dot{\beta}' \cdot h\left(\dot{\beta}' - \beta'\right) d\dot{\beta}' d\alpha'^h. \tag{7.80}$$

In the next step, we have to consider the filtered projection values $p'^f(\beta', \alpha'^h)$ in terms of the coordinate system of planes parallel to the central plane. We do this by bearing in mind the simple geometric relationships between the angles measured on the central plane and the angles describing the planes inclined to it, i.e.:

$$\beta' = \beta \tag{7.81}$$

and

$$\alpha'^h = \alpha^h. \tag{7.82}$$

The coordinates of a point in the rotated coordinate system (x', y') projected onto a similarly rotated system in the (x, y) plane can also be determined, using the following relationships:

$$s' = s \tag{7.83}$$

and

$$\frac{u'}{R'_f} = \frac{u}{R_f}. \tag{7.84}$$

Note also that the distance between the radiation source and the principal axis of the projection system, measured on the (x', y') plane, is:

$$\left(\mathrm{R}'_f\right)^2 = (\mathrm{R}_f)^2 + \dot{z}^2. \tag{7.85}$$

It is also worth noting that in both the (x, y) and the (x', y') coordinate systems, the linear velocity of the radiation source rotating around the principal axis of the projection system is a constant:

$$\varpi_{\text{Focus}} \cdot \mathrm{R}_f = \varpi'_{\text{Focus}} \cdot \mathrm{R}'_f. \tag{7.86}$$

Using the definition of angular velocity $\varpi_{\text{Focus}} = \frac{d\alpha^h}{dt}$, we can easily obtain the relationship between the angular increments $d\alpha^h$ in both systems:

$$d\alpha^h \cdot \mathrm{R}_f = d\alpha^{h\prime} \cdot \mathrm{R}'_f, \tag{7.87}$$

which, after combining with Eq. 7.85, gives us the following relationship:

$$d\alpha^{h\prime} = \frac{d\alpha^h \cdot \mathrm{R}_f}{\sqrt{\mathrm{R}_f^2 + \dot{z}^2}}. \tag{7.88}$$

Using Eqs. 7.81 7.84 and 7.88, Eq. 7.80 can be converted to the following form:

$$d\breve{\mu}(x, y, z) = \frac{\mathrm{R}_f}{2 \cdot \dot{u}^2} \cdot \int_{\beta_{\max}}^{\beta_{\max}} p^h\left(\dot{\beta}, \alpha^h, \dot{z}\right) \cdot \cos\dot{\beta} \cdot h^{RL}\left(\beta - \dot{\beta}\right) d\dot{\beta} d\alpha^h, \tag{7.89}$$

where

$$\dot{\beta} = \arctan\left(\frac{x\cos\alpha^h + y\sin\alpha^h}{\mathrm{R}_f + x\sin\alpha^h - y\cos\alpha^h}\right), \tag{7.90}$$

$$\dot{u}^2 = \left(x\cos\alpha^h + y\sin\alpha^h\right)^2 + \left(\mathrm{R}_f + x\sin\alpha^h - y\cos\alpha^h\right)^2 + (z_0 - z_p)^2. \tag{7.91}$$

We can now carry out the three-dimensional back-projection by integrating both sides of Eq. 7.89 with respect to the angle of rotation of the projection system α^h. The image reconstruction method for a slice at a distance z_p from the point $z = 0$ can thus be illustrated by the equation:

$$\breve{\mu}(x, y, z_p) = \frac{\mathrm{R}_f}{2} \int_{\alpha_p^h \ \pi}^{\alpha_p^h + \pi} \frac{1}{\dot{u}^2} \cdot \int_{\beta_{\max}}^{\beta_{\max}} p^h\left(\dot{\beta}, \alpha^h, \dot{z}\right) \cdot \cos\dot{\beta} \cdot h^{RL}\left(\beta - \dot{\beta}\right) d\dot{\beta} d\alpha^h, \tag{7.92}$$

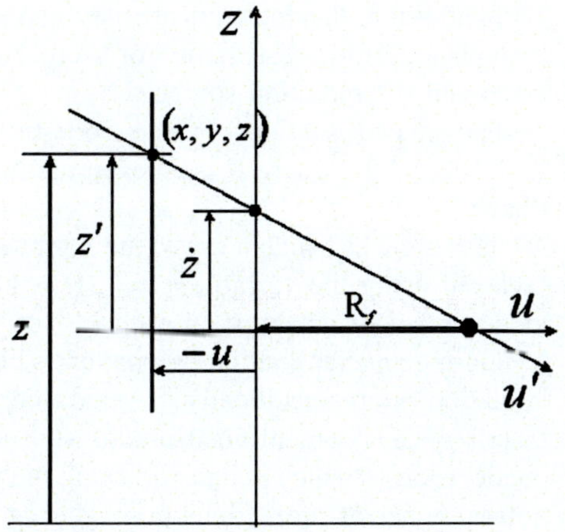

Fig. 7.34 A method of determining $\dot{z}$

where

$$\alpha_p^h = \frac{2\pi \cdot z_p}{\lambda}. \tag{7.93}$$

The final problem to be solved is the determination of the value of $\dot{z}$. This variable represents the inclination of the fan with respect to the perpendicular plane of symmetry of the projection system, measured along the z-axis. A method of determining this value is shown in Fig. 7.34.

The value of $\dot{z}$ is calculated by simply using the relationship:

$$\dot{z} = \frac{\mathrm{R}_f \cdot z'}{\mathrm{R}_f - u}, \tag{7.94}$$

where z' is the equivalent to the z-coordinate but in the local coordinate system (x, y, z') and is found using the simple relationship:

$$z' = \lambda \cdot \frac{\alpha^h}{2\pi} - z_p. \tag{7.95}$$

The quantities $\dot{\beta}$ and $\dot{u}^2$ are calculated using Eqs. 7.90 and 7.91.

When the scanner gantry is tilted, as is often to the case when scanning the head, the basic Feldkamp algorithm has to be modified. Descriptions of practical solutions to this algorithmic problem can be found in the articles [1, 19, 20, 57, 72].

7.3.4 Discrete Implementation of the Feldkamp Algorithm

In the cone-beam spiral scanner, the reconstruction algorithm only makes use of projections obtained at particular angles and measured only at particular points on the partial drum-shaped screen.

In addition, the detectors are assumed to be arranged on the screen in a way that ensures a uniform distribution of useful rays in the planes that contain the detector rows and the radiation source.

Fan-shaped sections of the cone-beam strike individual rows of detectors $k = 1, 2, \ldots, \mathrm{K}$, where K is an even number of rows. Each row has an identical arc shape.

The angle at which a ray of the fan-beam strikes a detector in a particular row is indexed using the variable $\eta = -(\mathrm{H}-1)/2, \ldots, 0, \ldots, (\mathrm{H}-1)/2$, where H is an odd number of detectors in each row of the array.

During an examination of a patient's body using spiral tomography, the beam of radiation (more specifically its middle) only passes through a specific point on the z-axis once. As mentioned previously, only a limited number of projections are made, each of which is indexed using the variable $\theta = 0, \ldots, \Theta - 1$ where Θ is the total number of projections made during the scan.

Therefore, the reconstruction algorithm only makes use of the projection values $\hat{p}^h(\eta, \theta, k); \eta = -(\mathrm{H}-1)/2, \ldots, 0, \ldots, (\mathrm{H}-1)/2; \theta = 0, \ldots, \Theta - 1; k = 1, 2, \ldots, \mathrm{K}$.

When setting the parameters for an examination, the positions on the z-axis, where the cross-sections are to be reconstructed, are established. We will concentrate on one of these, located at z_p. If the first projection takes place at an angle $\alpha^h{}_0 = 0$, the angle at which the middle of the cone-beam passes through the point $z = z_p$ is determined by Eq. 7.93.

Considering these factors, we can proceed with the reconstruction procedure as expressed entirely by Eq. 7.92.

Step I In this stage of the process, all of the projection values $\hat{p}^h(\eta, \theta, k)$; $\eta = -(\mathrm{H}-1)/2, \ldots, 0, \ldots, (\mathrm{H}-1)/2; \theta = 0, \ldots, \Theta - 1; k = 1, 2, \ldots, \mathrm{K}$, are subjected to geometric correction, using the relationship:

$$\hat{p}^h_{corr}(\eta, \theta, k) = \hat{p}^h(\eta, \theta, k) \cdot \cos(\eta \Delta_\beta). \tag{7.96}$$

Step II All of the fan-beam projections $\hat{p}^h_{\mathrm{corr}}(\eta, \theta, k); \theta = 0, \ldots, \Theta - 1$; $k = 1, 2, \ldots, \mathrm{K}$ can then be processed directly using a Ram-Lak filter, as explained in Chap. 6:

$$\hat{p}^h(\eta, \theta, k) = \Delta_\beta \cdot \sum_{\dot{\eta}=\ (\mathrm{H}\ \ 1)/2}^{(\mathrm{H}\ \ 1)/2} \hat{p}^h_{\mathrm{corr}}(\dot{\eta}, \theta, k) \cdot \hat{h}^{\mathrm{RL}}((\eta - \dot{\eta}) \cdot \Delta_\beta). \tag{7.97}$$

Step III Often there is no ray that actually passes exactly through a particular discrete point in space, or voxel, (i, j, n) and so there is no projection value available to the reconstruction algorithm. This means that the missing projection value has to be interpolated based on adjacent filtered measurements $\hat{p}^h(\eta, \theta, k)$, using a technique such as bilinear interpolation:

$$\hat{p}^h(\beta_{ij}(\theta), \theta, \dot{z}_{ijn}(\theta))$$

$$= \left(k^{\uparrow} - \frac{\dot{z}_{ijn}}{\dot{\Delta}_z^h}\right) \cdot \left(\left(\eta^{\uparrow} - \frac{\beta_{ij}}{\Delta_\beta}\right) \cdot \hat{p}^h(\eta^{\downarrow}, \theta, k^{\downarrow}) + \left(\frac{\beta_{ij}}{\Delta_\beta} - \eta^{\downarrow}\right) \cdot \hat{p}^h(\eta^{\uparrow}, \theta, k^{\downarrow})\right)$$

$$+ \left(\frac{\dot{z}_{ijn}}{\dot{\Delta}_z^h} - k^{\downarrow}\right) \cdot \left(\left(\eta^{\uparrow} - \frac{\beta_{ij}}{\Delta_\beta}\right) \cdot \hat{p}^h(\eta^{\downarrow}, \theta, k^{\uparrow}) + \left(\frac{\beta_{ij}}{\Delta_\beta} - \eta^{\downarrow}\right) \cdot \hat{p}^h(\eta^{\uparrow}, \theta, k^{\uparrow})\right). \tag{7.98}$$

The quantities β_{ij} and $\dot{z}_{ijn}$ represent the coordinates of the discrete point (i, j, n) expressed as parameters of the projection carried out at the angle θ.

The geometric relationships in Fig. 7.35 can be used to find the value of $\dot{z}_{ijn}$. Using the diagram below, it can easily be shown that $\dot{z}_{ijn}$ is calculated as follows:

$$\dot{z}_{ijn}(\theta) = \frac{R_f \cdot (z_0 - z_p)}{R_f - u_{ij}} \tag{7.99}$$

where

$$z_0 = \lambda \cdot \frac{\theta \cdot \Delta_\alpha^h}{2\pi} \tag{7.100}$$

and

$$u_{ij} = -i\Delta_{xy} \cdot \sin(\theta \cdot \Delta_\alpha^h) + j\Delta_{xy} \cdot \cos(\theta \cdot \Delta_\alpha^h), \tag{7.101}$$

where Δ_{xy} is the interval between individual points on the reconstructed image; Δ_z is the interval between the reconstructed slices.

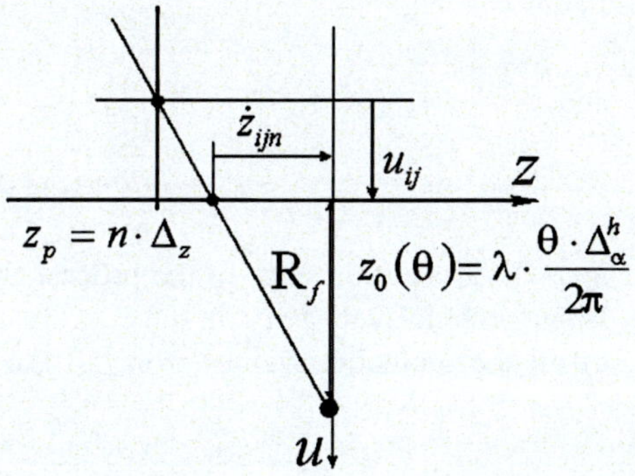

Fig. 7.35 Geometric relationships used in the determination of $\dot{z}_{ijn}$

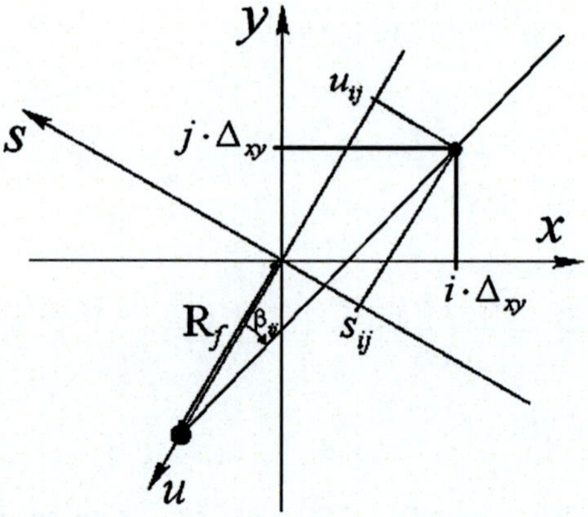

Fig. 7.36 Geometric relationships used in the determination of β_{ij}

The value of β_{ij} for the image point (i, j) in any slice at an angle of rotation α_0^h of the cone-beam projection system can be determined using Fig. 7.36.

The value of β_{ij} is easily determined from the formula for the sine of the angle indicated in the right-angled triangle in Fig. 7.36:

$$\beta_{ij}(\theta) = \arcsin\left(\frac{s_{ij}}{R_f - u_{ij}}\right), \tag{7.102}$$

where

$$s_{ij} = i\Delta_{xy} \cdot \cos\left(\theta\Delta_\alpha^h\right) + j\Delta_{xy} \cdot \sin\left(\theta\Delta_\alpha^h\right), \tag{7.103}$$

and u_{ij} has already been determined in Eq. 7.101.

To obtain the final form of Eq. 7.98 we only have to determine the four projection values $\hat{p}^h\left(\eta^\downarrow, \theta, k^\downarrow\right)$, $\hat{p}^h\left(\eta^\uparrow, \theta, k^\downarrow\right)$, $\hat{p}^h\left(\eta^\downarrow, \theta, k^\uparrow\right)$, $\hat{p}^h\left(\eta^\uparrow, \theta, k^\uparrow\right)$ taking part in the bilinear interpolation. Their indices are defined as follows:

$$k^\downarrow = Trunc\left(\dot{z}_{ij}, \dot{\Delta}_z\right), k^\uparrow = k^\downarrow + 1, \tag{7.104}$$

and

$$\eta^\downarrow = Trunc\left(\beta_{ij}, \Delta_\beta\right), \eta^\uparrow = \eta^\downarrow + 1. \tag{7.105}$$

Step IV It is at this stage of the process that the three-dimensional back-projection is performed. Every point in the coordinate space is given a value equal to the sum of all the projection values from all the rays passing through the point. For the projections $\hat{\dot{p}}^h(\beta_{ij}, \theta, \dot{z}_{ijn})$ made at angle θ; $\theta = 0, \ldots, \Theta - 1$, the operation can be written:

$$\hat{\mu}(i, j, z_p) \cong \frac{R_f}{2} \Delta_\alpha^h \cdot \sum_\theta \frac{1}{u_{ijn}^2} \cdot \hat{\dot{p}}(\beta_{ij}, \theta, \dot{z}_{ijn}), \tag{7.106}$$

where, from Fig. 7.35, we can show that:

$$u_{ijn}^2 = s_{ij}^2 + (R_f - u_{ij})^2 + (z_0 - z_p)^2, \tag{7.107}$$

where u_{ij} is calculated from Eq. 7.101.

A flowchart of the discrete version of the Feldkamp algorithm is given in Fig. 7.37.

7.3.5 The Advanced Single-Slice Rebinning Algorithm—ASSR

The *advanced single-slice rebinning algorithm* (ASSR) is one of the more complex reconstruction methods [4, 5, 29 31]. It is a development of a technique known as *single-slice rebinning* [46]. The premise behind the operation of ASSR is that image distortion can be reduced by adjusting the position of the imaged slice to match the spiral path of the X-ray tube. This involves calculating the appropriate angle of inclination of the plane with respect to the z-axis. The size of the angle depends on the position at which the reconstruction is performed. This algorithm, unlike the similar solutions described in [21, 40], uses a rebinning strategy.

By analysing the components of the motion of the projection system shown in Fig. 7.27, we can represent the spiral path of the moving tube using the following relationship:

$$\mathbf{focus}(\alpha^h) = \begin{bmatrix} x(\alpha^h) \\ y(\alpha^h) \\ z(\alpha^h) \end{bmatrix} = \begin{bmatrix} -R_f \cdot \sin \alpha^h \\ R_f \cdot \cos \alpha^h \\ \lambda \frac{\alpha^h}{2\pi} \end{bmatrix}. \tag{7.108}$$

On the other hand, any point on the partial cylindrical screen is related to the (x, y, z) coordinate system by the following vector equation:

$$\begin{aligned} \mathbf{screen}(\beta, \alpha^h, \dot{z}) &= \begin{bmatrix} x \\ y \\ z \end{bmatrix} \\ &= \begin{bmatrix} -R_f \cdot \sin \alpha^h \\ R_f \cdot \cos \alpha^h \\ \lambda \frac{\alpha^h}{2\pi} \end{bmatrix} + (R_f + R_d) \cdot \begin{bmatrix} \sin(\alpha^h + \beta) \\ -\cos(\alpha^h + \beta) \\ 0 \end{bmatrix} + \dot{z} \cdot \begin{bmatrix} 1 \\ 0 \\ 0 \end{bmatrix}. \end{aligned} \tag{7.109}$$

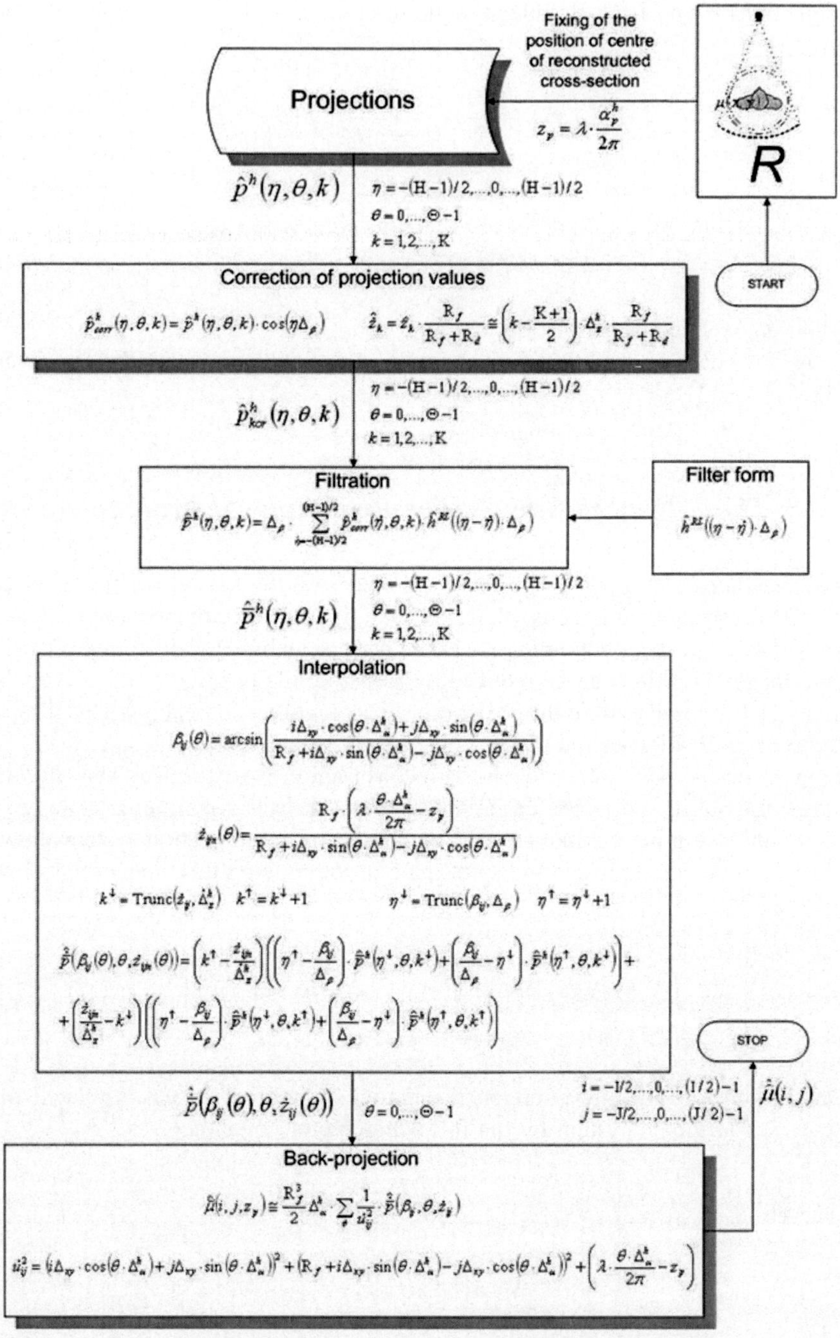

Fig. 7.37 A flowchart of the Feldkamp algorithm

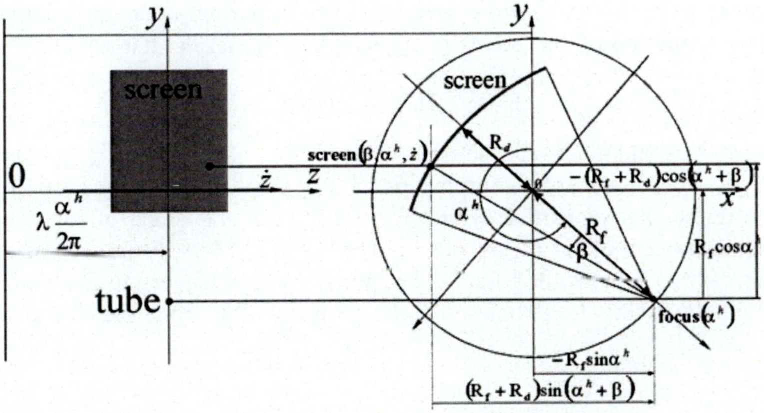

Fig. 7.38 Trigonometric relationships in a cone beam projection system with a partial cylindrical screen

These trigonometric relationships can easily be determined using Fig. 7.38, which shows the cone-beam projection system with a partial cylindrical screen.

It is much more useful, however, to represent the screen mathematically as a flat screen with coordinates (w, v). Whilst retaining the cylindrical design of the screen in practice, we can assume the existence of a corresponding flat screen:

$$\mathbf{screen}\left(w,\alpha^h,v\right)=\begin{bmatrix}x\\y\\z\end{bmatrix}=\begin{bmatrix}\mathrm{R}_d\cdot\sin\alpha^h\\-\mathrm{R}_d\cdot\cos\alpha^h\\\lambda\frac{\alpha^h}{2\pi}\end{bmatrix}+w\cdot\begin{bmatrix}-\cos\alpha^h\\-\sin\alpha^h\\0\end{bmatrix}+v\cdot\begin{bmatrix}0\\0\\1\end{bmatrix}. \tag{7.110}$$

As with the previous equation, this is based on a diagrammatic description (see Fig. 7.39, which illustrates how to calculate the various components of the vector **screen**).

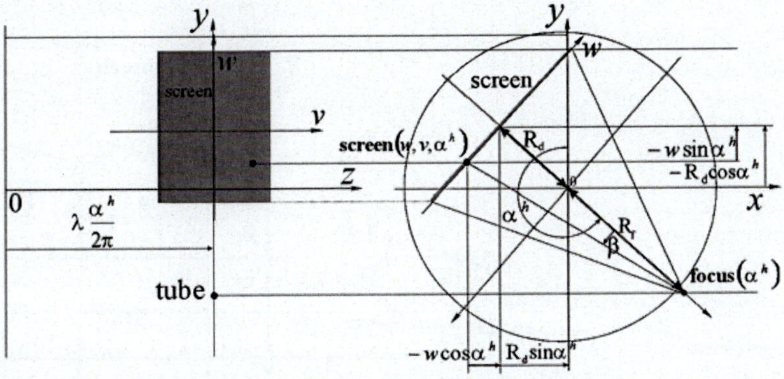

Fig. 7.39 Trigonometric relationships in a cone beam projection system with a flat screen

Equation 7.110 can be written equivalently in normal notation to indicate the condition imposed on the points in space, which lie on the flat screen:

$$R_d - x \sin \alpha^h + y \cos \alpha^h = 0. \tag{7.111}$$

Figures 7.40a and 7.40b can be used to derive relationships that allow us to calculate the coordinates of the projection of any point in the (x, y, z) space onto a screen (either flat or partial cylindrical), at a particular angle of rotation of the projection system α^h.

For the coordinates on a flat screen, we need to consider the geometry in the (x, y) plane. Using the Thales theorem, we can see from Fig. 7.40a that the

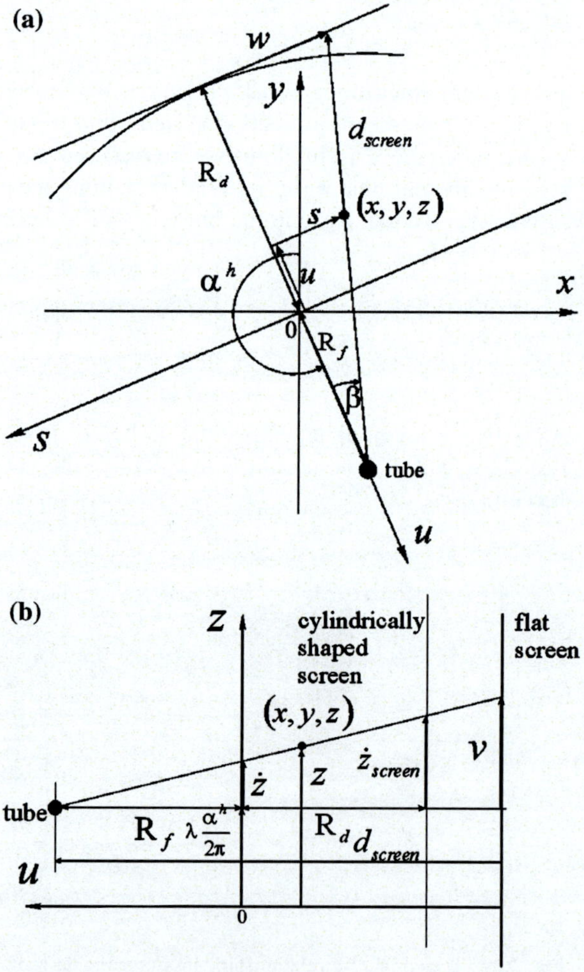

Fig. 7.40 Determining the coordinates of the projection of a given point onto the screen: **a** in the (x, y) plane; **b** in the plane that contains the ray passing through the point (x, y, z)

following relationship is appropriate for the projection of a point in space onto a flat screen:

$$\frac{w}{R_f + R_d} = \frac{-s}{R_f - u}. \tag{7.112}$$

The quantities s and u represent the coordinates of a point in the (x, y) system rotated by an angle α^h. Using the basic relationships given in Table 4.3, we can obtain the final form of the equation of the w-coordinate of the projection of the point (x, y) onto a flat screen:

$$w = \frac{-\left(x \cos \alpha^h + y \sin \alpha^h\right) \cdot \left(R_f + R_d\right)}{R_f + x \sin \alpha^h - y \cos \alpha^h}. \tag{7.113}$$

Figure 7.40b shows how to determine the v-coordinate of the projection onto the screen of the same point in space (x, y, z). This time, however, we consider the (x, z) plane. Here we can observe the triangle in the z-direction, for which the following holds true:

$$\frac{R_f + R_d}{R_f - u} = \frac{v}{z - \lambda \frac{\alpha^h}{2\pi}}. \tag{7.114}$$

Using the equation for the u-coordinate given in Table 4.3, we obtain the final form of the equation for the v-coordinate of the projection of the point onto the flat screen:

$$v = \frac{\left(z - \lambda \frac{\alpha^h}{2\pi}\right) \cdot \left(R_f + R_d\right)}{R_f + x \sin \alpha^h - y \cos \alpha^h}. \tag{7.115}$$

For a cylindrically shaped screen, the coordinates $(\beta, \dot{z})$ identify the ray passing through the point in space (x, y, z), at a projection angle α^h. For practical reasons, it is important to be able to find the relationships between the coordinates of the projection of any point (x, y, z) onto both types of screen.

Using Fig. 7.40a it is easy to find the relationship between the value of the w-coordinate on the flat screen and the angle β between the ray and the principal axis of the beam:

$$w = -\left(R_f + R_d\right) \tan \beta. \tag{7.116}$$

We can also use Fig. 7.40a to obtain the second of the required relationships:

$$\cos \beta = \frac{R_f + R_d}{d_{screen}}. \tag{7.117}$$

We can then use Fig. 7.40a to derive the following ratio:

$$\frac{\dot{z}_{screen}}{v} = \frac{R_f + R_d}{d_{screen}}, \tag{7.118}$$

which, combined with Eq. 7.117, immediately gives:

$$v = \frac{\dot{z}_{\mathrm{screen}}}{\cos\beta} = \frac{\dot{z}}{\cos\beta}\frac{\mathrm{R}_f + \mathrm{R}_d}{\mathrm{R}_f}. \tag{7.119}$$

The following pair of equations, obtained by rearranging equations (7.116) and (7.119), allows us to calculate the coordinates of the projection of the point (x, y, z) onto a cylindrically shaped screen:

$$\beta = -\arctan\frac{w}{\mathrm{R}_f + \mathrm{R}_d} \tag{7.120}$$

and

$$\dot{z} = v \cdot \cos\beta \cdot \frac{\mathrm{R}_f}{\mathrm{R}_f + \mathrm{R}_d} = \frac{v(\mathrm{R}_f + \mathrm{R}_d)}{\sqrt{(\mathrm{R}_f + \mathrm{R}_d)^2 + w^2}} \cdot \frac{\mathrm{R}_f}{\mathrm{R}_f + \mathrm{R}_d}. \tag{7.121}$$

The main distinguishing feature of the ASSR reconstruction algorithm is its abandonment of interpolation in the z-direction in the first stage of the process, in favour of finding the reconstruction plane that best matches the path that the projection system traces around the test object. The position of the reconstruction plane is defined by the parameter α_p^h, which corresponds to the place on the z-axis at which the reconstruction plane has a point in common with the spiral path of the moving X-ray tube. For simplicity, we will begin by assuming that $\alpha^h = \alpha_p^h = 0$. The position of the reconstruction plane in the (x, y, z) space satisfying this assumption is shown in Fig. 7.41.

The inclination of the reconstruction plane with respect to the x-axis, and thus the middle ray of the fan-beam at the point $\alpha^h = \alpha_p^h$, is represented by υ. In order to optimise the positioning of the plane, we allow any value for this angle, that is, where $\upsilon \neq 0$. The points on the plane can be described by the following relationship:

$$x \cdot \tan\upsilon - z = 0. \tag{7.122}$$

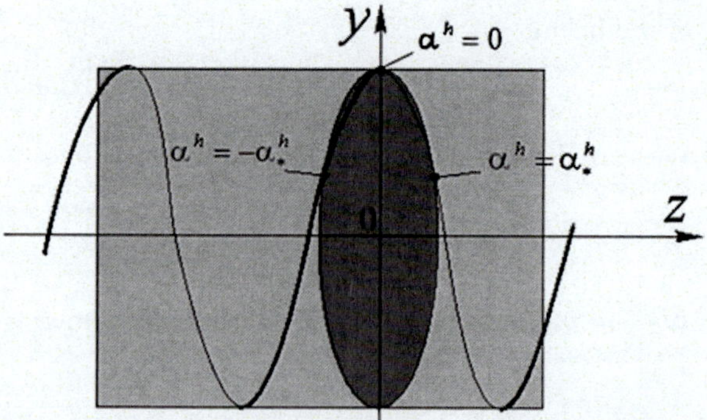

Fig. 7.41 The location of the reconstruction plane in (x, y, z) space in the ASSR reconstruction method

By calculating the variable z from this equation, it is easy to determine the cross-section of the cylinder (defined by Eq. 7.108), which contains the reconstruction plane. This cross-section is the ellipse calculated using the following vector equation:

$$\mathbf{ellipse}\left(\alpha^h\right) = \begin{bmatrix} x \\ y \\ z \end{bmatrix} = \begin{bmatrix} -R_f \sin\alpha^h \\ R_f \cos\alpha^h \\ x \tan\upsilon \end{bmatrix} = R_f \cdot \begin{bmatrix} -\sin\alpha^h \\ \cos\alpha^h \\ -\tan\upsilon \cdot \sin\alpha^h \end{bmatrix} \tag{7.123}$$

for $\alpha^h \in [-\pi, \pi]$.

The rotation of the reconstruction plane about the y-axis is shown in Fig. 7.42.

Up to now, in order to facilitate the derivation of the various geometric relationships, we have introduced a number of simplifications to the design of the projection system. However, when considering the actual operation of real scanners, we have to take into account several additional factors. The first of these is the fact that the reconstruction plane might not actually be situated at the origin of the coordinate system, i.e. $\alpha_p^h \neq 0$. This broadening of the problem means that (7.123) now becomes:

$$\mathbf{ellipse}\left(\alpha^h\right) = \begin{bmatrix} x \\ y \\ z \end{bmatrix} = \mathbf{O} + R_f \cdot \begin{bmatrix} -\sin\alpha^h \\ \cos\alpha^h \\ -\tan\upsilon \cdot \sin\left(\alpha^h - \alpha_p^h\right) \end{bmatrix}, \tag{7.124}$$

where

$$\mathbf{O} = \begin{bmatrix} 0 \\ 0 \\ \lambda\frac{\alpha_p^h}{2\pi} \end{bmatrix}. \tag{7.125}$$

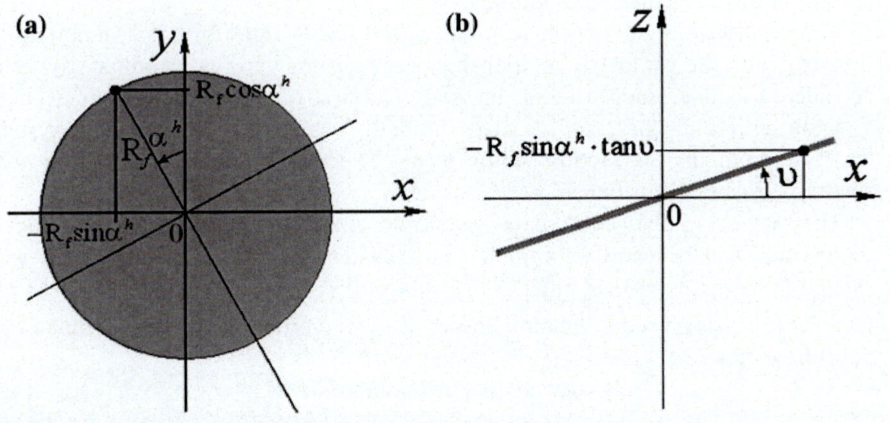

Fig. 7.42 The geometry of the reconstruction plane rotated about the y axis: **a** the reconstructed slice before rotation; **b** the reconstructed slice after rotation about the y axis

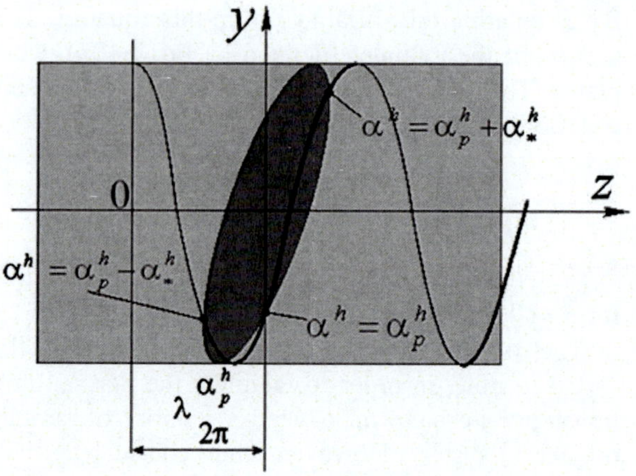

Fig. 7.43 Location of the reconstructed slice when α_p^h / 0

We can now represent the condition that the points lying in the reconstruction plane must satisfy, in a way similar to Eq. 7.122:

$$x \cos \alpha_p^h \cdot \tan \upsilon + y \sin \alpha_p^h \cdot \tan \upsilon + \lambda \frac{\alpha_p^h}{2\pi} - z = 0. \tag{7.126}$$

The imaging of a single slice takes place in the plane described by Eq. 7.126, for points inside the cylindrical path of the projection system. Of course, the image is reconstructed from projections made in this case by only those selected rays in the conical beam, which lie exactly in the plane at three positions, that is for: $\alpha^h = \alpha_p^h$, $\alpha^h = \alpha_p^h + \alpha_*^h$ and $\alpha^h = \alpha_p^h - \alpha_*^h$. The location of this reconstructed slice is illustrated by Fig. 7.43.

In order to obtain the other projection values needed for the reconstruction we need to use an approximation. In this algorithm, we calculate the necessary values using a fan-beam-based longitudinal approximation and further discussion will be based on this particular methodology.

Before proceeding to the presentation of the ASSR algorithm, it is important to first deal with the geometric relationships between the various coordinate systems considered in this reconstruction method. The first of the orthogonal coordinate systems represents the (x, y, z) space globally, whilst the second, local system (x', y', z') contains the reconstruction plane. The relationship between these two spaces is illustrated in Fig. 7.44.

The original global coordinate system (x, y, z), rotated around the z-axis, is represented by the triad (s, u, r). If we consider that the (s, u, r) system was rotated through an angle α_p^h (due to our choice of reconstruction plane at $\alpha^h = \alpha_p^h$) then the following vector equation allows us to convert between the coordinates of both these spaces:

$$\begin{bmatrix} x \\ y \\ z \end{bmatrix} = s \cdot \mathbf{s} + u \cdot \mathbf{u} + r \cdot \mathbf{r}, \tag{7.127}$$

Fig. 7.44 The global and local coordinate systems

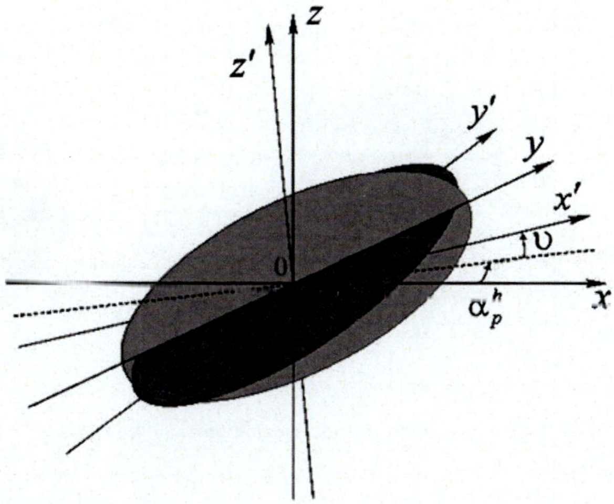

where the base vectors **s**, **u** and **r** are expressed as follows:

$$\mathbf{s} = \begin{bmatrix} \cos\alpha_p^h \\ \sin\alpha_p^h \\ 0 \end{bmatrix}, \ \mathbf{u} = \begin{bmatrix} -\sin\alpha_p^h \\ \cos\alpha_p^h \\ 0 \end{bmatrix}, \ \mathbf{r} = \begin{bmatrix} 0 \\ 0 \\ 1 \end{bmatrix}. \tag{7.128}$$

If the (s, u, r) system is rotated through a further angle α_p, the base vectors **s**, **u** and **r** become:

$$\mathbf{s}(\alpha_p) = \begin{bmatrix} \cos\left(\alpha_p^h + \alpha_p\right) \\ \sin\left(\alpha_p^h + \alpha_p\right) \\ 0 \end{bmatrix}, \ \mathbf{u}(\alpha_p) = \begin{bmatrix} -\sin\left(\alpha_p^h + \alpha_p\right) \\ \cos\left(\alpha_p^h + \alpha_p\right) \\ 0 \end{bmatrix}, \ \mathbf{r}(\alpha_p) = \begin{bmatrix} 0 \\ 0 \\ 1 \end{bmatrix}. \tag{7.129}$$

The local coordinate system defining the reconstruction plane is represented by (x', y', z'). However, the (x', y', z') system rotated around the z'-axis is represented by (s', u', r') (which means that x' and y' lie in the reconstruction plane). The geometrical relationships between these coordinates are shown in Fig. 7.45.

It is important to note that because we are searching for the optimum position of the reconstruction plane with respect to the spiral path of the moving projection system, the reconstruction plane is rotated around the y-axis and the (x', y', z') system is rotated through an angle α_p^h around the z-axis. Therefore, in order to convert the coordinates of a point (x', y', z') in the system into coordinates in the (x, y, z) system, we need to perform a two-stage process. The first of these converts the points in the (x', y', z') space into auxiliary coordinates (x'', y'', z''), which means that the original system is rotated by an angle $-\upsilon$ about the y''-axis (this is shown in Fig. 7.46a):

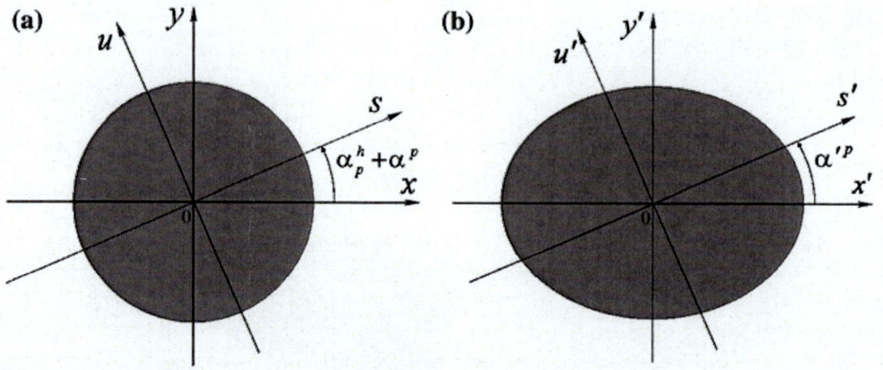

Fig. 7.45 Coordinate systems rotated through the angle $\alpha_p^h + \alpha_p$: **a** the global system; **b** the local system

$$\begin{bmatrix} x'' \\ y'' \\ z'' \end{bmatrix} = \begin{bmatrix} x' \cos \upsilon - z' \sin \upsilon \\ y' \\ x' \sin \upsilon + z' \cos \upsilon \end{bmatrix}. \tag{7.130}$$

The second spatial transformation converts the points in the (x'', y'', z'') system, rotated by the angle α_p^h about the z-axis, into the global coordinate system (x, y, z) (see Fig. 7.46b):

$$\begin{bmatrix} x \\ y \\ z \end{bmatrix} = \begin{bmatrix} x'' \cos \alpha_p^h - y'' \sin \alpha_p^h \\ x'' \sin \alpha_p^h + y'' \cos \alpha_p^h \\ z'' \end{bmatrix}. \tag{7.131}$$

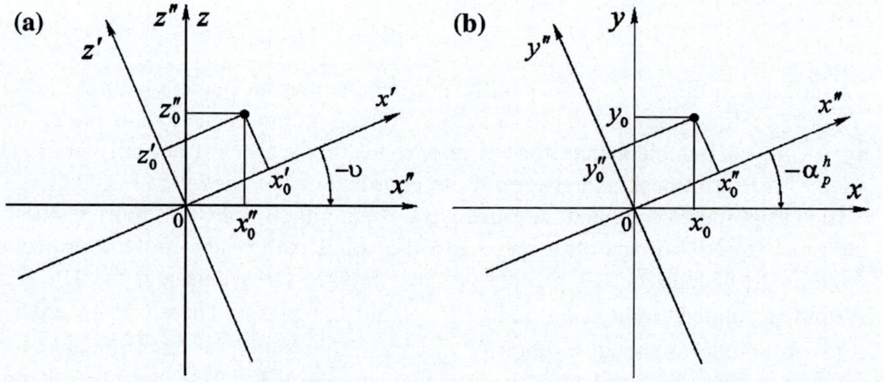

Fig. 7.46 The two stage transformation of the space where the reconstruction takes place into the global space: **a** the transition from (x', y', z') coordinates to auxiliary coordinates (x'', y'', z''); **b** the transition from (x'', y'', z'') coordinates to global coordinates (x, y, z)

Combining the transformations (7.130) and (7.131), we obtain the direct transform of the (x', y', z') space into the (x, y, z) space, which is represented by the matrix equation:

$$\begin{bmatrix} x \\ y \\ z \end{bmatrix} = x' \cdot \mathbf{x}' + y' \cdot \mathbf{y}' + z' \cdot \mathbf{z}', \tag{7.132}$$

where the base vectors $\mathbf{x}'$, $\mathbf{y}'$ and $\mathbf{z}'$ are expressed as follows:

$$\mathbf{x}' = \begin{bmatrix} \cos\upsilon \cdot \cos\alpha_p^h \\ \cos\upsilon \cdot \sin\alpha_p^h \\ \sin\upsilon \end{bmatrix}, \ \mathbf{y}' = \begin{bmatrix} -\sin\alpha_p^h \\ \cos\alpha_p^h \\ 0 \end{bmatrix}, \ \mathbf{z}' = \begin{bmatrix} -\sin\upsilon \cdot \cos\alpha_p^h \\ -\sin\upsilon \cdot \sin\alpha_p^h \\ \cos\upsilon \end{bmatrix}. \tag{7.133}$$

If we use a parallel projection system, the vector equation representing the relationship between the global coordinate system and the local system of the reconstruction plane is as follows:

$$x \cdot \mathbf{x} + y \cdot \mathbf{y} + z \cdot \mathbf{z} = \mathbf{O} + x' \cdot \mathbf{x}' + y' \cdot \mathbf{y}' + z' \cdot \mathbf{z}'. \tag{7.134}$$

For the reconstruction plane, that is, where $z' = 0$, Eq. 7.134 takes the form:

$$x \cdot \mathbf{x} + y \cdot \mathbf{y} + z \cdot \mathbf{z} = \mathbf{O} + x' \cdot \mathbf{x}' + y' \cdot \mathbf{y}'. \tag{7.135}$$

So far, we have only considered the central ray of the fan-shaped beam of radiation in the reconstruction plane. In order for the remaining rays to be regarded as elements of the hypothetical parallel beam, we need to consider an additional rotation of the coordinate system (x', y', z') about the z'-axis. If the angle of this rotation is represented by α'^p, then we need to combine a third transformation (from the (s', u', r') space to the (x, y, z) space) with the two discussed previously:

$$\begin{bmatrix} x \\ y \\ z \end{bmatrix} = s' \cdot \mathbf{s}' + u' \cdot \mathbf{u}' + r' \cdot \mathbf{r}', \tag{7.136}$$

where the base vectors in this vector equation have the following form:

$$\mathbf{s}' = \begin{bmatrix} \cos\upsilon \cdot \cos\alpha_p^h \cdot \cos\alpha'^p - \sin\alpha_p^h \cdot \sin\alpha'^p \\ \cos\upsilon \cdot \sin\alpha_p^h \cdot \cos\alpha'^p + \cos\alpha_p^h \cdot \sin\alpha'^p \\ \sin\upsilon \cdot \cos\alpha'^p \end{bmatrix}, \tag{7.137}$$

$$\mathbf{u}' = \begin{bmatrix} -\cos\upsilon \cdot \cos\alpha_p^h \cdot \sin\alpha'^p - \sin\alpha_p^h \cdot \cos\alpha'^p \\ -\cos\upsilon \cdot \sin\alpha_p^h \cdot \sin\alpha'^p + \cos\alpha_p^h \cdot \cos\alpha'^p \\ -\sin\upsilon \cdot \sin\alpha'^p \end{bmatrix}, \tag{7.138}$$

$$\mathbf{r}' = \begin{bmatrix} -\sin\upsilon \cdot \cos\alpha_p^h \\ -\sin\upsilon \cdot \sin\alpha_p^h \\ \cos\upsilon \end{bmatrix}. \tag{7.139}$$

In the ASSR reconstruction method, we need to determine the ray in the (s, u, r) system (more specifically in the (s, u) plane, when $r = 0$) equivalent to the ray passing through in the (s', u', r') system (when $r' = 0$), i.e. in the reconstruction plane. What we are looking for is the projection of a ray with parameters $(s'\alpha'^p)$ onto the (s, u) plane, in the form of a ray with the parameters (s, α^p). The relationship linking the parameters of the two rays can be found by noticing that their projections onto the (x, y) plane lie on the same straight line. To simplify matters, if we assume that the plane of the projection in the global (x, y, z) coordinate system is $z = 0$, then the required relationship is determined using the matrix equation:

$$\begin{bmatrix} 1 & 0 & 0 \\ 0 & 1 & 0 \\ 0 & 0 & 1 \end{bmatrix} (\mathbf{O} + s' \cdot \mathbf{s}' + u' \cdot \mathbf{u}') = \begin{bmatrix} x \\ y \\ z \end{bmatrix} = s \cdot \mathbf{s} + u \cdot \mathbf{u}. \tag{7.140}$$

It is important to note that each of the actual rays considered is either parallel to the s-axis or the s'-axis. Thus, the point (s_1, u_1) corresponds to the point $(s'_1, 0)$, and the point $(s_1, 0)$ corresponds, in turn, to another point on the ray in the (s', u') plane, such as the point defined by the pair (s'_1, u'_2). It is possible therefore to make Eq. 7.140 independent of the variables u' and u, which consequently leads to the following:

$$s = \frac{s' \cdot \cos \upsilon}{\sqrt{\cos^2 \alpha'^p + \cos^2 \upsilon \cdot \sin^2 \alpha'^p}}, \tag{7.141}$$

$$\cos \alpha^p = \frac{\cos \alpha'^p}{\sqrt{\cos^2 \alpha'^p + \cos^2 \upsilon \cdot \sin^2 \alpha'^p}}, \tag{7.142}$$

$$\sin \alpha^p = \frac{\sin \alpha'^p \cdot \cos \upsilon}{\sqrt{\cos^2 \alpha'^p + \cos^2 \upsilon \cdot \sin^2 \alpha'^p}} \tag{7.143}$$

and (for converting the coordinates in the opposite direction):

$$s' = \frac{s}{\sqrt{\sin^2 \alpha^p + \cos^2 \upsilon \cdot \cos^2 \alpha^p}}, \tag{7.144}$$

$$\cos \alpha'^p = \frac{\cos \alpha^p \cdot \cos \upsilon}{\sqrt{\sin^2 \alpha^p + \cos^2 \upsilon \cdot \cos^2 \alpha^p}}, \tag{7.145}$$

$$\sin \alpha'^p = \frac{\sin \alpha^p}{\sqrt{\sin^2 \alpha^p + \cos^2 \upsilon \cdot \cos^2 \alpha^p}}. \tag{7.146}$$

At the same time, it is worth using Eqs. 7.141 7.146 to determine the following trigonometric relationship for use later:

$$\sqrt{\sin^2 \alpha^p + \cos^2 \upsilon \cdot \cos^2 \alpha^p} \cdot \sqrt{\cos^2 \alpha'^p + \cos^2 \upsilon \cdot \sin^2 \alpha'^p} = \cos \upsilon. \tag{7.147}$$

After these preliminary discussions concerning the spatial factors relating to the projections and the location of the reconstruction plane, we are now ready to formulate the actual ASSR reconstruction procedure represented in Fig. 7.47.

At this point, we will examine the successive signal processing stages of the ASSR method.

7.3.5.1 Adjusting the Reconstruction Plane

After selecting the angle of rotation α_p^h of the spiral projection system so that the central ray of the beam intersects the z-axis at the midpoint of reconstructed slice,

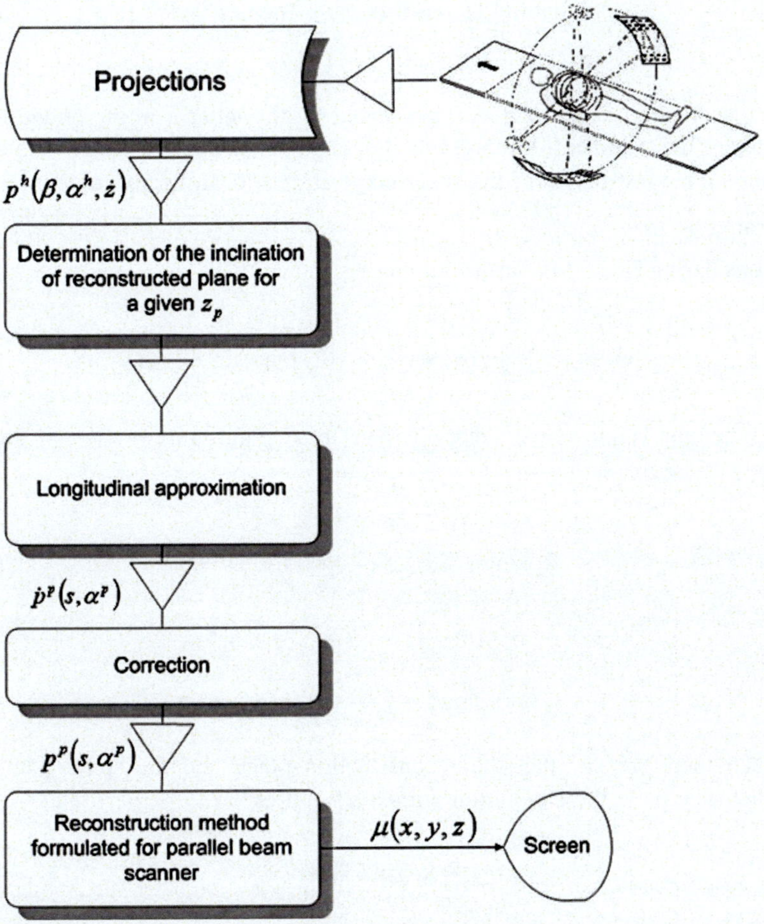

Fig. 7.47 A flowchart of the ASSR reconstruction method

we then have to determine the inclination of the plane of the slice. This angle of inclination is represented by the symbol υ.

In determining the optimum value for the angle υ, it is useful first to impose the condition $\alpha_p^h = 0$. The next step is to propose a selection criterion for the optimum angle. One possible optimisation criterion [29 31] is represented by the following formula:

$$\upsilon^{opt} = \min_{\upsilon}\left(\int_{a\pi}^{a\pi} \left|\mathbf{ellipse}(\alpha^h) - \mathbf{focus}(\alpha^h)\right| d\alpha^h\right). \tag{7.148}$$

Due to the symmetry of the integrand about $\alpha^h = 0$, the above equation can also be written equivalently:

$$\upsilon^{opt} = \min_{\upsilon}\left(\int_{0}^{a\pi} \left|\mathbf{ellipse}(\alpha^h) - \mathbf{focus}(\alpha^h)\right| d\alpha^h\right). \tag{7.149}$$

The appearance of the quantity represented by the letter a in the above formula requires some comment. It represents the range of the angle α^h taken into account during the reconstruction of the slice image at $\alpha_p^h = 0$. If, for example, $a = 1$ then this range is $\left[\alpha_p^h - \pi, \alpha_p^h + \pi\right]$.

Considering Eq. 7.149 further, it can be shown that:

$$\left|\mathbf{ellipse}(\alpha^h) - \mathbf{focus}(\alpha^h)\right| = \left|R_f \tan\upsilon \sin\alpha^h - \lambda\frac{\alpha^h}{2\pi}\right|. \tag{7.150}$$

The functions $R_f \tan\upsilon \sin\alpha^h$ and $\lambda\frac{\alpha^h}{2\pi}$ have three points in common in the range $\left[\alpha_p^h - \pi, \alpha_p^h + \pi\right]$ if:

$$R_f \tan\upsilon \sin\alpha^h - \lambda\frac{\alpha^h}{2\pi} \geq 0 \text{ for } \alpha^h = 0 \tag{7.151}$$

and

$$R_f \tan\upsilon \sin\alpha^h - \lambda\frac{\alpha^h}{2\pi} \leq 0 \text{ for } \alpha^h = a\pi. \tag{7.152}$$

We can therefore say that the reconstruction plane and the spiral path of the moving tube have three common points: $\alpha^h = 0$, $\alpha^h = \pm\alpha_*^h$, if:

$$1 \leq \frac{\alpha^h}{2\pi} R_f \tan\upsilon \leq \frac{a\alpha^h}{\sin(a\alpha^h)}. \tag{7.153}$$

This is illustrated in Fig. 7.48.

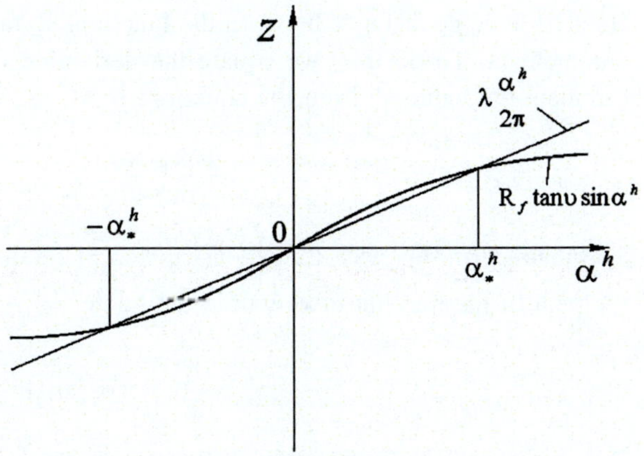

Fig. 7.48 Graphs of $R_f \tan \upsilon \sin \alpha^h$ and $\lambda\frac{\alpha^h}{2\pi}$, assuming the condition in (7.153) is fulfilled

The determination of α_*^h should then permit us to calculate the angle of inclination of the reconstruction plane using the formula:

$$\tan \upsilon = \frac{\lambda \alpha_*^h}{2\pi R_f \sin \alpha_*^h}. \tag{7.154}$$

Before we do this, however, we need to have chosen the value of α_*^h in such a way as to minimise the value of the integral in Eq. 7.149. By inspecting Fig. 7.48 and assuming the best fit of the reconstruction plane to the spiral path of the moving tube, we can conclude intuitively that in order to meet the optimisation criterion (7.149), we should use the following formula representing the average distance between the functions $R_f \tan \upsilon \sin \alpha^h$ and $\lambda\frac{\alpha^h}{2\pi}$:

$$\Delta z_{\mathrm{mean}} = \int_0^{a\pi} \left| \frac{\lambda \alpha_*^h \sin \alpha^h}{2a\pi^2 \sin \alpha_*^h} - \frac{\lambda \alpha^h}{2a\pi^2} \right| \mathrm{d}\alpha^\mathrm{h}. \tag{7.155}$$

Because of the difference between the two areas of integration (before and after $\alpha^h = \alpha_*^h$), Eq. 7.155 can be converted to the following form:

$$\Delta z_{\mathrm{mean}} = \frac{\lambda}{2a}\pi^2 \left(\int_0^{\alpha_*^h} \left(\frac{\alpha_*^h \sin \alpha^h}{\sin \alpha_*^h} - \alpha^h \right) \mathrm{d}\alpha^\mathrm{h} + \int_{\alpha_*^\mathrm{h}}^{a\pi} \left(\alpha^\mathrm{h} - \frac{\alpha_*^\mathrm{h} \sin \alpha^\mathrm{h}}{\sin \alpha_*^\mathrm{h}} \right) \mathrm{d}\alpha^\mathrm{h} \right). \tag{7.156}$$

By evaluating Eq. 7.156, we obtain the following simplified equation:

$$\Delta z_{\mathrm{mean}} = \frac{\lambda}{2a\pi^2} \left(\frac{\alpha_*^h}{\sin \alpha_*^h} (1 + \cos(a\pi) - 2\cos \alpha_*^h) + \frac{1}{2} a^2 \pi^2 - \left(\alpha_*^h\right)^2 \right). \tag{7.157}$$

Treating the right-hand side of Eq. 7.157 as a function of α_*^h, we can determine the value of α_*^h for which the function is a minimum. This is identical to obtaining the smallest average distance between the functions $R_f \tan\upsilon \sin\alpha^h$ and $\lambda\frac{\alpha^h}{2\pi}$, for a given parameter a. To do this, we equate the derivative of Δz_{mean} to zero, that is we calculate the value α_*^h from the equation:

$$\frac{\mathrm{d}\Delta z_{\text{mean}}}{\mathrm{d}\alpha_*^{\text{h}}} = 0. \tag{7.158}$$

To obtain α_*^h in this way, the reconstruction plane must lie as close as possible to the path of the moving tube, within the range $\left[\alpha_p^h - \pi, \alpha_p^h + \pi\right]$ of course:

$$\alpha_*^h = \frac{1}{2}(1 + \cos(a\pi)). \tag{7.159}$$

By combining Eq. 7.159 and Eq. 7.154, we obtain the following value for the optimum angle of inclination of the reconstruction plane:

$$\upsilon = \arctan\left(\frac{\lambda \cdot \arccos\left(\frac{1}{2}(1 + \cos(a\pi))\right)}{2\pi R_f \sin\left(\arccos\left(\frac{1}{2}(1 + \cos(a\pi))\right)\right)}\right). \tag{7.160}$$

7.3.5.2 Longitudinal Approximation

Longitudinal approximation uses the fact that both the real ray obtained physically from the projection and the ray from the approximated projection are in the same plane parallel to the z-axis. If that plane is represented by the symbol A, then this property can be written as follows:

$$A \parallel \mathbf{z} = \begin{bmatrix} 0 \\ 0 \\ 1 \end{bmatrix}. \tag{7.161}$$

The position of plane A with respect to the reconstruction plane is shown in Fig. 7.49.

The vectors $A \parallel \mathbf{u}'(\alpha'^p)$ and $\mathbf{O} + s' \cdot \mathbf{s}'(\alpha'^p) \in A$ uniquely identify plane A, which means that all of the points in the plane satisfy the equation:

$$(\mathbf{u}'(\alpha'^p) \times \mathbf{z})\left(\begin{bmatrix} x \\ y \\ z \end{bmatrix} - (\mathbf{O} + s' \cdot \mathbf{s}'(\alpha'^p))\right) = 0. \tag{7.162}$$

The point in the plane A of most interest is where the plane intersects with the spiral path of the moving X-ray tube. This point can be determined from the following matrix equation:

$$(\mathbf{u}'(\alpha'^p) \times \mathbf{z})\left(\mathbf{ellipse}(\alpha^h) - (\mathbf{O} + s' \cdot \mathbf{s}'(\alpha'^p))\right) = 0. \tag{7.163}$$

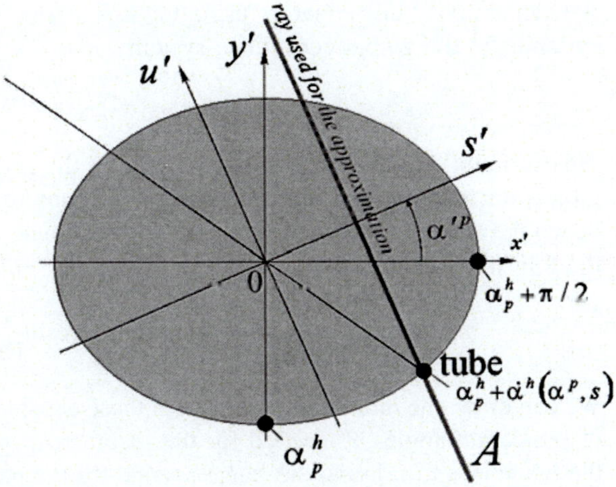

Fig. 7.49 The geometry of the longitudinal approximation

From relationships (7.124), (7.125) and (7.137) (7.139), we can see that the following equations are satisfied for this point:

$$\mathbf{ellipse}(\alpha^h) - (\mathbf{O} + s' \cdot \mathbf{s}'(\alpha'^p)) \\ = \begin{bmatrix} -\mathrm{R}_f \sin\alpha^h - s'\left(\cos\upsilon\cdot\cos\alpha_p^h\cdot\cos\alpha'^p - \sin\alpha_p^h\cdot\sin\alpha'^p\right) \\ \mathrm{R}_f\cos\alpha^h - s'\left(\cos\upsilon\cdot\sin\alpha_p^h\cdot\cos\alpha'^p + \cos\alpha_p^h\cdot\sin\alpha'^p\right) \\ -\mathrm{R}_f\tan\upsilon\sin\left(\alpha^h-\alpha_p^h\right) - \frac{\lambda\alpha^h}{2\pi} - s'\sin\upsilon\cdot\cos\alpha'^p \end{bmatrix} \tag{7.164}$$

and

$$\mathbf{u}'(\alpha'^p)\times\mathbf{z} = \begin{bmatrix} \mathrm{a} \\ \mathrm{a}\dfrac{\cos\upsilon\cdot\cos\alpha_p^h\cdot\sin\alpha'^p + \sin\alpha_p^h\cdot\cos\alpha'^p}{\cos\upsilon\cdot\sin\alpha_p^h\cdot\sin\alpha'^p - \cos\alpha_p^h\cdot\cos\alpha'^p} \\ 0 \end{bmatrix}, \tag{7.165}$$

where a is a real positive coefficient.

Taking into account the need to set the scalar product of the vectors in Eqs. 7.164 and 7.165 to zero, and defining:

$$\dot{\alpha}^h = \alpha^h - \alpha_p^h \tag{7.166}$$

as the angle of rotation of the projection system with respect to the point related to the place where the reconstruction is carried out, we obtain, after a series of operations, the following equation:

$$\mathrm{R}_f\left(\cos\alpha'^p\sin\dot{\alpha}^h - \sin\alpha'^p\cos\dot{\alpha}^h\cos\upsilon\right) + s'\cos\upsilon = 0. \tag{7.167}$$

We can simplify this equation using the Eqs. 7.144 7.146 and write it in terms of variables in the global coordinate system:

$$R_f \sin\left(\dot{\alpha}^h - \alpha^p\right) - s = 0. \quad (7.168)$$

This formula can then be used to determine the relative angle of rotation of the projection system, at which the path of the moving tube intersects the plane in which the longitudinal approximation will take place. The result is represented by the following relationship:

$$\dot{\alpha}^h(\alpha^p, s) = \alpha^p - \arcsin\frac{s}{R_f}. \quad (7.169)$$

We can draw one more conclusion from these considerations. It concerns the range of projection angles α^h needed for the reconstruction process. If α^p varies within the range $[-a\pi, a\pi]$, and the range needed for the parameter s for each projection value is $[-R, R]$, then it is necessary to perform the projections at the angles $\alpha^h \in \left[\alpha_p^h - a\pi + \arcsin\frac{R}{R_f}, \alpha_p^h + a\pi - \arcsin\frac{R}{R_f}\right]$.

In order for the approximation of the projection values to have as small an error as possible, we have to try to select a ray for this operation, which deviates as little as possible from the virtual path of the ray of the calculated projection. To help us think about this more clearly, we can determine two geometric constructions, as indicated in Fig. 7.50.

The first of these constructions involves establishing the plane that intersects the surface of the reconstructed slice at the points **O**, **ellipse**$\left(\alpha^h - \frac{\pi}{2}\right)$ and **ellipse**$\left(\alpha^h + \frac{\pi}{2}\right)$, and that contains the position of the tube, **focus**(α^h). The line

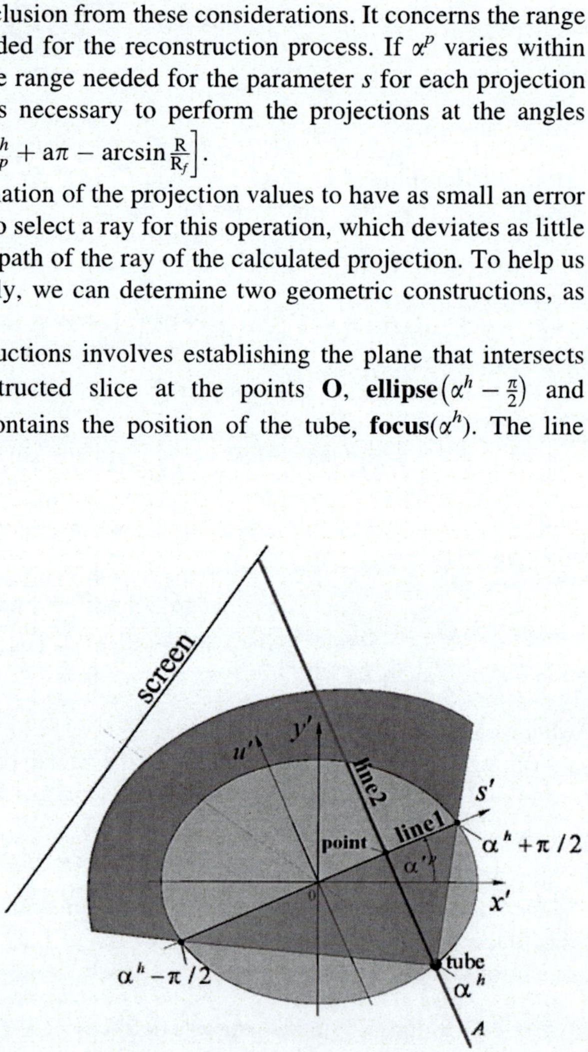

Fig. 7.50 Determining the optimum ray in a fan, for purposes of approximation

representing the intersection of this plane with the reconstructed slice is the set of points satisfying the equation:

$$\begin{aligned}\mathbf{line}_1 &= \mathbf{O} + \mathrm{a}_1\left(\mathbf{ellipse}\left(\alpha^h + \frac{\pi}{2}\right) - \mathbf{ellipse}\left(\alpha^h - \frac{\pi}{2}\right)\right) \\ &= \mathbf{O} - 2\mathrm{a}_1\mathrm{R}_f\begin{bmatrix}\cos\alpha^h \\ \sin\alpha^h \\ \tan\upsilon\cdot\cos\left(\alpha^h - \alpha_p^h\right)\end{bmatrix}\end{aligned}, \tag{7.170}$$

where a_1 is any real coefficient.

The second construction is the plane containing the point $\mathbf{focus}(\alpha^h)$ and the line at a distance $s' \cdot \mathbf{s}(\alpha'^p)$ from the centre of the coordinate system O, represented by the vector $\mathbf{u}'(\alpha'^p)$. The points of intersection of this plane with the ellipse of the reconstructed slice lie along the straight line with the equation:

$$\mathbf{line}_2 = \mathbf{O} + s' \cdot \mathbf{s}'(\alpha'^p) + \mathrm{a}_2\mathbf{u}'(\alpha'^p), \tag{7.171}$$

where a_2 is any real coefficient.

The point of intersection of these two lines satisfies the following vector equation:

$$\mathbf{O} + \mathrm{a}_1\left(\mathbf{ellipse}\left(\alpha^h + \frac{\pi}{2}\right) - \mathbf{ellipse}\left(\alpha^h - \frac{\pi}{2}\right)\right) = \mathbf{O} + s' \cdot \mathbf{s}'(\alpha'^p) + \mathrm{a}_2\mathbf{u}'(\alpha'^p). \tag{7.172}$$

Subtracting the vector $\mathbf{O}$ from both sides of this equation and multiplying both sides by $\mathbf{s}'(\alpha'^p)(\mathbf{s}'(\dot{\alpha}^p) \cdot \mathbf{s}'(\dot{\alpha}^p) = 1; \mathbf{u}'(\alpha'^p) \cdot \mathbf{s}'(\alpha'^p) = 0)$, we obtain an equation that represents the parameter a_1:

$$\begin{aligned}s' &= \mathrm{a}_1\left(\mathbf{ellipse}\left(\alpha^h + \frac{\pi}{2}\right) - \mathbf{ellipse}\left(\alpha^h - \frac{\pi}{2}\right)\right) \cdot \mathbf{s}'(\alpha'^p) \\ &= -2\mathrm{a}_1\mathrm{R}_f\frac{\cos\dot{\alpha}^h\cos\alpha'^p + \sin\dot{\alpha}^h\sin\alpha'^p\cos\upsilon}{\cos\upsilon}.\end{aligned} \tag{7.173}$$

Substituting the value $-2\mathrm{a}_1\mathrm{R}_f$, determined from relationship (7.173), into Eq. 7.171, we obtain a formula from which we can calculate the coordinates of the point in the reconstructed slice where $\mathbf{line}_1$ and $\mathbf{line}_2$ intersect:

$$\mathbf{point} = \begin{bmatrix} x \\ y \\ z \end{bmatrix} = \mathbf{O} + \frac{s'\cos\upsilon}{\cos\dot{\alpha}^h\cos\alpha'^p + \sin\dot{\alpha}^h\sin\alpha'^p\cos\upsilon}\begin{bmatrix}\cos\alpha^h \\ \sin\alpha^h \\ \tan\upsilon\cdot\cos\left(\dot{\alpha}^h\right)\end{bmatrix}. \tag{7.174}$$

Using matrix Eq. 7.174, we can easily calculate the coordinates (x, y, z) of the point **point** and then, using Eqs. 7.113 and 7.115, determine where it is projected onto the screen:

$$w_{\mathbf{point}} = \frac{R_f + R_d}{R_f} \cdot \frac{-s' \cdot \cos \upsilon}{\cos \dot{\alpha}^h \cos \alpha'^p + \sin \dot{\alpha}^h \sin \alpha'^p \cos \upsilon} \tag{7.175}$$

and

$$v_{\mathbf{point}} = \frac{R_f + R_d}{R_f} \cdot \left(\frac{s' \cos \dot{\alpha}^h \sin \upsilon}{\cos \dot{\alpha}^h \cos \alpha'^p + \sin \dot{\alpha}^h \sin \alpha'^p \cos \upsilon} - \lambda \frac{\dot{\alpha}^h}{2\pi} \right). \tag{7.176}$$

Converting these equations into the global coordinate system:

$$w_{\mathbf{point}} = -\frac{R_f + R_d}{R_f} \cdot \frac{-s}{\cos\left(\alpha^h - \alpha_p^h - \alpha^p\right)} \tag{7.177}$$

and

$$v_{\mathbf{point}} = \frac{R_f + R_d}{R_f} \cdot \left(\frac{s \cdot \cos\left(\alpha^h - \alpha_p^h\right) \cdot \tan \upsilon}{\cos\left(\alpha^h - \alpha_p^h - \alpha^p\right)} - \lambda \frac{\dot{\alpha}^h - \alpha_p^h}{2\pi} \right). \tag{7.178}$$

The projection value measured when parallel X-rays pass through the reconstruction plane of a test object with attenuation function $\mu(x, y, z)$ can be determined from the formula:

$$p'(s', \alpha'^p) = \int \mu(x, y, z) \cdot \delta(x' \cos \alpha'^p + y' \sin \alpha'^p - s') \mathrm{d}x' \mathrm{d}y'. \tag{7.179}$$

The geometric relationships used to formulate this equation are shown in Fig. 7.51.

To avoid having to transfer the results of the reconstruction procedure to the global coordinate system, the projection values from Eq. 7.179 should be defined earlier, through the exclusive use of quantities related to the target (x, y, z) system.

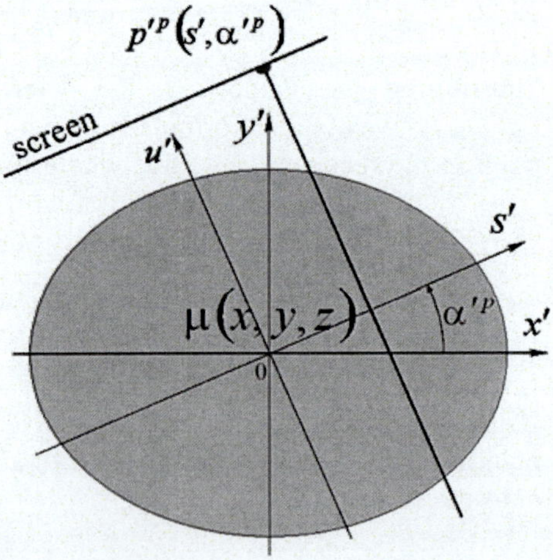

Fig. 7.51 Determining a parallel projection value in the reconstruction plane

First, we need to convert the argument of the Dirac delta. We can do this by using vector Eq. 7.135 to obtain the system of equations:

$$\begin{cases} x = x' \cos\alpha_p^h \cos\upsilon - y' \sin\alpha_p^h \\ y = x' \sin\alpha_p^h \cos\upsilon + y' \cos\alpha_p^h \end{cases}. \tag{7.180}$$

Hence, the variables x' and y' can be expressed as follows:

$$\begin{cases} x' = x\frac{\cos\alpha_p^h}{\cos\upsilon} + y\frac{\sin\alpha_p^h}{\cos\upsilon} \\ y' = -x\sin\alpha_p^h + y\cos\alpha_p^h \end{cases}. \tag{7.181}$$

Using these relationships together with Eqs. 7.144 7.146, we can modify the Dirac function appearing in the integration in Eq. 7.179:

$$\delta(x'\cos\alpha'^p + y'\sin\alpha'^p - s') = \delta\left(\frac{x\cos\left(\alpha_p^h + \alpha^p\right) + y\sin\alpha\left(\alpha_p^h + \alpha^p\right) - s}{\sqrt{\cos^2\alpha^p + \cos^2\upsilon\sin^2\alpha^p}}\right). \tag{7.182}$$

And finally, after using the Dirac delta scaling property, we obtain the equation:

$$\delta(x'\cos\alpha'^p + y'\sin\alpha'^p - s') = \sqrt{\cos^2\alpha^p + \cos^2\upsilon\sin^2\alpha^p} \cdot \delta\left(x\cos\left(\alpha_p^h + \alpha^p\right) + y\sin\alpha\left(\alpha_p^h + \alpha^p\right) - s\right). \tag{7.183}$$

The second of these essential changes concerns the variables with respect to which the integration is carried out. When converting the variables of integration to x and y, we need to calculate the Jacobian:

$$\frac{\partial(x', y')}{\partial(x, y)} = \frac{1}{\cos\upsilon}. \tag{7.184}$$

After performing both these conversions, the integral Eq. 7.179 becomes:

$$p'^p(s', \alpha'^p) = \int \mu(x, y, z) \cdot \frac{\sqrt{\cos^2\alpha^p + \cos^2\upsilon\sin^2\alpha^p}}{\cos\upsilon} \cdot \delta\left(x\cos\left(\alpha_p^h + \alpha^p\right) + y\sin\alpha\left(\alpha_p^h + \alpha^p\right) - s\right)dxdy. \tag{7.185}$$

However, it would still be difficult to carry out any kind of reconstruction procedure using projection values calculated like this. This is because the density of the hypothetical detectors on the virtual screen varies depending on the angle of incidence of the parallel beam. To allow for this, we need to deform the ellipse of the reconstructed slice into a circle as observed from the point of view of the projection system. This is done by using a geometric factor to convert all the projection values determined from Eq. 7.185:

$$\tilde{p}^{p}(s,\alpha^{p}) = \frac{\cos\upsilon}{\sqrt{\cos^{2}\alpha^{p} + \cos^{2}\upsilon\sin^{2}\alpha^{p}}} \cdot p'^{p}(s',\alpha'^{p})$$
$$= \int \mu(x,y,z)\cdot\delta\left(x\cos\left(\alpha_{p}^{h}+\alpha^{p}\right) + y\sin\alpha\left(\alpha_{p}^{h}+\alpha^{p}\right) - s\right)\mathrm{d}x\mathrm{d}y. \quad (7.186)$$

A small point that is also worth considering is the fact that the real rays used for the interpolation actually pass through the various tissues along a longer path than that of the interpolated rays. This means that we have to make another correction, which can be written as follows:

$$p^{p}(s,\alpha^{p}) = \mathrm{CORRECTION}\cdot\tilde{p}^{p}(s,\alpha^{p}), \quad (7.187)$$

where CORRECTION is a correction factor.

It only remains to determine the correction factor CORRECTION. Once again, it is important to remember here that both the interpolated ray and the real ray lie in the same plane, parallel to the z-axis. The interpolation error is proportional to the value of the angle. If both rays pass through almost the same tissues, the projection values associated with these rays will be related to the corresponding path lengths through the tissues. Owing to this, we can derive the angle-dependent correction factor by using the cosine of the angle:

$$\mathrm{CORRECTION} = \frac{p^{p}(s,\alpha^{p})}{\tilde{p}^{p}(s,\alpha^{p})} = \frac{u}{\tilde{u}} = \cos\varepsilon, \quad (7.188)$$

where ε is the angle between the real and the virtual ray.

The geometry of this method of determining the correction factor is shown in Fig. 7.52.

We still have to decide, however, how to actually calculate the value of the cosine correction factor. To do this, notice first that the direction and sense of the

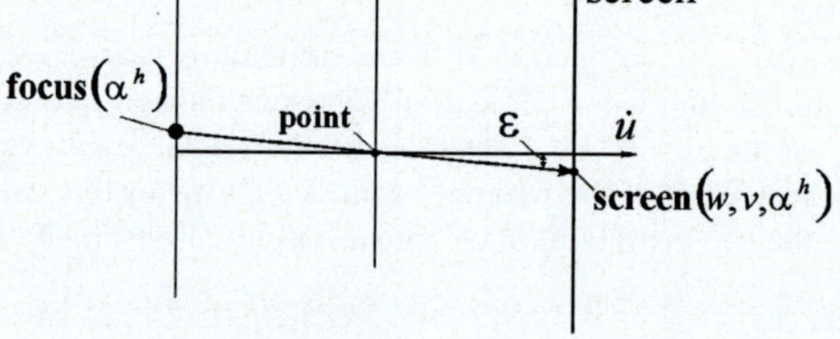

Fig. 7.52 The geometry of the cosine correction factor

virtual interpolated ray are defined by the vector $\mathbf{u}'(\alpha'^p)$, and for the real ray they are defined by the difference between the vectors **screen** (w, v, α^h) and **focus** (α^h). The scalar product of these two vectors is expressed as follows:

$$\left(\mathbf{screen}\left(w, v, \alpha^h\right) - \mathbf{focus}\left(\alpha^h\right)\right) \cdot \mathbf{u}'\left(\alpha'^p\right) = \left\|\mathbf{screen}\left(w, v, \alpha^h\right) - \mathbf{focus}\left(\alpha^h\right)\right\| \cdot \left\|\mathbf{u}'\left(\alpha'^p\right)\right\| \cdot \cos\varepsilon, \tag{7.189}$$

where ε is the angle between the vector $\mathbf{u}'(\alpha'^p)$ and the vector **screen** (w, v, α^h) – **focus** (α^h).

Consequently, from Eq. 7.189, we calculate the cosine correction factor of the interpolation as follows:

$$\cos\varepsilon = \frac{\left(\mathbf{screen}\left(w, v, \alpha^h\right) - \mathbf{focus}\left(\alpha^h\right)\right)}{\left\|\mathbf{screen}\left(w, v, \alpha^h\right) - \mathbf{focus}\left(\alpha^h\right)\right\|} \cdot \mathbf{u}'\left(\alpha'^p\right), \tag{7.190}$$

where $\|\mathbf{u}'(\alpha'^p)\| = 1$.

Using the relationships (7.108), (7.110) and (7.137) (7.139) in Eq. 7.190, we obtain the following formula:

$$\cos\varepsilon = \frac{\begin{bmatrix} w\cos\alpha^h - (\mathrm{R}+\mathrm{R_d})\sin\alpha^h \\ w\sin\alpha^h - (\mathrm{R}+\mathrm{R_d})\cos\alpha^h \\ v \end{bmatrix}}{\sqrt{w^2 + v^2 + (\mathrm{R}+\mathrm{R}_d)^2}} \cdot \frac{\begin{bmatrix} -\sin\left(\alpha^p + \alpha_p^h\right)\cos\upsilon \\ \cos\left(\alpha^p + \alpha_p^h\right)\cos\upsilon \\ -\sin\alpha^p\sin\upsilon \end{bmatrix}}{\sqrt{\sin^2\alpha^p + \cos^2\upsilon\sin^2\alpha^p}}. \tag{7.191}$$

After rearranging Eq. 7.191, we obtain a computable formula for the required factor:

$$\begin{aligned} \mathrm{CORRECTION} &= \cos\varepsilon \\ &= \frac{w\sin\left(\dot{\alpha}^h - \alpha^p\right)\cos\upsilon + (\mathrm{R}+\mathrm{R_d})\cos\left(\dot{\alpha}^h - \alpha^p\right)\cos\upsilon - v\sin\alpha^p\sin\upsilon}{\sqrt{w^2+v^2+(\mathrm{R}+\mathrm{R}_d)^2}\cdot\sqrt{\sin^2\alpha^p + \cos^2\upsilon\sin^2\alpha^p}}, \end{aligned} \tag{7.192}$$

where $\dot{\alpha}^h = \alpha^h - \alpha_p^h$ still holds true.

7.3.5.3 Reconstruction by Convolution/Filtration and Back-Projection

Now that we have $p^p(s, \alpha^p)$, we can proceed to the final signal processing stages of the ASSR reconstruction method, that is, the use of any reconstruction method originally devised for a parallel projection system.

During the final operation, the back-projection of the filtered values $p^p(s, \alpha^p)$, we need to bear in mind that the parameter a may have a value other than 1. This means we have to convert the relationship defining the back-projection operation to the following form:

$$\mu(x, y) = \frac{\int_{a\pi}^{a\pi} p^p(s, \alpha^p) d\alpha^p}{2a}. \quad (7.193)$$

In addition, if the gantry of the scanner is tilted, the reconstruction algorithm needs to take this into account. A practical solution to this problem is described in the article [31].

7.3.6 Discrete Implementation of the ASSR Algorithm

In a spiral cone-beam projection system, the ASSR algorithm can only make use of projections obtained at certain angles and measured only at particular points on the partial cylindrical-shaped screen.

The beam of radiation formed by the collimator reaches the individual detector rows $k = 1, 2, \ldots, \mathrm{K}$, where K is an even number of rows placed on the screen. In any given row, selected rays in the beam strike the detectors, each of which is indexed by the variable $\eta = -(\mathrm{H}-1)/2, \ldots, 0, \ldots, (\mathrm{H}-1)/2$, where H is an odd number of detectors in each row of the array (number of channels).

During a spiral tomography examination, the radiation beam (actually its centre) only passes once through any point on the z-axis. In practice, only a limited number of projections are carried out, each of which is indexed by the variable $\theta = 0, \ldots, \Theta - 1$, where $\Theta - 1$ is the total number of projections made during the examination.

So, we can sum up by saying that the reconstruction algorithm has available to it the projection values $\hat{p}^h(\eta, \theta, k)$, in the ranges: $\eta = -(\mathrm{H}-1)/2, \ldots, 0, \ldots, (\mathrm{H}-1)/2; \theta = 0, \ldots, \Theta - 1; k = 1, 2, \ldots, \mathrm{K}$.

Before using the algorithm, we need to determine the location of the middle of the reconstructed slice on the z-axis, a basic parameter for the examination. This position is represented by z_p or by the angle of rotation of the projection system α_p^h at the moment the centre of symmetry of the cone-beam intersects with it. A way of converting z_p into α_p^h is given by Eq. 7.93.

Next, using Eq. 7.160, we calculate the angle through which the reconstructed slice is rotated about the y-axis when the projection system is at an angle α_p^h. This angle is represented by the symbol υ.

Having determined the initial parameters α_p^h and υ, we are ready to perform the reconstruction procedures using a rebinning strategy. That means relating the results of the projections made in the cone-beam system to the raster of the parallel-beam system as defined by the pair $\left(s_l, \alpha_\psi^p\right)$, where

$$s_l = l \cdot \Delta_s, \quad (7.194)$$

where $l = -(L-1)/2, \ldots, 0, \ldots, (L-1)/2$ is the index of the detectors in the parallel-beam system; L is the maximum number of detectors on the screen in the parallel-beam system; Δ_s is the distance between the detectors in the parallel-beam system, and

$$\alpha^p_\psi = \psi \cdot \Delta^p_\alpha, \tag{7.195}$$

where $\psi = 0, \ldots, \Psi - 1$ is the index of the projections in the parallel-beam system; Δ^p_α is the maximum number of projections.

The indices ordering the projections made in the hypothetical parallel-beam system have the following relationships with the parameters of the cone-beam projection:

$$\mathrm{L} = 2\left(\mathrm{R}\ div\ \Delta^p_s\right) + 1 \tag{7.196}$$

and

$$\Psi = Trunc\left(\mathrm{a} \cdot 2\pi, \Delta^p_\alpha\right). \tag{7.197}$$

The procedure for obtaining the individual parallel projection values $p^p(s_l, \alpha^p_\psi)$ with indices in the ranges: $l = -(L-1)/2, \ldots, 0, \ldots, (L-1)/2$ and $\psi = 0, \ldots, \Psi - 1$ is as follows.

Step I For each value of l and ψ, we calculate the optimum angular position of the projection system (along the lines of Eq. 7.169) for performing longitudinal approximation. We can calculate this position using the relationship:

$$\alpha^h_{l\psi} = \psi\Delta^p_\alpha - \arcsin\frac{l\Delta^p_s}{\mathrm{R}_f} + \alpha^h_p \tag{7.198}$$

and we can calculate the position of virtual detectors on a flat screen (using Eqs. 7.177) and (7.178), which would measure the projection values best suited for further processing, using the following two equations:

$$w_{l\psi} = \frac{\mathrm{R}_f + \mathrm{R}_d}{\mathrm{R}_f} \cdot \frac{-l\Delta_s}{\cos\left(\alpha^h_{l\psi} - \alpha^h_p - \psi\Delta_\alpha\right)} \tag{7.199}$$

and

$$v_{l\psi} = \frac{\mathrm{R}_f + \mathrm{R}_d}{\mathrm{R}_f} \cdot \left(\frac{l\Delta^p_s \cdot \cos\left(\alpha^h_{l\psi} - \alpha^h_p\right) \cdot \tan \upsilon}{\cos\left(\alpha^h_{l\psi} - \alpha^h_p - \psi\Delta^p_\alpha\right)} - \lambda \frac{\dot{\alpha}^h_{l\psi} - \alpha^h_p}{2\pi} \right). \tag{7.200}$$

As $w_{l\psi}$ and $v_{l\psi}$ apply to a flat screen, they need to be converted into the coordinates of the real partial cylindrical screen, using the following two equations (see Eqs. 7.120 and 7.121):

$$\beta_{l\psi} = -\arctan\frac{w_{l\psi}}{\mathrm{R}_f + \mathrm{R}_d} \tag{7.201}$$

and

$$\dot{z}_{l\psi} = v_{l\psi} \cdot \cos\beta \cdot \frac{\mathrm{R}_f}{\mathrm{R}_f + \mathrm{R}_d}. \tag{7.202}$$

It is highly unlikely that amongst the rays in the cone-beams there are any that have parameters that exactly match these calculated values. The solution to this is to interpolate these parameters from others in the neighbourhood. It is useful, however, to define them first using their relative values, calculated as shown below:

$$\eta_{l\psi} = \frac{\beta_{l\psi}}{\Delta^h_\beta}, \tag{7.203}$$

$$\theta_{l\psi} = \frac{\alpha^h_{l\psi}}{\Delta^h_\alpha} \tag{7.204}$$

and

$$k_{l\psi} = \frac{\mathrm{K}+1}{2} + \frac{\dot{z}_{l\psi}}{\Delta^h_z} \cdot \frac{\mathrm{R}_f + \mathrm{R}_d}{\mathrm{R}_f}. \tag{7.205}$$

In order to carry out trilinear interpolation, we must next define what we mean by the neighbourhood referred to above, using the following set of eight projection values:

$$\begin{gathered}\hat{p}^h\left(\eta^\uparrow_{l\psi}, \theta^\uparrow_{l\psi}, k^\uparrow_{l\psi}\right);\ \hat{p}^h\left(\eta^\downarrow_{l\psi}, \theta^\uparrow_{l\psi}, k^\uparrow_{l\psi}\right);\ \hat{p}^h\left(\eta^\uparrow_{l\psi}, \theta^\downarrow_{l\psi}, k^\uparrow_{l\psi}\right);\ \hat{p}^h\left(\eta^\downarrow_{l\psi}, \theta^\downarrow_{l\psi}, k^\uparrow_{l\psi}\right);\\ \hat{p}^h\left(\eta^\uparrow_{l\psi}, \theta^\uparrow_{l\psi}, k^\downarrow_{l\psi}\right);\ \hat{p}^h\left(\eta^\downarrow_{l\psi}, \theta^\uparrow_{l\psi}, k^\downarrow_{l\psi}\right);\ \hat{p}^h\left(\eta^\uparrow_{l\psi}, \theta^\downarrow_{l\psi}, k^\downarrow_{l\psi}\right);\ \hat{p}^h\left(\eta^\downarrow_{l\psi}, \theta^\downarrow_{l\psi}, k^\downarrow_{l\psi}\right),\end{gathered} \tag{7.206}$$

where $\eta^\downarrow_{l\psi} = Trunc(\eta_{l\psi}, 1)$; $\eta^\uparrow_{l\psi} = \eta^\downarrow_{l\psi} + 1$; $\theta^\downarrow_{l\psi} = Trunc(\theta_{l\psi}, 1)$; $\theta^\uparrow_{l\psi} = \theta^\downarrow_{l\psi} + 1$; $k^\downarrow_{l\psi} = Trunc(k_{l\psi}, 1)$; $k^\uparrow_{l\psi} = k^\downarrow_{l\psi} + 1$.

The next step in the process is to begin the interpolation of the projection values $\hat{p}^p(l, \psi) = \dot{p}^p\left(s_l, \alpha^p_\psi\right)$. We can do this using trilinear interpolation as follows:

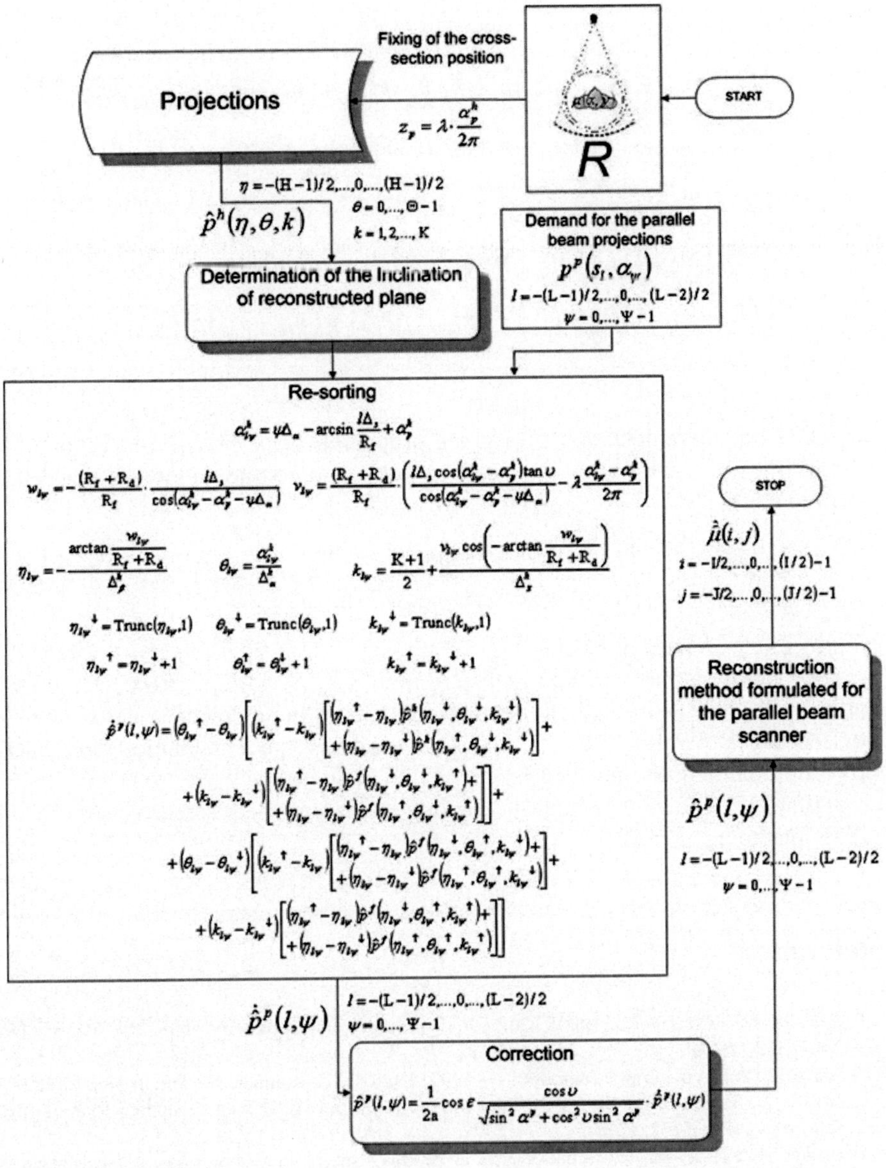

Fig. 7.53 A flowchart of the discrete version of the ASSR image reconstruction method for cone beam projections

$$
\begin{aligned}
\hat{p}^p(l,\psi) = & \left(\theta^{\uparrow}_{l\psi} - \theta_{l\psi}\right) \\
& \cdot\left[\left(k^{\uparrow}_{l\psi} - k_{l\psi}\right)\left[\left(\eta^{\uparrow}_{l\psi} - \eta_{l\psi}\right)\hat{p}^h\left(\eta^{\downarrow}_{l\psi}, \theta^{\downarrow}_{l\psi}, k^{\downarrow}_{l\psi}\right) + \left(\eta_{l\psi} - \eta^{\downarrow}_{l\psi}\right)\hat{p}^h\left(\eta^{\uparrow}_{l\psi}, \theta^{\downarrow}_{l\psi}, k^{\downarrow}_{l\psi}\right)\right]\right. \\
& \left. + \left(k_{l\psi} - k^{\downarrow}_{l\psi}\right)\left[\left(\eta^{\uparrow}_{l\psi} - \eta_{l\psi}\right)\hat{p}^f\left(\eta^{\downarrow}_{l\psi}, \theta^{\uparrow}_{l\psi}, k^{\downarrow}_{l\psi}\right) + \left(\eta_{l\psi} - \eta^{\downarrow}_{l\psi}\right)\hat{p}^f\left(\eta^{\uparrow}_{l\psi}, \theta^{\uparrow}_{l\psi}, k^{\downarrow}_{l\psi}\right)\right]\right] + \\
& \cdot\left(\theta_{l\psi} - \theta^{\downarrow}_{l\psi}\right) \cdot \\
& + \left[\left(k^{\uparrow}_{l\psi} - k_{l\psi}\right)\left[\left(\eta^{\uparrow}_{l\psi} - \eta_{l\psi}\right)\hat{p}^h\left(\eta^{\downarrow}_{l\psi}, \theta^{\downarrow}_{l\psi}, k^{\uparrow}_{l\psi}\right) + \left(\eta_{l\psi} - \eta^{\downarrow}_{l\psi}\right)\hat{p}^h\left(\eta^{\uparrow}_{l\psi}, \theta^{\downarrow}_{l\psi}, k^{\uparrow}_{l\psi}\right)\right]\right. \\
& \left. + \left(k_{l\psi} - k^{\downarrow}_{l\psi}\right)\left[\left(\eta^{\uparrow}_{l\psi} - \eta_{l\psi}\right)\hat{p}^f\left(\eta^{\downarrow}_{l\psi}, \theta^{\uparrow}_{l\psi}, k^{\uparrow}_{l\psi}\right) + \left(\eta_{l\psi} - \eta^{\downarrow}_{l\psi}\right)\hat{p}^f\left(\eta^{\uparrow}_{l\psi}, \theta^{\uparrow}_{l\psi}, k^{\uparrow}_{l\psi}\right)\right]\right]
\end{aligned}
\tag{7.207}
$$

Step II After the calculation of a given projection value $\hat{p}^p(l,\psi)$, in accordance with Eqs. 7.186 and 7.187 we need to subject it to the following correction operation:

$$
\hat{p}^p(l,\psi) = \frac{1}{2\text{a}} \cos\varepsilon \frac{\cos\upsilon}{\sqrt{\cos^2\alpha^p + \cos^2\upsilon \sin^2\alpha^p}} \cdot \hat{p}^p(l,\psi), \tag{7.208}
$$

where $\cos\varepsilon$ is determined using Eq. 7.192.

The parallel projection values $\hat{p}^p(l,\psi)$; $l = -(\text{L}-1)/2, \ldots, 0, \ldots, (\text{L}-1)/2$ and $\psi = 0, \ldots, \Psi - 1$ obtained like this can be used in any reconstruction method devised for a parallel projection system, such as the convolution and back-projection method discussed in Sect. 5.4.

Figure 7.53 shows the signal processing stages for the discrete version of the ASSR method.

References

1. Aradate H, Nambu K (1990) Computed tomography apparatus. Japanese Patent No. 2,825,352 (1990)
2. Arenson JS, Levinson R, Fruendlich D (1993) Dual sclice scanner. US Patent No. 5,228,069
3. Bresler Y, Skrabacz CJ (1989) Optimal interpolation in helical scan computed tomography. Proc ICASSP 3:1472 1475
4. Bruder H, Kachelrieß M, Schaller S et al (2000a) Single slice rebinning reconstruction in spiral cone beam computed tomography. IEEE Trans Med Imaging 9:873 887
5. Bruder H, Kachelrieß M, Schaller S et al (2000b) Performance of approximate cone beam reconstruction in multislice spiral computed tomography. Proc SPIE Med Imaging Conf 3979:541 555
6. Chen L, Liang Y, Heuscher DJ (2003) General surface reconstruction for cone beam multislice spiral computed tomography. Med Phys 30(10):2804 2821
7. Crawford CR, King KF (1990) Computer tomography scanning with simultaneous patient translation. Med Phys 17(6):967 981

8. Danielsson PE, Edholm P, Ericsson J et al (1997) Toward exact 3D reconstruction for helical scanning of long object. A new detector arrangement and new completeness condition. In: Proceedings of international meeting on Fully 3D image reconstruction, pp 141 144
9. Danielsson PE, Edholm P, Ericsson J et al (1999) The original PI method for helical cone beam CT. In: Proceedings of international meeting on Fully 3D image reconstruction, pp 3 6
10. Defrise M, Clack R (1994) A cone beam reconstruction algorithm using shift variant filtering and cone beam backprojection. IEEE Trans Med Imaging 13:186 195
11. Defrise M, Noo F, Kudo H (2000) A solution to the long object problem in helical cone beam tomography. Phys Med Biol 45:623 643
12. Dinwiddle KL, Friday RG, Racz JA et al (1980) Tomographic scanning apparatus having detector signal digitizing means mounted to rotate with detectors. US Patent No 4,190,772
13. Feldkamp LA, Davis LC, Kress JW (1984) Practical cone beam algorithm. J Opt Soc Am A 1:612 619
14. Filipczak PA (1961) Slip ring assembly for high voltages. US Patent No. 2,979,685
15. Fuchs T, Krause J, Schaller S et al (2000) Spiral interpolation algorithms for multislice spiral CT part II: measurement and evaluation of slice sensivity profiles and noise at a clinical multislice system. IEEE Trans Med Imaging 19(9):835 847
16. Grangeat P (1991) Mathematical framework of cone beam 3D reconstruction via the first derivative of the Radon transform. In: Herman GT, Louis AK, Natterer F (eds) Mathematical methods in thomography. Lecture Notes in Mathematics 1497. Springer, Berlin
17. Gullberg GT, Zeng GL, Christian PE et al (1991) Single photon emission computed tomography of the heart using cone beam geometry and noncircular detector rotation. In: Proceedings of 11th international conference on Information processing in medical imaging, pp 123 138
18. Gullberg GT, Zeng GL (1992) A cone beam filtered backpropagation reconstruction algorithm for cardiac single photon emission computed tomography. IEEE Trans Med Imaging 11(1):91 101
19. Hein IA, Taguchi K, Mori I et al (2003a) Tilted helical Feldkamp cone beam reconstruction algorithm for multislice CT. Proc SPIE Int Symp Med Imaging 5032:1901 1910
20. Hein IA, Taguchi K, Silver MD (2003b) Feldkamp based cone beam reconstruction for gantry tilted helical multislice CT. Med Phys 30(12):3233 3242
21. Heuscher DJ (1999) Helical cone beam scans using oblique 2D surface reconstructions. In: Proceedings of international meeting on Fully 3D image reconstruction, pp 204 207
22. Heuscher DJ, Lindstrom WW, Tuy HK (1996) Multiple detector ring spiral scanner with relatively adjustable helical paths. US Patent No. 5,485,492
23. Hsieh J (2000) Tomographic reconstruction for tilted helical multislice CT. IEEE Trans Med Imaging 19(9):864 872
24. Hsieh J, Hu H (2001) A frequency domain compensation scheme for multi slice helical CT reconstruction with tilted gantry. Proc SPIE 4322:105 112
25. Hu H (1996) An improved cone beam reconstruction algorithm for the circular orbit. J Scanning Microsc 18:572 581
26. Hu H (1999) Multi slice helical CT: scan and reconstruction. Med Phys 26(1):5 18
27. Hu H, Shen Y (1998) Helical CT reconstruction with longitudinal filtration. Med Phys 25:2130
28. Kachelrieß M, Kalender WA (2002) Extended parallel backprojection for cardiac cone beam CT for up to 128 slices. Radiology 225(P):310
29. Kachelrieß M, Schaller S, Kalender WA (2000a) Advanced single slice rebinning in cone beam spiral CT. Med Phys 27(4):754 773
30. Kachelrieß M, Schaller S, Kalender WA (2000b) Advanced single slice rebinning in cone beam spiral CT. Proc SPIE Med Imaging Conf 3979:494 505
31. Kachelrieß M, Fuchs T, Schaller S et al (2001) Advanced single slice rebinning for tilted spiral cone beam CT. Med Phys 28(6):1033 1041

32. Kachelrieß M, Knaup M, Kalender WA (2004) Extended parallel backprojection for standard three dimensional and phase correlated four dimensional axial and spiral cone beam CT with arbitrary pitch, arbitrary cone angle, and 100% dose usage. Med Phys 31:1623 1641
33. Kak AC, Slanley M (1988) Principles of computerized tomographic imaging. IEEE Press, New York
34. Kalender WA (2003) Computed tomography: fundamentals, system technology, image quality. Wiley, New York (2003)
35. Kalender WA, Seissler W, Klotz E et al (1990) Spiral volumetric CT with single breath hold technique, continuous transport, and continuous scanner rotation. Radiology 176:181 183
36. Kirillov AA (1961) On a problem of I. M. Gel'fand. Sov Math Dokl 2:268 269
37. Kudo H, Saito T (1994) Derivation and implementation of a cone beam reconstruction algorithm for nonplanar orbits. IEEE Trans Med Imaging 13:196 211
38. Kudo H, Noo F, Defrise M (1998) Cone beam filtered backpropagation algorithm for truncated helical data. Phys Med Biol 43:2885 2909
39. Kudo H, Noo F, Defrise M (2000) Quasi exact filtered backpropagation algorithm for long object problem in helical cone beam tomography. IEEE Trans Med Imaging 19:902 921
40. Larson GL, Ruth CC, Crawford CR (1998) Nutating slice image reconstruction. Patent Appl WO 98/44847
41. Lee SW, Wang G (2003) A Grangeat type half scan algorithm for cone beam CT. Med Phys 30:689 700
42. Lewitt RM (1983) Reconstruction algorithms: transform methods. Proc IEEE 71(3):390 408
43. Liang Y, Kruger RA (1996) Dual slice spiral versus single slice spiral scanning: comparison of the physical performance of two computed tomography scanners. Med Phys 23:205 220
44. Nishimura H, Miyazaki O (1988) CT system for spirally scanning subject on a movable bed synchronized to X ray tube revolution. US Patent No. 4,789,929
45. Noo F, Heuscher DJ (2002) Image reconstruction from cone beam data on a circular short scan. Proc SPIE 4684:50 59
46. Noo F, Defrise M, Clackdoyle R (1999) Single slice rebinning method for helical cone beam CT. Phys Med Biol 44:561 570
47. Pelc NJ, Glover GH (1986) Method for reducing image artifacts due to projection measurement inconsistencies. US Patent No. 4,580,219
48. Proska R, Köhler T, Grass M, Timmer J (2000) The n Pi method for helical cone beam CT. IEEE Trans Med Imaging 19:848 863
49. Schaller S, Flohr T, Steffen P (1997) New, efficient Fourier reconstruction method for approximate image reconstruction in spiral cone beam CT at small cone angles. Proc SPIE Med Imaging Conf 3032:213 224
50. Schaller S, Noo F, Sauer F et al (1999) Exact radon rebinning algorithm for long object problem in helical cone beam CT. In: Proceedings of international meeting on Fully 3D image reconstruction, pp 11 14
51. Schaller S, Noo F, Sauer F et al (2000) Exact Radon rebinning algorithm using local region of interest for helical cone beam CT. IEEE Trans Med Imaging 19:361 375 (2000a)
52. Schaller S, Flohr T, Klingenbeck K et al (2000b) Spiral interpolation algorithms for multislice spiral CT Part I: theory. IEEE Trans Med Imaging 19(9):822 834
53. Schaller S, Stierstiorfer K, Bruder H et al (2001) Novel approximate approach for high quality image reconstruction in helical cone beam CT at arbitrary pitch. Proc SPIE Med Imag Conf 4322:113 127
54. Slavin PE (1969) X ray helical scanning means for displaying an image of an object within the body being scanned. US Patent No. 3,432,657
55. Smith BD (1985) Image reconstruction from cone beam reconstructions: Necessary and sufficient conditions and reconstruction methods. IEEE Trans Med Imaging MI 4:14 25
56. Smith BD, Chen JX (1992) Implementation, investigation, and improvement of a novel cone beam reconstruction method. IEEE Trans Med Imaging MI 11:260 266
57. Taguchi K (1995) X ray computed tomography apparatus. US Patent No. 5,825,842

58. Taguchi K, Aradate H (1998) Algorithm for image reconstruction in multi slice helical CT. Med Phys 25:550 561
59. Tam KC (2000) Exact local regio of interest reconstruction in spiral cone beam filtered backpropagation CT: theory. Proc SPIE Med Imaging 3979:506 519
60. Tam KC, Samarasekera S, Sauer F (1998) Exact cone beam CT with a spiral scan. Phys Med Biol 43:847 855
61. Turbell H, Danielsson PE (1999) An improved PI method for reconstruction from helical cone beam projections. Proc Nucl Sci Symp 2:865 868
62. Turbell H, Danielsson PE (2000) Helical cone beam tomography. Int J Imaging Syst Technol 11(1):91 100
63. Tuy HK (1983) An inversion formula for cone beam reconstruction. SIAM J Appl Math 43:546 552
64. Wang G, Cheng PC (1995) Rationale of Feldkamp type cone beam CT. In: Proceedings of 4th international conference on Young Computer Scientist
65. Wang G, Vannier MW (1994) Longitudinal resolution in volumetric X ray computerized tomography analytical comparison between conventional and helical computerized tomography. Med Phys 21(3):429 433
66. Wang G, Vannier MW (1997a) Optimal pitch in spiral computed tomography. Med Phys 24:1635 1639
67. Wang G, Vannier MW (1997b) Low contrast resolution in volumetric x ray CT analytical comparison between conventional and spiral CT. Med Phys 24(3):373 376
68. Wang G, Lin T H, Cheng P et al (1991) A general cone beam reconstruction algorithm for X ray microtomography. J Scanning Microsc 13(I):126 128
69. Wang G, Lin T H, Cheng P et al (1993) A polygonal general cone beam reconstruction algorithm. IEEE Trans Med Imaging 12(3):486 496
70. Wang G, Lin T H, Cheng P et al (1994) Half scan cone beam X ray microtomography formula. J Scanning Microsc 16:216 220
71. Weng Y, Zeng GL, Gullberg GT (1993) A reconstruction algorithm for helical cone beam SPECT. IEEE Trans Nucl Sci 40:1092 1101
72. Yan M, Cishen Z (2005) Tilted plane Feldkamp type reconstruction algorithm for spiral cone beam CT. Med Phys 32(11):3455 3467
73. Yan X, Leahy R (1992) Cone beam tomography with circular, elliptical and spiral orbits. Phys Med Biol 37:493 506
74. Zeng GL, Gullberg GT (1992) A cone beam tomography algorithm for orthogonal circle endline orbit. Phys Med Biol 37:563 577
75. Zeng GL, Clark R, Gullberg GT (1994) Implementation of Tuy's cone beam inversion formula. Phys Med Biol 39:493 507

Chapter 8
Algebraic Reconstruction Techniques

The group of algorithms known by their initials algebraic reconstruction techniques (ARTs) is the second most popular family of reconstruction methods. However, ART techniques belong in turn to a broader methodology, which makes use of finite series expansion [4, 5, 15, 16, 18].

All approaches related to this methodology are characterised by a simplification carried out at the very beginning of the reconstruction process [5]. This simplification relies on the assumption that the reconstructed image consists of a finite number of elements. In this group of methods (unlike analytical methods), this kind of discretisation takes place before the introduction of a discrete form of algorithm. At the conceptual stage, the area of interest is divided into blocks of identical size, each of which is defined as having a uniform radiation attenuation coefficient and the geometrical centre of each block will be considered as corresponding to one pixel of the reconstructed digital image. The topology of the reconstructed image is shown in Fig. 8.1.

As can be seen from Fig. 8.1, each block in the image is identified horizontally by the coordinate $i = 1,\ldots,I$ and vertically by $j = 1,\ldots,J$. Thus, within each block of the image, the uniform attenuation coefficient can be represented by μ_{ij}.

One very important characteristic, which may persuade us to use algebraic algorithms, is that they enable us in becoming independent of the geometry of the projection system. Here, we will assume that projections are made using a parallel-beam system [1], although any other system can be considered just as easily.

Therefore, as we did when we considered analytical reconstruction methods, each projection value obtained at an angle α^p_ψ and measured at a point on the screen a distance s_l away from the axis of the projection will be represented by the discrete form of the projection function:

$$\hat{p}^p(l,\psi) \equiv p^p\left(l\Delta^p_s, \psi\Delta^p_\alpha\right), \tag{8.1}$$

where l is the detector number, in the matrix; ψ is the projection number, Δ^p_s is the distance between the individual detectors on the screen, Δ^p_α is the angle through which the tube-screen arrangement is rotated after each projection.

R. Cierniak, *X Ray Computed Tomography in Biomedical Engineering*,
DOI: 10.1007/978 0 85729 027 4 8,

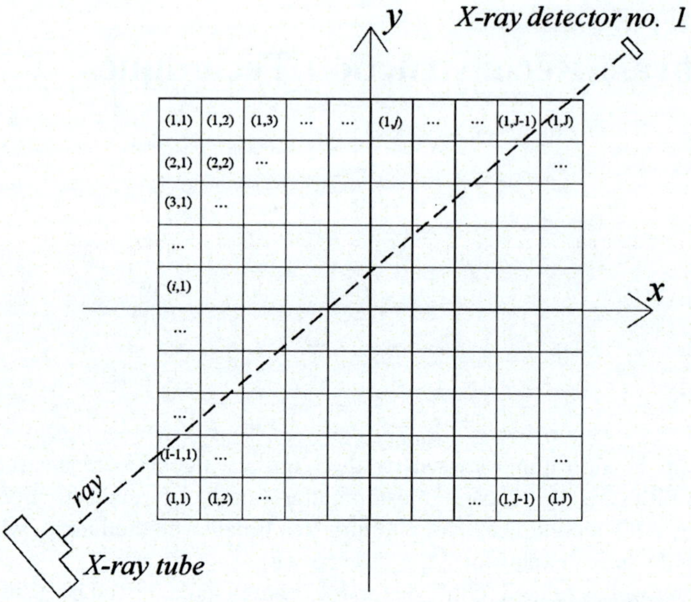

Fig. 8.1 Projection system geometry of the algebraic image reconstruction method

Assuming this approach to the topology of the reconstructed image and having available a set of projections $\psi = 1,\ldots,\Psi - 1$, each measured at points on the screen $l = -\mathrm{L}/2,\ldots,0,\ldots,(\mathrm{L}/2) - 1$ (where Ψ is the maximum number of projections and L is an even number of detectors on the screen), we are now able to formulate the image reconstruction problem for algebraic methods.

8.1 Formulation of the Algebraic Problem of Image Reconstruction from Projections

Before we consider this problem further, perhaps it is appropriate to return to the Radon transform defined earlier, in this case in its discrete form:

$$\hat{p}^p(l, \psi) \equiv R(\mu(x, y)). \tag{8.2}$$

The algebraic approach, in addition to this, assumes that a given attenuation coefficient distribution $\mu(x, y)$ can be represented approximately as a finite, linear combination of basis functions and constant coefficients [5, 18], which can be written as follows:

$$\mu(x, y) \cong \hat{\mu}(i, j) = \sum_{i=1}^{\mathrm{I}} \sum_{j=1}^{\mathrm{J}} \mu_{ij} \varrho_{ij}(x, y), \tag{8.3}$$

where $\varrho_{ij}(x,y)$ is the elements of a set of basis functions; μ_{ij} is a constant coefficient within the block (i,j); $i = 1,\ldots,\mathrm{I}; j = 1,\ldots,\mathrm{J}$.

A basis function in its simplest form might be

$$\varrho_{ij}(x,y) = \begin{cases} 1 & \text{when } (x,y) \text{ is in the block } (i,j) \\ 0 & \text{when } (x,y) \text{ is outside block } (i,j) \end{cases}, \tag{8.4}$$

but there are also other forms of this function [15].

Taking into consideration formula (8.3), we can represent Eq. 8.2 by the following relationship:

$$\hat{p}^p(l,\psi) = R(\mu(x,y)) \cong R\left(\sum_{i=1}^{\mathrm{I}}\sum_{j=1}^{\mathrm{J}} \mu_{ij}\varrho_{ij}(x,y)\right). \tag{8.5}$$

Given the linearity property of the Radon transform, this formula can be converted to:

$$\hat{p}^p(l,\psi) \cong \sum_{i=1}^{\mathrm{I}}\sum_{j=1}^{\mathrm{J}} \mu_{ij} R\left(\varrho_{ij}(x,y)\right). \tag{8.6}$$

So, for the algebraic method, the result of a projection carried out at an angle $\alpha^p = \psi\Delta_\alpha^p$ and measured at a point of the screen $s = l\Delta_s^p$, in a parallel-beam projection system, can be written

$$\hat{p}^p(l,\psi) \cong \sum_{i=1}^{\mathrm{I}}\sum_{j=1}^{\mathrm{J}} \mu_{ij}\chi_{ij}(l,\psi), \tag{8.7}$$

where the substitution

$$\chi_{ij}(l,\psi) = R\left(\varrho_{ij}(x,y)\right) \tag{8.8}$$

can be interpreted physically as the contribution of a given image block with parameters (i,j) to the formation of the projection value identified by the pair (l,ψ), measured at the screen. A description of one of the heuristic methods for determining the value $\chi_{ij}(l,\psi)$ is given below.

Bearing this in mind, i.e. the non-zero width of the radiation detector, it is easy to ascertain the set of image blocks that have an influence on the formation of the projection value $\hat{p}^p(l,\psi)$. As can be seen from Fig. 8.2a, as the ray passes through the test object (the image), all the squares through which part of the ray passes are taken into consideration. The next step is to consider the contribution made by each image block to the way in which each ray (l,ψ) passes through in the course of making a series of projections. This contribution can be calculated, for example, by counting the sub-blocks of a given block (i,j) through which the ray l of projection ψ passes, as illustrated in Fig. 8.2b (10 sub blocks).

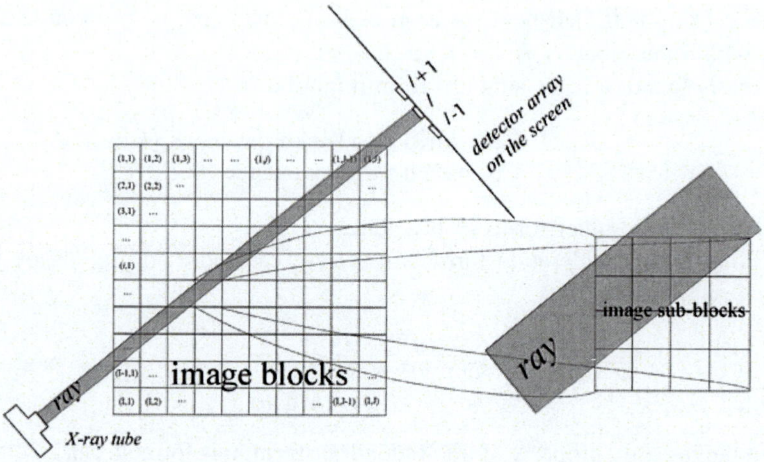

Fig. 8.2 The determination of $\chi_{ij}(l,\psi)$: **a** determination of the set of image blocks taking part in the formation of the projection value, **b** a way of determining the contribution a given image block makes to the formation of a specific projection value

The value of each contribution $\chi_{ij}(l,\psi)$ varies between 0 and 1, where a value equal to 0 means that the ray (l,ψ) does not pass through the block (i,j) and a value of 1 means that the ray passes through only that block.

The determination and normalisation of the individual contributions $\chi_{ij}(l,\psi)$, for each projection value is as follows:

$$\chi_{ij}(l,\psi) = \frac{number\_of\_sub - blocks_{ij}(l,\psi)}{\sum_{Bl} number\_of\_sub - blocks}, \tag{8.9}$$

where $number\_of\_sub - blocks_{ij}(l,\psi)$ is the number of sub-blocks in the block through which the ray (l,ψ) passes; *number of sub − blocks* is the number of sub-blocks in each block; *Bl* is the number of blocks through which the ray (l,ψ) passes.

If we know the values of $\chi_{ij}(l,\psi)$ for all projection angles $\psi = 1,\ldots, \Psi - 1$, and for all screen coordinates $l = -L/2, \ldots, 0, \ldots, (L/2) - 1$ then formula (8.7) allows us to formulate a system of linear equations and so solve the reconstruction problem using algebraic methods. This system of equations is solved with respect to μ_{ij} using various methods belonging to the whole class of ART algorithms. As the dimensionality (I × J) of the array μ_{ij} does not allow us to rewrite Eq. 8.7 in vector form, we need to transform this matrix into vector μ with dimensions $I \cdot J$. One possible way of implementing this transformation is the successive placing of the columns $j = 1,\ldots, J$ of array μ_{ij} into the vector μ. If we do the same with the projection matrix, we are able to rewrite the equation as

$$\mathbf{p} = \chi \mu, \tag{8.10}$$

where **p** is the projection vector with dimensions $L \cdot \Psi$; χ is the matrix of values $\chi_{ij}(l, \psi)$ with dimensions $L \cdot \Psi \times I \cdot J$.

At this point, the image reconstruction problem has been reduced to solving the matrix equation (8.10), that is, to estimate the value of matrix μ based on the value of matrix **p**.

The biggest advantage of the algebraic approach to the reconstruction task is that it is independent of the actual geometry of the projection system. To use an ART algorithm for projection systems other than parallel-beam systems, all we need to do is to recalculate the matrix χ. The biggest disadvantage of the approach is the complexity of the calculation caused by the enormous size of the matrix χ. For example, if we have a system with 512 radiation detectors and we make 100 projections during one revolution of the projection system, for an image with dimensions $I \times J = 256 \times 256$, the number of calculations amounts to $51{,}200 \times 65{,}536$. Fortunately, the complexity of the calculation is significantly reduced by the fact that most of the values in the matrix χ will be 0.

8.2 Algebraic Reconstruction Algorithms

The algebraic assumptions described above, especially with respect to the topology of the reconstructed image, have become the basis for an entire class of reconstruction algorithms aimed at solving the system of linear equations (8.7).

We will begin our consideration of selected algebraic reconstruction methods with the earliest approach, the basic ART algorithm, and in subsequent sub-sections, we will consider increasingly sophisticated algorithms based on it.

8.2.1 Basic ART Algorithm

Kaczmarz [20] described the fundamentals of the algebraic reconstruction technique even before the emergence of computerised tomography. In Kaczmarz's [11] original version, ART was not concerned with the problem of reconstructing an image from projections at all. However, it was identical to an algorithmic approach published much later, specifically for computed tomography.

The basic ART reconstruction algorithm is the starting point for a number of methods that use iteration to find the solution to the system of equations [5, 17, 18, 19]

$$\hat{p}_k = \chi_k^T \mu, \tag{8.11}$$

where χ_k^T is kth row of matrix χ; p_k is kth element of matrix $\mathbf{p}$; $k = 1, \ldots, L \cdot \Psi$.

To make our task easier, we will assume that the number of blocks is equal to 2, that is $I \cdot J = 2$. For this case, the equation can be written as

Fig. 8.3 A graphical interpretation of Eq. 8.12

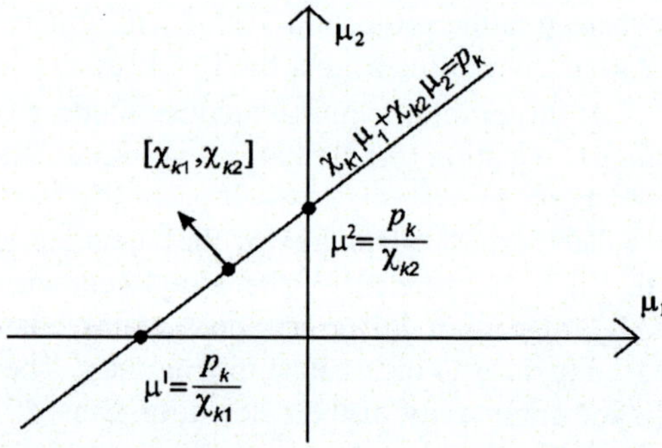

$$\chi_{k1}\mu_1 + \chi_{k2}\mu_2 = \hat{p}_k,\ k = 1,\ldots,\mathrm{L}\cdot\Psi. \tag{8.12}$$

As we can see, each of these $\mathrm{L}\cdot\Psi$ equations represents the equation of a straight line. This line can be interpreted as the set of all points on the plane (μ_1, μ_2), whose coordinates $\mu^t = [\mu_1^t, \mu_2^t]$; $t = 1, 2,\ldots,\infty$ satisfy one of Eq. 8.12. An example of one of the lines described by 8.12, together with an interpretation of its individual elements in coordinate system (μ_1, μ_2) is shown in Fig. 8.3.

We can see from Fig. 8.3 that in general, the vector χ_k is a vector normal to the hyperplane μ, that is $\chi_k \perp \mu$, the proof of which is given below.

Proof By considering the difference $\mu^{1\ \ 2}$ of the two vectors $\mu^1 = [\mu_1^1, \mu_2^1]$ and $\mu^2 = [\mu_1^2, \mu_2^2]$, fulfilling Eq. 8.11:

$$\hat{p}_k = \chi_k^{\mathrm{T}}\mu^1, \quad \text{and} \quad \hat{p}_k = \chi_k^{\mathrm{T}}\mu^2. \tag{8.13}$$

we obtain

// The difference of the vectors

$\mu^{1-2} \quad \mu^1 \quad \mu^2$

$\chi_k^{\mathrm{T}}\mu^{1-2} \quad \chi_k^{\mathrm{T}}(\mu^1 \quad \mu^2)$ Multiplying both sides by vector χ_k^{T}

$\chi_k^{\mathrm{T}}\mu^1 \quad \chi_k^{\mathrm{T}}\mu^2$

// Finally: The same $\hat{p}_k$ occurs in both instances

$\hat{p}_k \quad \hat{p}_k \quad 0$

If $\chi_k^T\mu^{1\ \ 2} = 0$, then the vector $\mu^{1\ \ 2}$, parallel to the line described by Eq. 8.12, is perpendicular to the vector χ_k. Thus, vector χ_k is perpendicular to the line. □

It is also worth noting that the scalar products occurring on the left side of each equation of the system of equations (8.12) can be written in their equivalent form:

$$\hat{p}_k = \chi_{k1}\mu_1 + \chi_{k2}\mu_2 = \|\chi_k\|\cdot\|\mu\|\cdot\cos\angle(\chi_k, \mu). \tag{8.14}$$

It follows that if individual rows χ_k of matrix χ are normalised, i.e. each of the components of the vector is divided by the length $\|\chi_k\|$ of the vector, then Eq. 8.14 can be presented in the following format:

$$\frac{\hat{p}_k}{\|\chi_k\|} = \frac{\chi_{k1}}{\|\chi_k\|}\mu_1 + \frac{\chi_{k2}}{\|\chi_k\|}\mu_2 = \|\mu\| \cdot \cos\angle(\chi_k, \mu). \tag{8.15}$$

Although, in this situation, the coefficients of the equation of the line have changed, it is clear from Fig. 8.4 that this does not affect its location on the plane.

However, the interpretation of $\frac{\hat{p}_k}{\|\chi_k\|}$ changes in a fundamental way. As follows from Eq. 8.15 and as shown in Fig. 8.5, the quantity $\frac{\hat{p}_k}{\|\chi_k\|}$ represents the shortest distance of the straight line from the origin of the coordinate system (μ_1, μ_2).

As a result of the normalisation of all the rows χ_k of matrix χ, the lengths of the vectors χ_k become $\|\chi_k\| = 1$ for all k rows. For simplicity, we will temporarily limit the number k to 2, which means that in the (μ_1, μ_2) plane we can draw two straight lines, represented by the equations:

$$\frac{\chi_{11}}{\|\chi_1\|}\mu_1 + \frac{\chi_{12}}{\|\chi_1\|}\mu_2 = \frac{\hat{p}_1}{\|\chi_1\|}, \tag{8.16}$$

$$\frac{\chi_{21}}{\|\chi_2\|}\mu_1 + \frac{\chi_{22}}{\|\chi_2\|}\mu_2 = \frac{\hat{p}_2}{\|\chi_2\|}. \tag{8.17}$$

The intersection of these two lines gives the solution of the system of equations for the pair (μ_1, μ_2). To arrive at this solution, we can start from any point on the plane $\mu^0 = [\mu_1^0, \mu_2^0]$, and project this point onto the line with index $k = 1$. Because $\|\chi_1\| = 1$, the length of the projection of vector μ^0 onto the line on which the vector χ_1 lies, is equal to $\frac{\chi_1^T}{\|\chi_1\|}\mu^0$. However, the smallest distance of vector μ^0 from the line, onto which we project it, is $\frac{\chi_1^T}{\|\chi_1\|}\mu^0 - \frac{\hat{p}_1}{\|\chi_1\|}$. To be able to make the projection, we must give direction to this scalar value by multiplying by the vector $\frac{\chi_1^T}{\|\chi_1\|}$, which gives us the vector $\left(\frac{\chi_1^T}{\|\chi_1\|}\mu^0 \frac{p_1}{\|\chi_1\|}\right)\frac{\chi_1^T}{\|\chi_1\|}$. Making this projection onto the

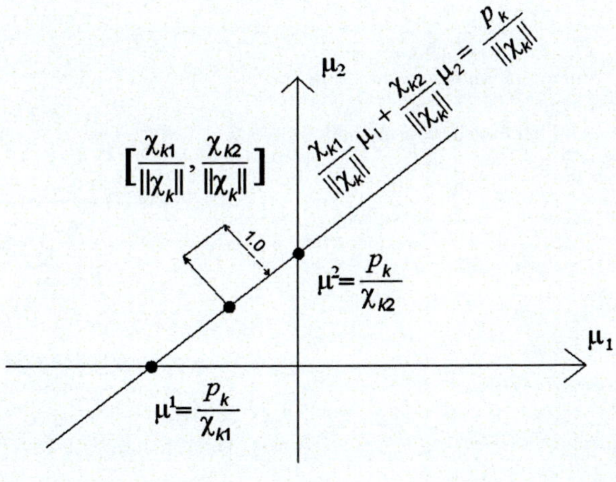

Fig. 8.4 A graphical interpretation of Eq. 8.15 after the normalisation of vector χ_k

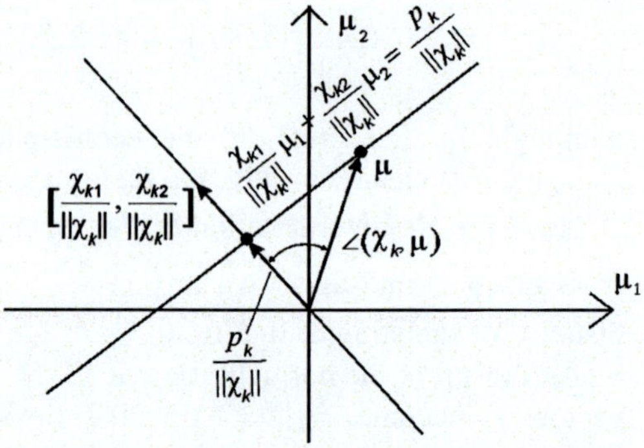

Fig. 8.5 A graphical interpretation of $\frac{\hat{p}_k}{\|\chi_k\|}$ from Eq. 8.15

line relies on the subtraction of the vector $\left(\frac{\chi_1^T}{\|\chi_1\| - \frac{p_1}{\|\chi_1\|}}\mu^0\right)\frac{\chi_1^T}{\|\chi_1\|}$ from the original value μ^0 to obtain the new value $\dot{\mu}^1$, located on the line. So, as a first step toward solving (8.10) we can rewrite

$$\dot{\mu}^1 = \mu^0 - \left(\frac{\chi_1^T}{\|\chi_1\| - \frac{\hat{p}_1}{\|\chi_1\|}}\mu^0\right)\frac{\chi_1^T}{\|\chi_1\|}\frac{\chi_1^T}{\|\chi_1\|} = \mu^0 - \frac{(\chi_1^T\mu^0 - \hat{p}_1)\chi_1^T}{\|\chi_1\|^2}. \tag{8.18}$$

A geometrical interpretation of one iteration in the ART reconstruction method is illustrated in Fig. 8.6.

After conditioning the vector $\dot{\mu}^1$ obtained in this way (a list of possible conditions is shown in Table 8.1), we use it as the input for the next step of the iteration. We will express the conditioning with the following function [18] $\mu^1 = \text{condition}(\dot{\mu}^1)$.

In subsequent steps of the ART iteration algorithm, we project the vectors μ^t onto successive hyperplanes defined by the vectors χ_k. This operation is described by the following general relationship:

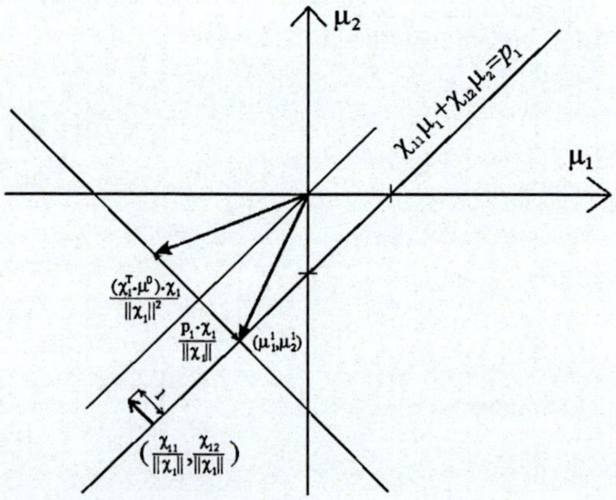

Fig. 8.6 A graphical interpretation of one iteration of the basic version of the ART reconstruction method

Table 8.1 Types of conditioning for the vectors $\dot{\mu}^t$

ART algorithm convention	Kind of relationship
Unconditioned algorithm	$\mu^t \quad condition(\dot{\mu}^t) \quad \dot{\mu}^t$
Partially conditioned algorithm	$\mu^t \quad condition(\dot{\mu}^t) \quad \begin{cases} 0 & \text{for } \dot{\mu}^t < 0 \\ \dot{\mu}^t & \text{for } \dot{\mu}^t \geq 0 \end{cases}$
Completely conditioned algorithm	$\mu^t \quad condition(\dot{\mu}^t) \quad \begin{cases} 0 & \text{for } \dot{\mu}^t < 0 \\ \dot{\mu}^t & \text{for } 0 \leq \dot{\mu}^t \leq 1 \\ 1 & \text{for } \dot{\mu}^t > 1 \end{cases}$

$$\dot{\mu}^{t+1} = \mu^t - \frac{(\chi_k^{\mathrm{T}} \mu^t - \hat{p}_k)\chi_k^{\mathrm{T}}}{\|\chi_k\|^2}, \tag{8.19}$$

where $t = 0, 1, \ldots$; χ_k and $\hat{p}_k$ are used in a periodic way, i.e.: $\hat{p}_t = \hat{p}_k, \chi_t = \chi_k$ when $k = (t \, mod \, \mathrm{I} \cdot \mathrm{J}) + 1$.

As with the first iteration, the values of the elements of the vector $\dot{\mu}^{t+1}$ are conditioned on the basis of the transformations shown in Table 8.1. After applying the condition, the vectors automatically become the vectors μ^{t+1} and during this process converge towards the optimal solution. In order to increase the accuracy of the method defined by (8.10), further iterations of the algorithm run cyclically along successive rows of the matrix χ. After reaching the last row, the calculations begin again at the first row, etc.

It is also worth stressing that the algorithm works in such a way that, at any given moment, only one of the $\mathrm{I} \cdot \mathrm{J}$ equations is satisfied and by combining Eqs. 8.11 and 8.19, we can rewrite

$$\hat{p}_{t+1} = \chi_k^{\mathrm{T}} \dot{\mu}^{t+1} = \chi_k^{\mathrm{T}} \mu^{t+1} - \frac{\chi_k^{\mathrm{T}} \mu^t - \hat{p}_k}{\|\chi_k\|^2} \chi_k^{\mathrm{T}} \chi_k. \tag{8.20}$$

This means that the $k = (t \, mod \, \mathrm{I} \cdot \mathrm{J}) + 1th-$ equation is satisfied with the tth iteration of the algorithm.

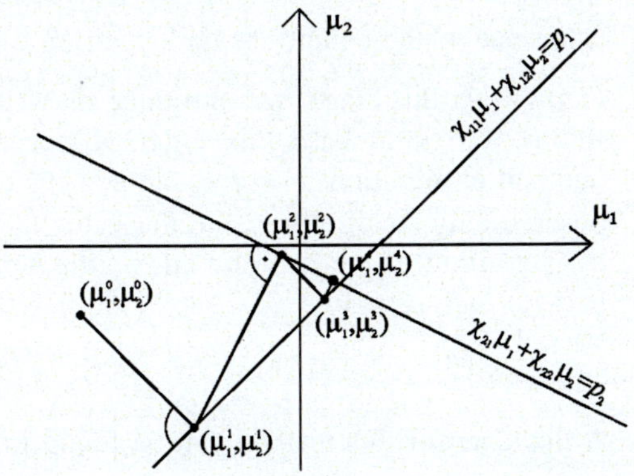

Fig. 8.7 A geometrical interpretation of successive iterations of the ART algorithm for a case where the lines are almost perpendicular

One reason why it is worth using this algorithm is the existence of lots of zeros in matrix χ. This redundancy in χ causes an overwhelming number of mutually perpendicular vectors χ_k in the $\mathrm{I} \cdot \mathrm{J}$-dimensional space and so greatly speeds up the algorithm. A geometrical interpretation of the ART method, for two dimensions only, is given in Fig. 8.7.

Finally, it is worth adding that the basic ART algorithm is rather slow in converging to a solution because of the difficulty in matching a criterion for stopping the iterative process [24]. Because the algorithm results in successive approximations to the solution, there are no guarantees of achieving the solution exactly. The stopping criterion might take into account the degree of saturation of the solution (i.e. a lack of progress in consecutive iterations) or there could be a rigid criterion where the number of iterations was pre-determined.

8.2.2 Practical Approach to the Basic ART Algorithm

Step I The first step of the algorithm is to establish the initial value of the vector $\mu^0 \in \mathbb{R}^{\mathrm{I} \cdot \mathrm{J}}$, representing the reconstructed image. We also give an initial value $t = 0$ to the parameter controlling the iteration of the algorithm.

Step II Here, we calculate the vector $\dot{\mu}^{t+1}$ from the vector μ^0, the values p_k and the kth row of matrix χ, using the iteration relationship:

$$\dot{\mu}^{t+1} = \mu^t - \frac{\left(\chi_k^{\mathrm{T}} \mu^t - \hat{p}_k\right) \chi_k^{\mathrm{T}}}{\|\chi_k\|^2},$$

where $k = (t \, mod \, \mathrm{I} \cdot \mathrm{J}) + 1$.

Step III The next step in the iteration of the vector μ^{t+1} representing the image is to take the components of the vector obtained after making the transformation:

$$\mu^{t+1} = condition\left(\dot{\mu}^{t+1}\right),$$

using one of the conditions contained in Table 8.1.

Step IV At this stage, we introduce the criterion for stopping the iterating algorithm. We could base this criterion, for example, on choosing an acceptable number of iterations $t = t_{\max}$ and/or on establishing a situation in which we observe only small changes in the value of the vector μ^{t+1} in successive steps of the algorithm. If the criterion allows the iteration process to continue, then we go back to *Step II* and let:

$$\mu^t \longleftarrow \mu^{t+1}. \tag{8.21}$$

A flowchart of this method can be found in Fig. 8.8.

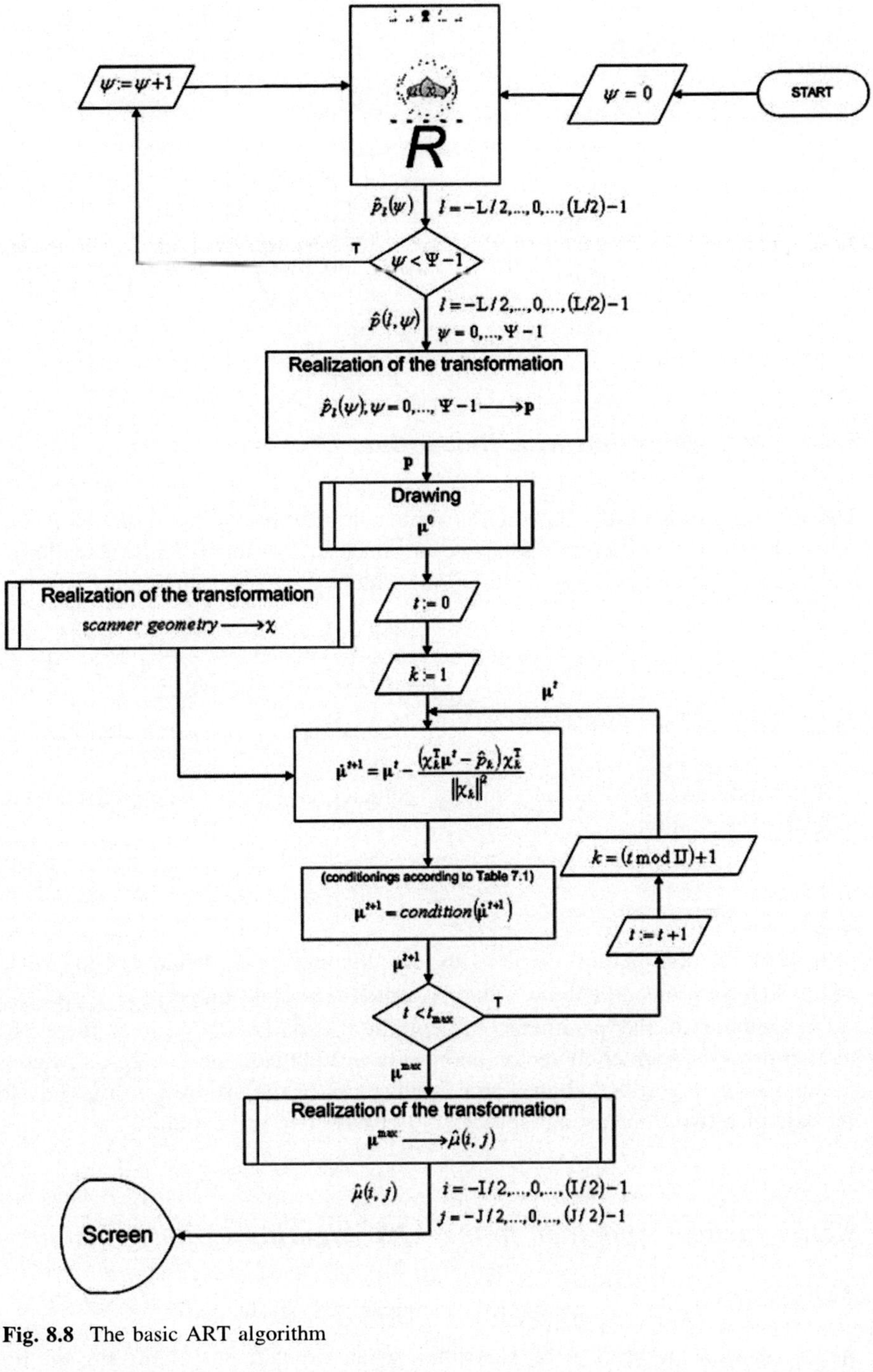

Fig. 8.8 The basic ART algorithm

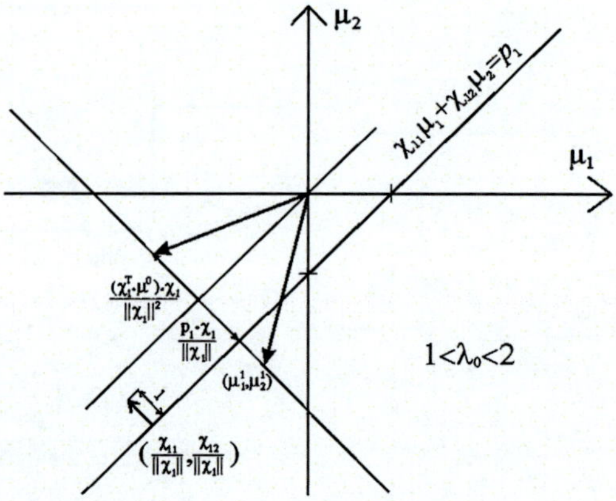

Fig. 8.9 Geometric relationships in the method with relaxation

8.2.3 ART Algorithm with Relaxation

The ART algorithm with relaxation is similar in operation to the basic ART algorithm. However, the difference is that we introduce an additional parameter called the relaxation parameter to the basic iteration formula (8.19), as follows [5, 8]:

$$\dot{\mu}^{t+1} = \mu^t - \lambda_t \frac{(\chi_k^{\mathrm{T}} \mu^t - \hat{p}_k)\chi_k^{\mathrm{T}}}{\|\chi_k\|^2}, \tag{8.22}$$

where λ_t is the tth element of a sequence of relaxation parameters $\{\lambda_t\}_{t=0}^{\infty}$; $k = (t \bmod \mathrm{I} \cdot \mathrm{J}) + 1$.

The condition placed on the values of sequence $\{\lambda_t\}_{t=0}^{\infty}$ can be expressed by the following inequality:

$$\upsilon_1 \leq \lambda_t \leq 2 - \upsilon_2, \tag{8.23}$$

where $\upsilon_1, \upsilon_2 > 0$.

In essence, this method involves the lengthening or shortening of the vector with which we project the initial vector μ^t onto the straight line $\hat{p}_{t+1} = \chi_{t+1}^{\mathrm{T}} \dot{\mu}^{t+1}$. If the magnitude of the parameter lies within the range $0 < \lambda_t < 1$, there is a shortening of the correction vector, and if it is within the range $1 < \lambda_t < 2$, there is a lengthening. Figure 8.9 shows the consequences of the use of λ_t in Eq. 8.24 for the case of a two-dimensional space (μ_1, μ_2) with two projections.

8.2.4 Practical Approach to the ART Algorithm with Relaxation

A systematic account of the algorithm is presented below.

Step I As with the basic ART algorithm, when we start this algorithm, the first step is to determine the initial value of the vector $\boldsymbol{\mu}^0 \in \mathbb{R}^{\mathrm{I \cdot J}}$, representing the image reconstructed from the projections. We also assign an initial value $t = 0$ to the parameter controlling the iteration of the algorithm.

Step II We now determine the vector $\dot{\mu}^{t+1}$ from the vector μ^0, the values p_k and the kth row of matrix χ, using the iteration relationship:

$$\dot{\mu}^{t+1} = \mu^t - \lambda_t \frac{(\chi_k^T \mu^t - \hat{p}_k)\chi_k^T}{\|\chi_k\|^2},$$

where $k = (t \bmod \mathrm{I} \cdot \mathrm{J}) + 1$; λ_t is the tth element of a sequence of relaxation parameters $\{\lambda_t\}_{t=0}^{\infty}$ (this value changes during the iteration process); where $\upsilon_1 \leq \lambda_t \leq 2 - \upsilon_2$ for each t; $\upsilon_1 > 0$, $\upsilon_2 > 0$.

Step III The next step in the iteration of the vector μ^{t+1} representing the image is to take the components of the vector obtained after making the transformation:

$$\mu^{t+1} = condition\left(\dot{\mu}^{t+1}\right),$$

using one of the conditions contained in Table 8.1.

Step IV At this stage, we introduce the criterion for stopping the iterating algorithm. We could base this criterion, for example, on choosing an acceptable number of iterations $t = t_{\max}$ and/or on establishing a situation in which we observe only small changes in the value of the vector μ^{t+1} in successive steps of the algorithm. If the criterion allows the iteration process to continue, then we go back to *Step II* and let:

$$\mu^t \longleftarrow \mu^{t+1}.$$

A flowchart of this method can be found in Fig. 8.10.

8.2.5 Chaotic ART Algorithm

The chaotic ART algorithm is an asynchronous method of reconstructing an image from projections [6]. The description and proof of the convergence of this algorithm can be found in the paper [13]. We can begin a description of the relationships in this reconstruction method with the basic iteration formula:

$$\forall_k \dot{\mu}^{t,k} = \mu^{t \;\; 1} - \lambda \frac{(\chi_k^T \mu^{t \;\; 1} - \hat{p}_k)\chi_k^T}{\|\chi_k\|^2}, \tag{8.24}$$

where χ_1^T is the kth row of matrix χ; p_k is the kth element of matrix $\mathbf{p}$; $\mu \in \mathbb{R}^{\mathrm{I \cdot J}}$ is the matrix of the image divided into blocks; $0 < \lambda < 2$ is the relaxation parameter; $k \in K_t$ is an element of the set $K_t \subset \{1, 2, \ldots, \mathrm{I} \cdot \mathrm{J}\}$, which is a component part of the chaotic set $K = \{K_t\}_{t=0}^{\infty}$.

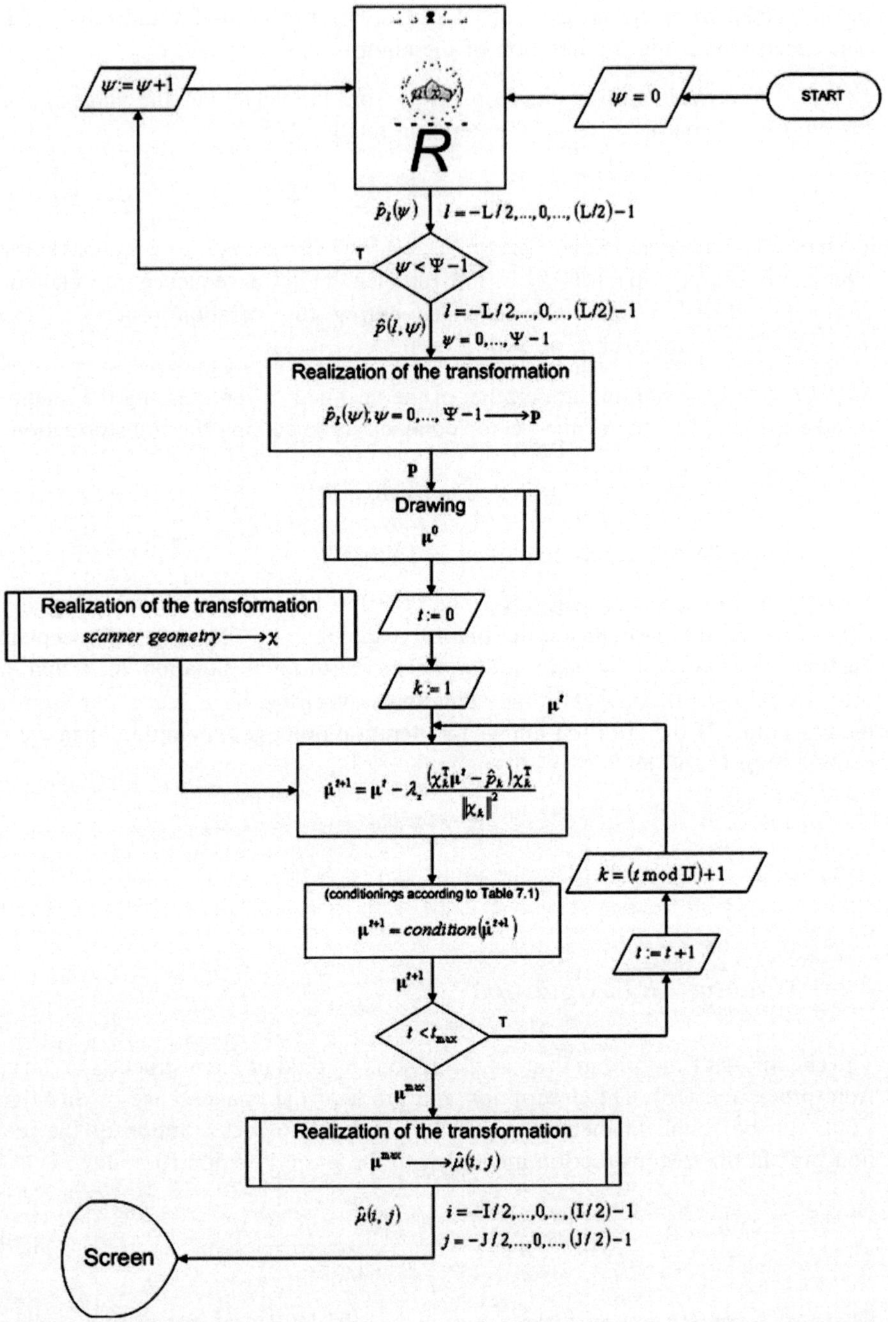

Fig. 8.10 ART algorithm with relaxation

The chaotic way in which the elements of the sets $K_t \subset \{1, 2, \ldots, \mathrm{I} \cdot \mathrm{J}\}$ are selected means that the following condition is satisfied:

$$\lim_{t \to \infty} \sup K_t = \{1, 2, \ldots, \mathrm{I} \cdot \mathrm{J}\}. \tag{8.25}$$

In other words, each of the rows of matrices χ and $\mathbf{p}$ occurs in the sets K_t in total an infinite number of times.

The next value of μ^t in the whole recursive sequence, as it approaches the optimal solution, is calculated on the basis of the weighted sum:

$$\mu^t = \sum_{k \in K_t} w_k^t \dot{\mu}^{t,k}, \tag{8.26}$$

where the weighting of this sum satisfies the equation:

$$\sum_{k \in K_t} w_k^t = 1. \tag{8.27}$$

The principal feature of the chaotic algorithm, differentiating it from the basic ART algorithm, is that the calculation of the next value of the solution is based on the whole set of rows of matrices χ and $\mathbf{p}$. In each step of the algorithm, a different set of these rows is chosen. In this case, this is done in a chaotic way.

8.2.6 Practical Approach to the Chaotic ART Algorithm

A systematic account of the algorithm is presented below.

Step I An arbitrary starting value is chosen for the matrix $\mu^0 \in \mathbb{R}^{\mathrm{I} \cdot \mathrm{J}}$.

Step II For each t, the sets $K_t \subset \{1, 2, \ldots, \mathrm{I} \cdot \mathrm{J}\}$ are selected chaotically. In the case of a finite number of iterations, it is necessary to ensure that all rows of the matrices χ and $\mathbf{p}$ occur in all the sets K_t, in total a sufficiently large number of times.

Step III Each iteration of the algorithm makes use of all the rows of the matrices χ and $\mathbf{p}$, whose indices belong to the current set K_t:

$$\dot{\mu}^{t,k} = \mu^{t\ 1} - \lambda \frac{(\chi_k^{\mathrm{T}} \mu^{t\ 1} - \hat{p}_k)\chi_k^{\mathrm{T}}}{\|\chi_k\|^2}.$$

Step IV With a set of values $\dot{\mu}^{t,k}$; $k \in K_t$ we can find a solution to the system of equations in the tth step:

$$\mu^t = \sum_{k \in K_t} w_k^t \dot{\mu}^{t,k},$$

where

$$\sum_{k \in K_t} w_k^t = 1.$$

Step V This repeats the sequence of actions starting from *Step III*, until $t = t_{\max}$.

A flowchart of this method can be found in Fig. 8.11.

8.3 Iterative Coordinate Descent Algorithm

The reconstruction algorithm known commercially as the adaptive statistical iterative reconstruction (ASIR) method is based on an approach presented comprehensively in [27] the iterative coordinate descent (ICD) algorithm. The main distinguishing feature of this method is that it takes into consideration the statistical nature of the X-ray intensity measurements obtained from the scanner. This results in an effective reduction in the level of noise in the reconstructed image and thus an improved low-contrast resolution of the scanners in which the reconstruction algorithm is applied. As we know, the low-contrast resolution depends on the radiation dose used during a scan. The greater the radiation intensity, the sharper the image is, and vice versa [14]. With this approach, it becomes possible to reduce the radiation dose absorbed by the patient while maintaining a reasonable value of low-contrast resolution for the apparatus.

The method discussed here actually makes use of two ways to describe the geometry of the projection system: that used in analytical reconstruction methods, and that used in algebraic techniques. However, we describe the algorithm here, in this chapter, because the main methodological burden of the algorithm is situated in the stage where the image reconstruction is carried out algebraically.

8.3.1 The Geometry of the Projection System in 3D Space

This approach to image reconstruction is related in principle to the projection system geometry discussed in the part of Sect. 7.3 concerned with the tube-detector-table system. The main difference in this algebraic method is its treatment of the geometry of the reconstructed image. The algorithm here is designed for spiral cone-beam scanners, so the geometry of the projection system has to be changed significantly as compared to that given in Sect. 8.1.

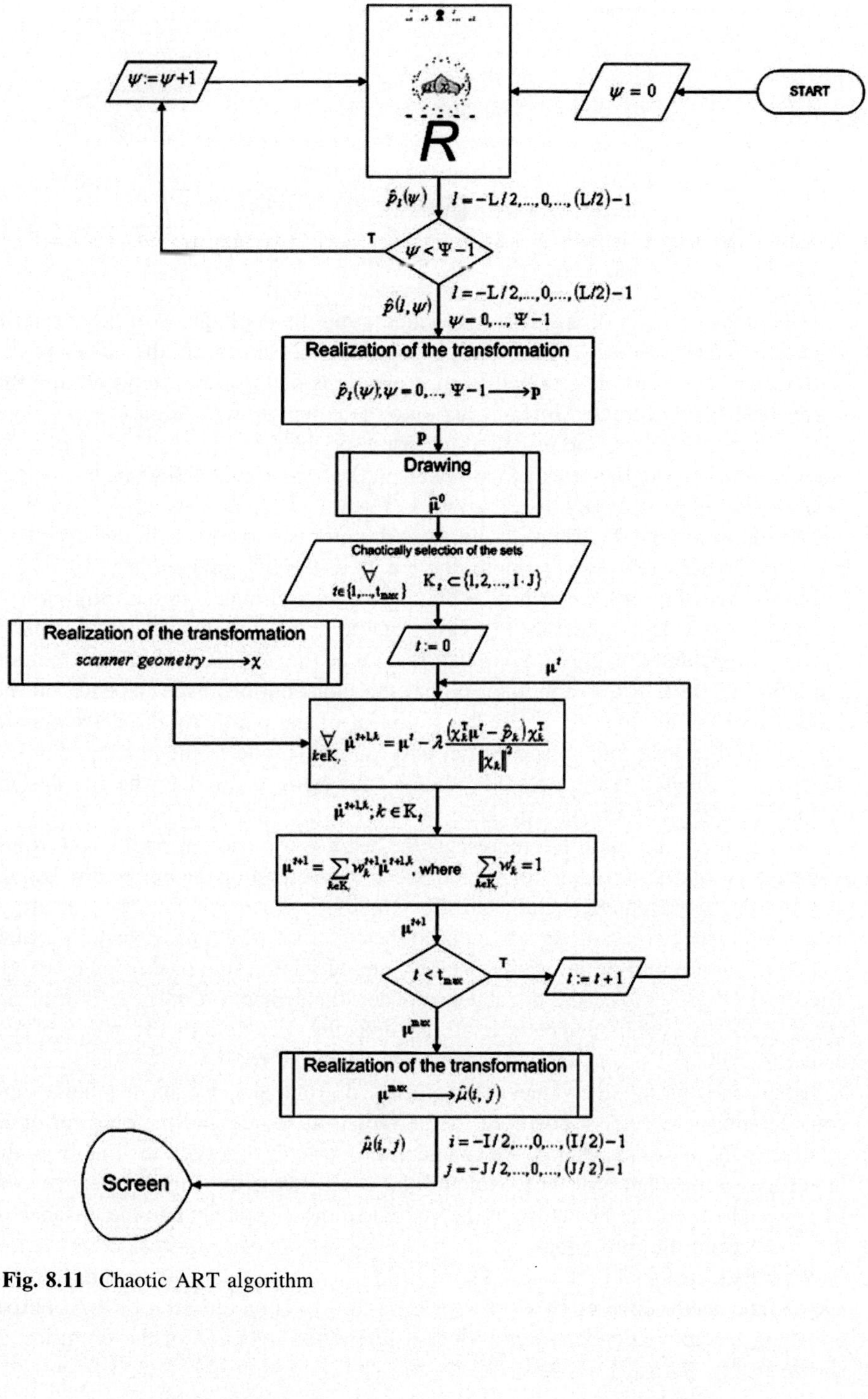

Fig. 8.11 Chaotic ART algorithm

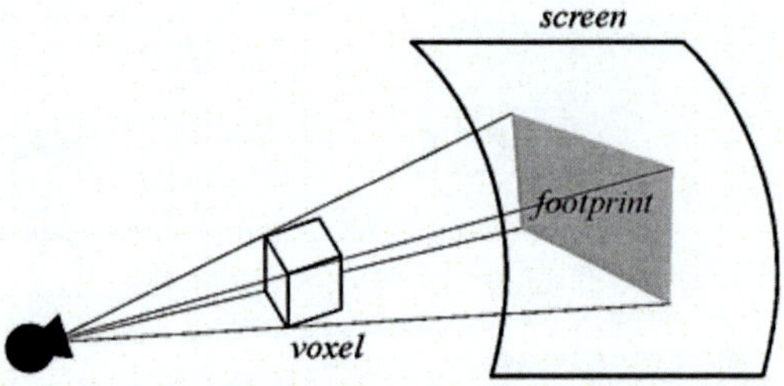

Fig. 8.12 A voxel projection onto the detector array

In the paper [27], a different way of calculating the coefficients of the χ matrix from that given in Sect. 8.1 has been proposed. In this approach, the values of the matrix elements χ are determined from projections of the cubes, representing the voxels of the reconstructed image, cast onto the detector array. Figure 8.12 shows such a voxel projection, the so-called footprint, on the detector array. Note that the index m determining the order of the voxels in the reconstructed 3D image changes as follows: $m = 1, \ldots, \mathrm{I}, \mathrm{I}+1, \ldots, \mathrm{I}\cdot\mathrm{J}, \mathrm{I}\cdot\mathrm{J}+1\ldots, \mathrm{I}\cdot\mathrm{J}\cdot\mathrm{N}$ (using the notation introduced in Sect. 3.4), where I and J are the numbers of pixels in the x y plane and N is the number of layers along the z axis in the 3D image.

In this algorithm, the contribution that a given voxel makes to the formation of the projection value, reflecting the value of the corresponding element of the χ matrix, is calculated using an approach known as the 3D distance-driven method [7]. What matters in this approach is that the contribution made depends on the surface area of the detector under the footprint of the pixel. As the detectors are 2D, we need to take into consideration two footprints, one in the plane parallel to the x y coordinate system and the other in the plane parallel to the y z system (x z). Examples of footprints in these two planes are shown in Fig. 8.13.

In Fig. 8.13, $\mathrm{D_c}$ and $\mathrm{D_r}$ represent the widths of the channels and rows, respectively of the detector for which we are calculating the projection value; $\mathrm{d_{wc}}$ and $\mathrm{d_{wr}}$ represent the widths of the voxel's footprint on the detector array, measured, respectively, along a tangent to the curve on which the detector channel is located (at the mid-point of the detector) and along the line of the detector row. The diagram also shows the distances between the projection of the centre of the voxel onto the screen and centre of the detector, i.e. $\mathrm{d_{vc}}$ (in the plane of the detector channel) and d_{vr} (in the plane of the detector row).

When calculating the values of $\mathrm{d_{wc}}$, $\mathrm{d_{wr}}$, $\mathrm{d_{vc}}$ and $\mathrm{d_{vr}}$, we have to take into consideration, the current positions of the radiation source and the detector array relative to the voxel m. That is, we consider the angle α_{xy} between the line from the tube focus to the centre of the voxel and the x- or y-axis, the angle α_z between the line from the focus to the centre of the voxel and the x y plane, and the distance of the voxel from the tube focus.

With these values $\mathrm{D_c}$, $\mathrm{d_{wc}}$, $\mathrm{d_{vc}}$, $\mathrm{D_r}$, $\mathrm{d_{wr}}$ and $\mathrm{d_{vr}}$ we can then calculate the area of a specific detector covered by the footprint of the voxel on the detector array. First, however, for convenience, we introduce a "flattened" version of the footprint, as shown in Fig. 8.14 [7].

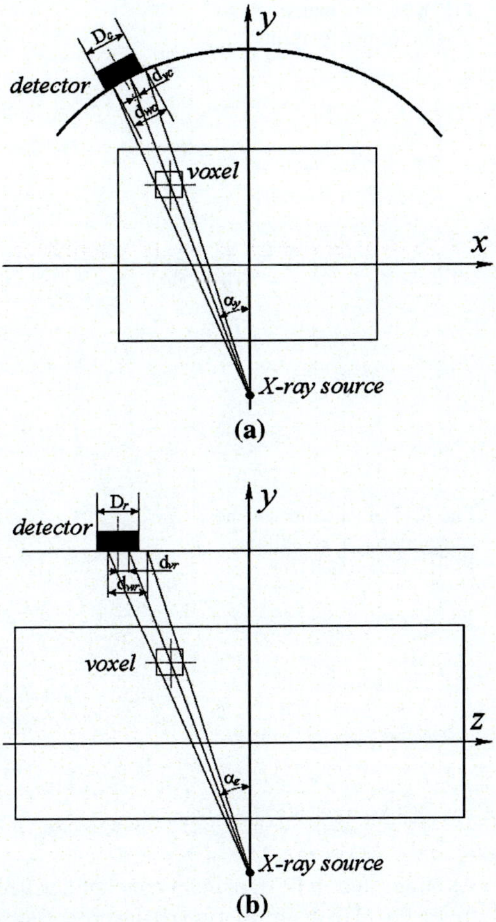

Fig. 8.13 Voxel footprint **a** aligned along the detector channels of the array, **b** aligned along the detector rows of the array

This simplified form of the voxel footprint makes it easier to approximate the shaded area shown in the diagram using the overlapping segments d_{wc} and d_{vc} in one direction, and d_{wr} and d_{vr} in the other. From Fig. 8.15, we can calculate the joint contribution of these segments in each of these dimensions, using the following formula [27]:

$$\Delta = \frac{D + d_w}{2} - |d_v|. \tag{8.28}$$

This measure obviously makes sense if there is partial coverage of the segments. However, we also need to take into account other instances, such as when the segments do not touch, or when one segment is completely contained inside another, using the following formula:

$$\Delta = \min\left[\max\left[0, \frac{D + d_w}{2} - |d_v|\right], \min\,[D, d_w]\right]. \tag{8.29}$$

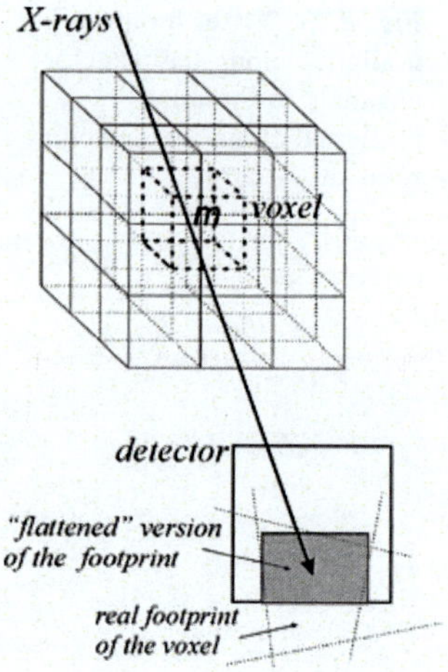

Fig. 8.14 A "flattened" version of the footprint

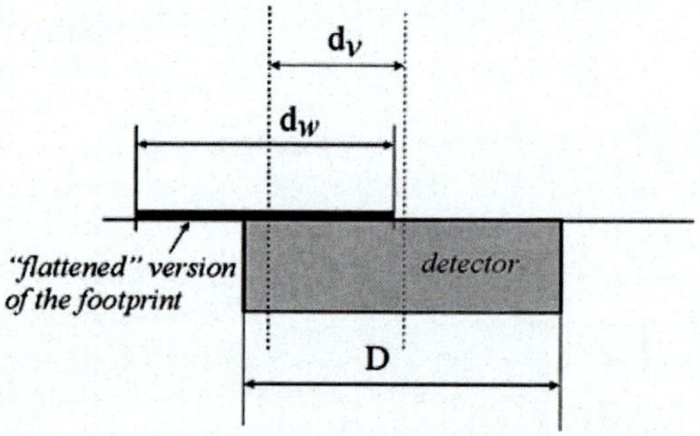

Fig. 8.15 Evaluation of the contribution of a voxel in overlapping a detector

As suggested in [27], using a concept derived from [7], the overall contribution of a given voxel to the formation of the projection value can be determined by the product of the areas covered, normalised by the respective D quantities in the channel and the row dimensions, multiplied by $\frac{\Delta_x}{\cos\alpha_{xy}\cdot\cos\alpha_z}$ (assuming that $\Delta_x = \Delta_y = \Delta_z$). This last factor corrects for the inclination of the beam passing from the tube focus through the centre of the voxel. So, finally, we have the matrix element χ for the kth projection measurement of the mth voxel in the reconstructed 3D image:

$$\chi_{km} = \frac{\Delta_x}{\cos\alpha_y \cdot \cos\alpha_z} \cdot \frac{\min\left[\max\left[0, \frac{\mathrm{D_r}+\mathrm{d_{wr}}}{2} + |\mathrm{d_{vr}}|\right], \min[\mathrm{D_r}, \mathrm{d_{wr}}]\right]}{\mathrm{D_r}} \cdot \frac{\min\left[\max\left[0, \frac{\mathrm{D_c}+\mathrm{d_{wc}}}{2} + |\mathrm{d_{vc}}|\right], \min[\mathrm{D_c}, \mathrm{d_{wc}}]\right]}{\mathrm{D_c}}. \tag{8.30}$$

Note also that in Eq. 8.30, α_y is used to represent a version of the angle α_{xy} restricted within the range ±45°, as follows:

$$\alpha_y = \left(\alpha_{xy} + \frac{\pi}{4}\right) mod\ \frac{\pi}{4} - \frac{\pi}{4}. \tag{8.31}$$

8.3.2 *Formulation of the Reconstruction Problem in Terms of Probability*

We will start this algorithm by assuming that the most appropriate statistical model to describe the number of photons leaving the X-ray tube in a given equal time interval is the Poisson distribution. This defines the probability of recording the number of X-ray photons λ at the focus of the tube as follows:

$$P(\Lambda = \lambda) = \frac{\lambda^{*\lambda}}{\lambda!} e^{\ \lambda^*}, \tag{8.32}$$

where λ^* is the expected value of a random variable Λ.

As we know from Chap. 4 (see Eq. 4.12), the projection value $\hat{p}$ measured at a given angle of rotation α_ψ of the projection system by a given detector l is determined by the following relationship:

$$\hat{p}(l, \psi) = \ln\left(\frac{I_0}{\mathrm{I}}\right) \tag{8.33}$$

where I_0 is the intensity of radiation emitted by the tube (it is assumed that this can be determined accurately, by preliminary calibration of the projection system); I is the intensity of the radiation after passing through the test object.

Transforming formula (8.33) and adjusting the indices by taking into account the algebraic reconstruction problem formulated in Eq. 8.11, we obtain

$$I_k = I_0 e^{\ \hat{p}_k}, \tag{8.34}$$

where

$$\hat{p}_k = \sum_{m=1}^{\mathrm{I \cdot J}} \chi_{km} \mu_m. \tag{8.35}$$

Assuming that the radiation intensity measured after passing through the test object is proportional to the number of photons recorded by the detector during the projection $\hat{p}_k$, and that this measurement also depends on the expected (average) attenuation coefficients μ^*_m, we obtain

$$I_k \propto \lambda_k^* = \lambda_0 e^{\sum_{m\ 1}^{\mathrm{I \cdot J}} \chi_{km} \mu_m^*}. \tag{8.36}$$

On the other hand, the number of radiation quanta passing through the patient's body and arriving at the detector during the projection $\hat{p}_k$ is dictated by the statistics from Eq. 8.32, which can be rewritten as follows

$$P(\Lambda_k = \lambda_k) = \frac{\lambda_k^{*\lambda_k}}{\lambda_k!} e^{\lambda_k^*}, \tag{8.37}$$

where λ^*_k is defined by relationship (8.36) and all the random variables Λ_k are independent.

The probability in Eq. 8.37 can be regarded as a conditional probability, by assuming that the expected value is equal to λ^*_k:

$$P(\Lambda_k = \lambda_k | \lambda_k^*) = \frac{\lambda_k^{*\lambda_k}}{\lambda_k!} e^{\lambda_k^*}. \tag{8.38}$$

Hence, if the expected number of recorded photons for each projection k is λ^*_k, the conditional probability of a given number of photons passing through during all the projections will be

$$P(\Lambda = \lambda | \lambda^*) = \prod_{k=1}^{L\cdot\Psi} \frac{\lambda_k^{*\lambda_k}}{\lambda_k!} e^{\lambda_k^*}, \tag{8.39}$$

where $\Lambda = [\Lambda_k]$; $\lambda = [\lambda_k]$; $\lambda^* = [\lambda_k^*]$.

Substituting relationship (8.36) into Eq. 8.39, we obtain the following formula:

$$P(\Lambda = \lambda | \lambda^*) = \prod_{k=1}^{L\cdot\Psi} \frac{\left(\lambda_0 e^{\sum_{m=1}^{I\cdot J} \chi_{km}\mu_m^*}\right)^{\lambda_k}}{\lambda_k!} e^{\lambda_0 e^{\sum_{m=1}^{I\cdot J} \chi_{km}\mu_m^*}} = P(\Lambda = \lambda | \mu^*), \tag{8.40}$$

where $\mu^* = [\mu_k^*]$.

The resulting probability measure is determined by the expected values of the attenuation coefficients μ_k^* in individual homogeneous blocks of the image. Based on Eq. 8.40, we can devise a class of reconstruction algorithms known in the literature as maximum-likelihood (ML) estimation methods [22]. In these methods, we manipulate the values of μ_k^* so as to maximise the probability defined in Eq. 8.40, for measured values of λ_k. Unfortunately, the use of this method often leads to instability in the reconstruction process [25]. One way to counteract these negative effects is to introduce a stabilising factor (referred to in the literature as a regularisation term) into the reconstruction method. This usually defines *a priori* the structure of the reconstructed image and is intended to inhibit oscillations in the reconstruction process and accelerate the convergence of the algorithm to a solution. The whole expression to be optimised at this point consists of two terms: the principal term (the basis for the maximum-likelihood method) and the regularisation term (*a priori* information about the reconstructed image). Reconstruction methods based on such a complex optimisation criterion are known in the literature as maximum *a posteriori* (MAP) methods [3, 9]. The theoretical basis for these methods is the Bayesian model, which in this case looks like this

$$P(\mu^* | \Lambda = \lambda) = \frac{P(\Lambda \cap \mu^*)}{P(\Lambda)} = \frac{P(\mu^* \cap \Lambda)}{P(\Lambda)} = \frac{P(\Lambda = \lambda | \mu^*)}{P(\Lambda)} P(\mu^*). \tag{8.41}$$

Equation (8.41) links the conditional probability $P(\Lambda = \lambda|\mu^*)$ with the conditional probability $P(\mu^*|\Lambda = \lambda)$. The relationship between the probabilities $P(\Lambda = \lambda|\mu^*)$ and $P(\mu^*|\Lambda = \lambda)$ can be represented in another way, by taking the logarithm of both sides. This gives us:

$$\ln P(\mu^*|\Lambda = \lambda) = \ln P(\Lambda = \lambda|\mu^*) + \ln P(\mu^*) - \ln P(\Lambda). \tag{8.42}$$

Furthermore, when considering that we are optimising by searching for the best solution using gradient methods, i.e. by differentiating the optimisation criterion with respect to the variables μ_k, we can eliminate the $\ln P(\Lambda)$ term on the right hand side of Eq. 8.42 [23]. As a result, estimating the values μ_k^* will take place *a posteriori* by solving the following optimisation problem:

$$\mu^*_{\max} = \arg\min_{\mu^*}(\ln P(\Lambda = \lambda|\mu^*) + \ln P(\mu^*)). \tag{8.43}$$

Let us consider, then, the first component of the optimisation criterion, which after substituting Eq. 8.39 becomes:

$$\begin{aligned}
&\ln P(\Lambda = \lambda|\lambda^*) \\
&= \sum_{k=1}^{L\cdot\Psi} \ln\left(\frac{\left(\lambda_0 e^{\sum_{m=1}^{I\cdot J}\chi_{km}\mu^*_m}\right)^{\lambda_k}}{\lambda_k!} e^{\lambda_0 e^{\sum_{m=1}^{I\cdot J}\chi_{km}\mu^*_m}}\right) \\
&= \sum_{k=1}^{L\cdot\Psi}\left(\lambda_k \ln\lambda_0 - \lambda_k\sum_{m=1}^{I\cdot J}\chi_{km}\mu^*_m - \ln(\lambda_k!) - \lambda_0 e^{\sum_{m=1}^{I\cdot J}\chi_{km}\mu^*_m}\right).
\end{aligned} \tag{8.44}$$

If at this point, we represent the projection values that would result from the determination of the expected values μ_m^* by

$$\hat{p}^*_k = \sum_{m=1}^{I\cdot J}\chi_{km}\hat{\mu}^*_m, \tag{8.45}$$

then Eq. 8.44 can be converted into the following form:

$$\ln P(\Lambda = \lambda|\lambda^*) = \sum_{k=1}^{L\cdot\Psi}\left(\lambda_k \ln\,\lambda_0 - \lambda_k\hat{p}^*_k - \ln\,(\lambda_k!) - \lambda_0 e^{\hat{p}^*_k}\right). \tag{8.46}$$

Expanding the $\lambda_0 e^{\hat{p}^*_k}$ component in Eq. 8.46 about the values:

$$\hat{p}_k = \ln\left(\frac{I_0}{I_k}\right) = \ln\left(\frac{\lambda_0}{\lambda_k}\right) \tag{8.47}$$

into a second-order Taylor series and taking into consideration $\Delta\hat{p}_k = \hat{p}^*_k - \hat{p}_k$, we obtain the following relationship:

$$\ln P(\Lambda = \lambda|\lambda^*) \approx \sum_{k=1}^{\mathrm{L}\cdot\Psi}\left(-\frac{\lambda_k}{2}\left(\hat{p}_k^* - \hat{p}_k\right)^2 + \lambda_k \ln\left(\lambda_0\right) - \ln\left(\lambda_k!\right) - \lambda_k\left(1 + \ln\frac{\lambda}{\lambda_k}\right)\right). \tag{8.48}$$

It should be stressed that the values $\hat{p}_k$ are associated with actual measurements of the intensity of the X-rays after passing through the test object.

A form of Eq. 8.48, which will be more useful later, is:

$$\ln P(\Lambda = \lambda|\lambda^*) \approx \sum_{k=1}^{\mathrm{L}\cdot\Psi}\left(-\frac{\lambda_k}{2}\left(\hat{p}_k^* - \hat{p}_k\right)^2 + fun(\lambda_k)\right), \tag{8.49}$$

where

$$fun(\lambda_k) = \lambda_k \ln\left(\lambda_0\right) - \ln\left(\lambda_k!\right) - \lambda_k\left(1 + \ln\frac{\lambda}{\lambda_k}\right). \tag{8.50}$$

is a function independent of $\hat{\mu}_k$.

By taking Eq. 8.45 into consideration, Eq. 8.49 can also be represented by the following matrix form:

$$\ln P(\Lambda = \lambda|\lambda^*) - \frac{1}{2}(\chi\mu^* - \mathbf{p})^{\mathrm{T}}\mathbf{D}(\chi\mu^* - \mathbf{p}) + fun(\lambda), \tag{8.51}$$

where $\mathbf{D}$ is a diagonal matrix:

$$\mathbf{D} = \begin{bmatrix} d_1 & 0 & \cdots & 0 \\ 0 & d_2 & \cdots & 0 \\ \vdots & \vdots & \ddots & \vdots \\ 0 & 0 & \cdots & d_{\mathrm{L}\cdot\Psi} \end{bmatrix} = \begin{bmatrix} \lambda_1 & 0 & \cdots & 0 \\ 0 & \lambda_2 & \cdots & 0 \\ \vdots & \vdots & \ddots & \vdots \\ 0 & 0 & \cdots & \lambda_{\mathrm{L}\cdot\Psi} \end{bmatrix}. \tag{8.52}$$

In addition, it is assumed [26] that

$$d_k = \lambda_k = \lambda_0 e^{\ \hat{p}_k} \cong \frac{1}{\sigma_{\hat{p}_k}}. \tag{8.53}$$

where $\sigma_{\hat{p}_k}$ are the variances of the projection measurements $\hat{p}_k$.

Therefore, having formulated the ML term, it is now time to determine the form of the regularisation term. A very popular image-processing tool for regularising optimisation criteria is Markov random fields (MRF).

To begin with, let us define the concept of the random field as a set of random variables $S = \{S_m, m \in M\}$, where $M = \{m = (x, y);\ 0 \le x \le \mathrm{I} - 1;\ 0 \le y \le \mathrm{J}-1\}$ [10]. The digital image $\mu = \{\mu_m, m \in M\}$ can be regarded as an implementation of the random field S, that is, as a set of random variables associated with the lattice M [12].

Defining the immediate neighbourhood of the pixel m as the set $N(m) \subset M^m$; $M^m = M - \{m\}$ as the set of all neighbouring sites of the pixel $m \in M$, a given random field is a Markov random field if

1 For all $m \in M$, $P(\mu_m) > 0$,

2. For all $m \in M$, $P\left(\mu_m \middle| \mu_{N(m)}\right) = P(\mu_m | \mu_m : m \in N(m))$, where $m \in M^m$ and $\mu_{N(m)} = \{\mu_m\}$.

This second condition is known as the Markovianity and it means that the probability that a pixel has a given value depends only on the image elements immediately adjacent to that pixel.

One of the properties of MRFs is that it can be defined by the global Gibbs distribution, which takes the following form

$$P(\mu_m) = \frac{1}{Z} e^{\ E(\mu_m)}, \tag{8.54}$$

where

$$Z = \sum_{\mu_m \in S} e^{\ E(\mu_m)}, \tag{8.55}$$

is known as the partition function or normalising constant and $E(\mu_m)$ is the energy function.

The Gibbs distribution is related to the concept of a set of cliques C, i.e. appropriate configurations of voxels connected to each other in a lattice, where the members of a clique are statistically dependent on each other. It is important that each pair of a given clique is immediately adjacent. There are several types of clique, depending on the number of pixels in the clique: i.e. first-order clique, second-order clique, etc., which are defined as:

$$C_1 \equiv M = \{m : m \in M\}, \tag{8.56}$$

for the first-order clique,

$$C_2 \equiv \{(m, m) : m, m \in M, m \neq m, m \in N(m), m \in N(m)\}, \tag{8.57}$$

for the second-order clique.

A clique of type C_2 with a 26-pixel neighbourhood in 3D space, is shown in Fig. 8.16.

In this case, the definition of the energy in Eq. 8.54 can be represented by:

$$E(\mu) = \sum_{c \in C} V_c(\mu_m : m \in C), \tag{8.58}$$

where the function $V_c(\cdot)$ defines the clique potentials in clique C.

We can see from formula (8.43) that we are interested in the logarithm of the probability (8.54). This is represented as follows (taking into consideration the expected values of the attenuation coefficients in the reconstructed image):

$$\ln P(\hat{\mu}_m^*) = -\ln Z - \sum_{c \in C} V_c(\hat{\mu}_m : m \in C). \tag{8.59}$$

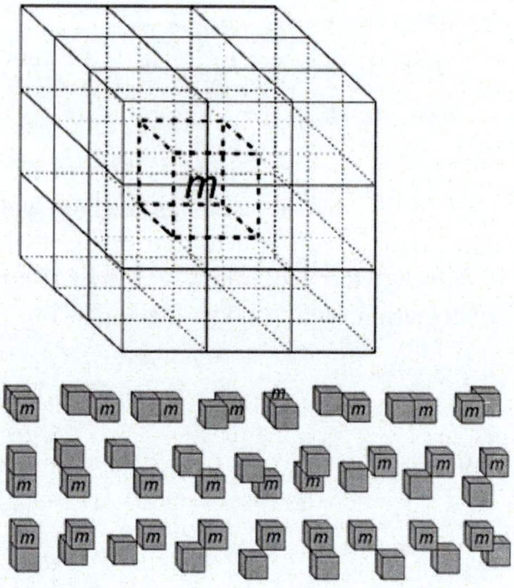

Fig. 8.16 A clique with 26 nearest neighbours

As gradient methods are used in the reconstruction algorithm, the $-\ln Z$ component can be omitted, as a normalising constant.

In the paper [2], formulating the generalised Gaussian MRF (GGMRF) reconstruction method, the following form of the logarithm of the probability from Eq. 8.59 (referring to the relationship resulting from the Gibbs distribution), has been proposed:

$$\ln P\left(\hat{\mu}_m^*\right) = -\frac{1}{fun(\sigma)} \sum_{m,m \in C} V_\sigma\left(\hat{\mu}_m^* - \hat{\mu}_m^*\right), \tag{8.60}$$

where $m, m = 1, \ldots, \mathrm{I} \cdot \mathrm{J}$; $fun(\cdot)$ is a monotone increasing function; σ is an empirically determined scalar and controls the reconstructed prior image in the neighbourhood of a given voxel, taking into consideration the noise model in the image (methods of estimating the value of σ are given in [21]); $V_\sigma(\cdot)$ is the potential function, penalising local differences between neighbouring voxels in the image.

In [2], it was assumed that $fun(\sigma) = a\sigma^a$ and $V_\sigma\left(\hat{\mu}_m^* - \hat{\mu}_m^*\right) = w_{mm}\rho\left(\hat{\mu}_m^* - \hat{\mu}_m^*\right)$, where

$$\rho\left(\hat{\mu}_m^* - \hat{\mu}_m^*\right) = \left|\hat{\mu}_m^* - \hat{\mu}_m^*\right|^a \tag{8.61}$$

for a ≥ 0.

In short, we can convert the logarithm from Eq. 8.60 into the following form:

$$\ln P\left(\hat{\mu}_m^*\right) = -\frac{1}{a\sigma^a} \sum_{m,m \in C} w_{mm}\left|\hat{\mu}_m^* - \hat{\mu}_m^*\right|^a, \tag{8.62}$$

where w_{mm} are normalised weighting coefficients chosen as the inverse of the distance between the voxels so that $\sum_{m,m \in C} w_{mm} = 1$.

The parameter a in Eq. 8.62 allows us to control the degree of edge preservation in the reconstructed image. It is of paramount importance for maintaining the sharpness of the image when smoothing it by means of the $\ln P(\hat{\mu}_m^*)$ term in the optimisation criterion (8.43). Parameter a in Eq. 8.62 plays a key role in the trade-off between edge sharpness preservation and image smoothness, i.e. noise reduction in the reconstructed image. Values of $a > 1$ allow us to preserve the convexity of the regularising function, making it much easier for the optimising algorithm (reconstructing the image) to find the global extremum. A value of $a = 2$ however causes substantial edge smoothing in the reconstructed image. Thus, parameter a should have a value within the limits $1 \leq a \leq 2$ such as $a = 1.2$.

To increase the ability to influence the property of the regularising term with respect to the above-mentioned trade-off between preserving the edges in the image and eliminating noise, a modified form of the potential function has been proposed [27]

$$\rho\left(\hat{\mu}_m^* - \hat{\mu}_m^*\right) = \frac{\left|\hat{\mu}_m^* - \hat{\mu}_m^*\right|^a}{1 + \left|\frac{\hat{\mu}_m^* \ \hat{\mu}_m^*}{d}\right|^{a \ b}}, \tag{8.63}$$

where a represents the degree of nearness and b the degree of distance, between the central pixel and a given pixel in the neighbourhood (in the literature b is named q), where $1 \leq b \leq a < 2$; d determines the approximate transition threshold between low and high contrast regions in the reconstructed image.

If a is fixed, a smaller value of b results in improved performance of the regularising term in preserving edges in the reconstructed image, since for large $\hat{\mu}_m^* - \hat{\mu}_m^*$ the values of the term become relatively constant. On the other hand, by manipulating the value of d we can move the property towards either smaller or greater values of $\hat{\mu}_m^* - \hat{\mu}_m^*$.

In the literature, the optimisation term based on the potential function given in Eq. 8.63 is referred to as q-generalised Gaussian MRF (q-GGMRF).

The optimisation problem as written in Eq. 8.43 can easily be transformed into a more convenient form for finding the minimum, that is for finding the optimal reconstructed image. Equation (8.43) can thus be converted into the following form:

$$\mu_{\max}^* = \arg\min_{\mu*}(-\ln P(\Lambda = \lambda|\mu^*) - \ln P(\mu^*)). \tag{8.64}$$

From our previous considerations based on Eq. 8.51 and 8.60, the reconstruction problem reduced to the optimisation problem defined by Eq. 8.51 can be written as follows:

$$\mu_{\max}^* = \arg\min_{\mu*}\left(\frac{1}{2}(\mathbf{p} - \chi\mu^*)^{\mathrm{T}}\mathbf{D}(\mathbf{p} - \chi\mu^*) + \frac{1}{fun(\sigma)}\sum_{m,m\in C} V_\sigma\left(\hat{\mu}_m^* - \hat{\mu}_m^*\right)\right). \tag{8.65}$$

8.3.3 Solving the Problem of Optimisation

As mentioned in Sect. 8.3.2, the functions defining the optimisation criterion are convex, so we can use a number of methods for finding optimal solutions to Eq. 8.65 and still be guaranteed to achieve a global minimum. The choice of a suitable optimisation method should be guided mainly by considerations of computational efficiency [27].

The first component of the optimisation criterion shown in Eq. 8.65 is approximately a quadratic function, which means that in this optimisation problem we can use a method known in the literature as the Newton iterative algorithm. To demonstrate the ability of this algorithm to find the minimum of a quadratic function, let us use a very simple example function: $fun(x) = x^2$. We will represent the value of the variable x in the tth iterative step of the algorithm by $x^{(t)}$. If we expand $fun(x)$ into a Taylor series about the value $x^{(t)}$, the search for the extremum of $fun(x)$ can be written as:

$$\begin{aligned} fun_{\min}(x) &= \min_x\left(Fun^{(t)}(x)\right) \\ &= \min_x\left(fun\left(x^{(t)}\right) + \left(x - x^{(t)}\right)fun'\left(x^{(t)}\right) + \frac{1}{2}\left(x - x^{(t)}\right)^2 fun''\left(x^{(t)}\right)\right), \end{aligned} \tag{8.66}$$

which represents the approximation of the function $fun(x)$ by the quadratic function $Fun(x)$ in the neighbourhood of the point $x^{(t)}$.

A necessary condition for the existence of an extremum of this function at x is that the derivative of the function at that point equals 0:

$$\frac{\mathrm{d}Fun^{(t)}(x)}{\mathrm{d}x} = 0, \tag{8.67}$$

hence

$$x^{(t)} - \frac{fun'\left(x^{(t)}\right)}{fun''\left(x^{(t)}\right)} = x^{(t)} - \frac{2x^{(t)}}{2} = 0. \tag{8.68}$$

In this way, we achieve convergence of the optimisation algorithm to the solution in one step. If $fun(x)$ is approximately quadratic, as with the optimisation criterion given in Eq. 8.65, the convergence will still be relatively fast. In that case, the value $x_{min}^{(t)}$ at which the function $Fun^{(t)}(x)$ is a minimum is only an approximation to the value at which $fun(x)$ actually has its minimum. Assuming that in subsequent iterative steps we choose $x_{\min}^{(t)}$ as the initial condition $x^{(t+1)}$ about which to expand the function $fun(x)$, we can write:

$$\left.\frac{dFun^{(t)}(x)}{dx}\right|_{x=x^{(t+1)}} = fun'\left(x^{(t)}\right) + \left(x - x^{(t)}\right)fun''\left(x^{(t)}\right)\Big|_{x=x^{(t+1)}} = 0. \tag{8.69}$$

Thus, by finding the roots of Eq. 8.69, we find successive approximations $x^{(t)}$; $t = 1, 2, \ldots$ to the value at which $\mathrm{fun}(x)$ is a minimum. This procedure for finding the minimum is shown graphically in Fig. 8.17.

The algorithm described comprehensively in [27] is not simply a direct application of Newton's method to the MAP method. This is because the Taylor series expansion only includes the ML term and not the a priori term. With this in mind, we will use the following relationship to find the optimal solution:

$$\hat{\mu}_m^{(t+1)} = \underset{\mu > 0}{\mathrm{argmin}} \left(\sum_{k=1}^{L \cdot \Psi} \frac{d_k}{2} \left(2\chi_{km} \left(\hat{p}_k - \chi_k^* \mu^{(t)} \right) \left(\mu_m^* - \mu_m^{*(t)} \right) + \chi_{km}^2 \left(\mu_m^* - \mu_m^{*(t)} \right)^2 \right) + \frac{1}{fun(\sigma)} \sum_{m,m \in C} V_\sigma \left(\hat{\mu}_m^* - \hat{\mu}_m^* \right) \right), \tag{8.70}$$

where: χ_k is the kth row of the matrix χ.

Note that we do not consider the Hessian matrix in the Taylor series expansion of the quadratic term in Eq. 8.70. This means that in this approach, as one image pixel is being improved by successive optimisation steps, the rest of the pixels remain fixed. This leads to a significant speeding up of the reconstruction process. To reduce any adverse effects introduced by this simplification, the sequence of choosing the pixels for modification is determined randomly. The modification to the algorithm for finding the optimal solution in multi-dimensional space is known as the Newton Raphson method [26, 27].

To change the individual image points, it now only remains for us to determine the value at which the function in the brackets in Eq. 8.70 is a minimum. To do this, we calculate the zero point of the derivative of the function with respect to $\overset{*}{\mu}_m$, giving us:

$$\sum_{k=1}^{K \cdot H \cdot \Theta} d_k \chi_{km} \left(\hat{p}_k - \chi_k^* \mu^{(t)} \right) + \sum_{k=1}^{K \cdot H \cdot \Theta} d_k \chi_{km}^2 \left(\mu_m^* - \mu_m^{*(t)} \right) + \frac{1}{fun(\sigma)} \sum_{m,m \in C} \varrho_\sigma \left(\hat{\mu}_m^* - \hat{\mu}_m^* \right) = 0, \tag{8.71}$$

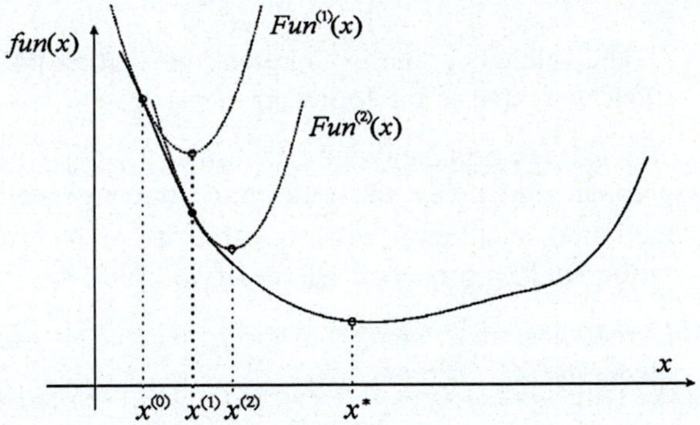

Fig. 8.17 Graphical interpretation of Newton's algorithm

where: $Q_\sigma(\cdot)$ is the first derivative of the potential function $V_\sigma(\cdot)$ and is called the influence function.

For the $\rho\left(\hat{\mu}_m^* - \hat{\mu}_m^*\right)$ function in Eq. 8.63, the influence function has the following form:

$$Q_\sigma\left(\hat{\mu}_m^* - \hat{\mu}_m^*\right)$$
$$= w_{mm} \frac{\left|\hat{\mu}_m^* - \hat{\mu}_m^*\right|^a}{1 + \left|\frac{\hat{\mu}_m^* \quad \hat{\mu}_m^*}{d}\right|^{a \quad b}} \left(a - \frac{a-b}{d_{a \quad b}} \frac{\left|\hat{\mu}_m^* - \hat{\mu}_m^*\right|^a}{1 + \left|\frac{\hat{\mu}_m^* \quad \hat{\mu}_m^*}{d}\right|^{a \quad b}} sign\left(\hat{\mu}_m^* - \hat{\mu}_m^*\right) \right). \tag{8.72}$$

To satisfy the assumptions for Eq. 8.70, we substitute $\hat{\mu}_m^* = \hat{\mu}_m^{*(t+1)}$ into Eq. 8.71 and continue the next step of iteration process for $\hat{\mu}_m^{*(t)} = \hat{\mu}_m^{*(t+1)}$.

8.4 Practical Approach to the Iterative Coordinate Descent Alogorithm

The discussions above form the basis for the formulation of a reconstruction algorithm from measurements made using a spiral projection system (scanner) with a conical beam of radiation.

The geometry of this type of scanner is discussed in detail in Sect. 7.3 and this will be the basis of our discussions here. In addition, as far as the geometry of the reconstructed image is concerned, everything established in Sect. 8.3.1 is also relevant here. The method given there for determining the elements of the matrix coefficients χ in the 3D image is particularly important. Therefore, the values of the elements χ_{km}; $k = 1, 2, \ldots, \mathrm{K} \cdot \mathrm{H} \cdot \Theta$ (K is the number of rows, H is the number of detectors in each row placed on the screen (channels), Θ is the total number of projections made during the examination); $m = 1, \ldots, \mathrm{I}, \mathrm{I}+1, \ldots, \mathrm{I} \cdot \mathrm{J}, \mathrm{I} \cdot \mathrm{J} + 1 \ldots, \mathrm{I} \cdot \mathrm{J} \cdot \mathrm{N}$ (I and J are the numbers of pixels in the x y plane and N is the number of slices of the spatial image along the z axis) are calculated *a priori* from the projection parameters, before the actual process of reconstruction.

From the measurements made by the scanner we obtain the individual projection values $\hat{p}_k$; $k = 1, \ldots, \mathrm{K} \cdot \mathrm{H} \cdot \Theta$.

The values χ_{km} and $\hat{p}_k$ represent the starting point for the reconstruction algorithm presented in the following steps:

Step I It is worth mentioning that since the objective functions in the optimisation problem are convex, to speed up the convergence of the algorithm to a solution, the initial condition $\mu^{*(t)}$ for $t = 0$ is determined using a standard algorithm such as the Feldkamp method, discussed in Chap. 6.

Step II The element $\mu_m^{*(t)}$ of the reconstructed image to be adjusted is selected randomly.

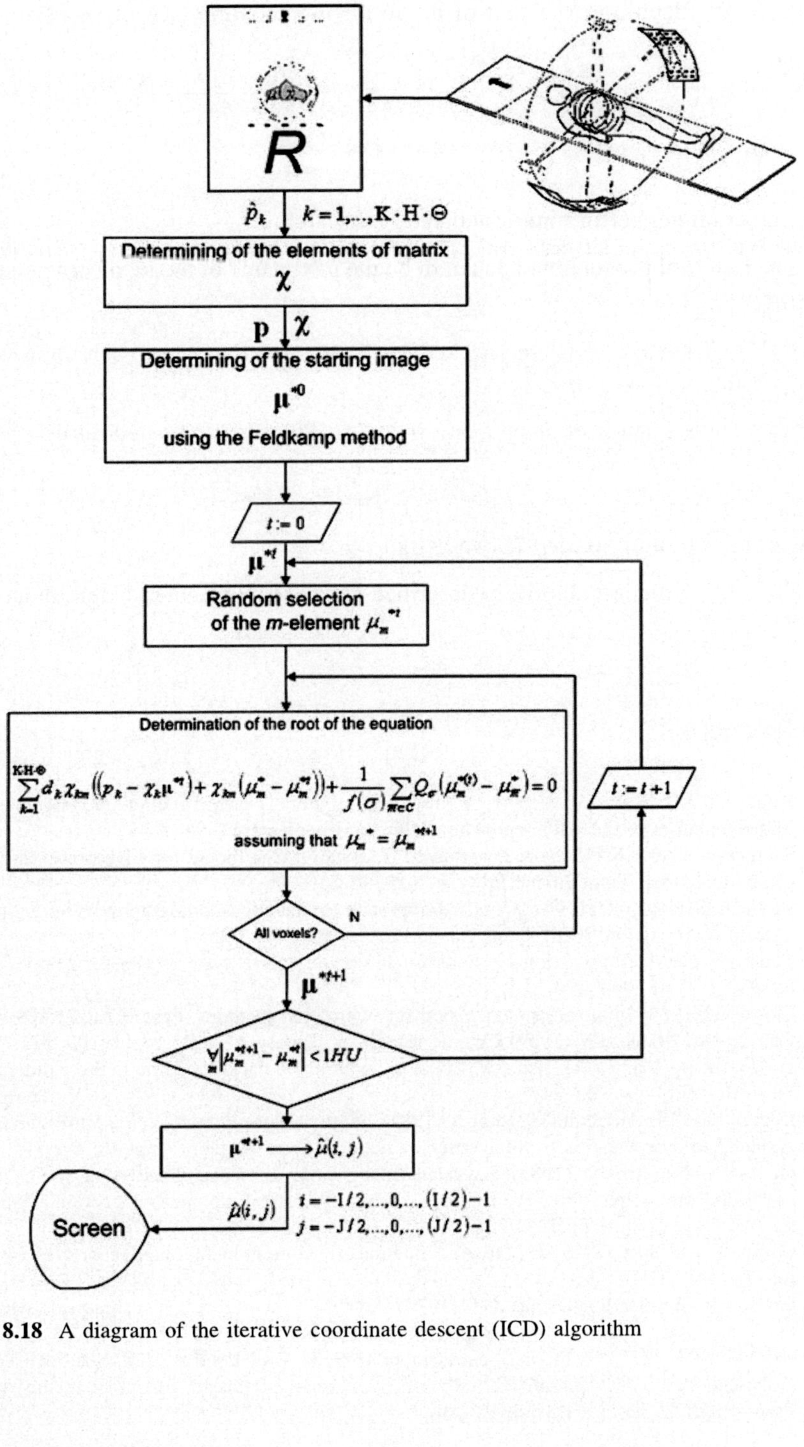

Fig. 8.18 A diagram of the iterative coordinate descent (ICD) algorithm

Step III We determine the root of the following equation (see Eq. 8.71):

$$\sum_{k=1}^{K \cdot H \cdot \Theta} d_k \chi_{km} \left(\hat{p}_k - \chi_k^* \mu^{(t)} \right) + \sum_{k=1}^{K \cdot H \cdot \Theta} d_k \chi_{km}^2 \left(\mu_m^* - \mu_m^{*(t)} \right) + \frac{1}{fun(\sigma)} \sum_{m,m \in C} Q_\sigma \left(\hat{\mu}_m^* - \hat{\mu}_m^* \right) = 0,$$

by, for example, performing a half-interval search.

The root of this equation is taken to be the next value of the reconstructed pixel, i.e. $\mu_m^{*(t+1)}$.

Step IV All the *m*-voxels are checked to see whether they have been improved. If not, we return to *Step II*.

Step V The sequence of steps from *Step II* to *Step IV* is repeated until

$$\forall_m \left| \mu_m^{*(t+1)} - \mu_m^{*(t)} \right| < 1HU,$$

where, on returning to *Step II*, we assign $t = t + 1$.

The reconstruction algorithm described above is represented diagrammatically in Fig. 8.18.

References

1. Andersen AH, Kak AC (1984) Simultaneous algebraic reconstruction technique: a new implementation of the ART algorithm. Ultrason Imaging 6:81 94
2. Bouman C, Sauer K (1993) A generalized Gaussian image model for edge preserving MAP estimation. IEEE Trans Image Process 2(3):296 310
3. Bouman C, Sauer K (1996) A unified approach to statistical tomography using coordinate descent optimization. IEEE Trans Image Process 5(3):480 492
4. Censor Y (1981) Row action methods for huge and sparse systems and their applications. SIAM Rev 23(3):444 464
5. Censor Y (1983) Finite series expansion reconstruction methods. Proc IEEE 71:409 419
6. Chazan D, Miranker W (1969) Chaotic relaxation. Linear Algebra Appl 2:199 222
7. DeMan B, Basu S (2004) Distance driven projection and backprojection in three dimensions. Phys Med Biol 49:2463 2475
8. Eggermont PPB, Herman GT, Lent A (1981) Iterative algorithms for large partitioned linear systems, with application to image reconstruction. Linear Algebra Appl 40:37 67
9. Geman S, McClure D (1985) Bayesian image analysis: an application to single photon emission tomography. in: Proceedings of the statistical computing section. American statistical association, pp 12 18
10. Geman S, McClure D (1987) Statistical methods for tomographic image reconstruction. Bull Int Stat Inst LII 4 5 21
11. Gordon R, Bender R, Herman GT (1970) Algebraic reconstruction techniques (ART) for three dimensional electron microscopy and X ray photography. J Theor Biol 29:471 481
12. Grimmett GR (1973) A theorem about random fields. Bull London Math Soc 5:81 84
13. Gubarieny N (1999) Generalized model of asynchronous iterations for image reconstruction. Proc Confer PPAM'99, Kazimierz Dolny

14. Hara AK, Paden RG, Silva AC, Kujak J, Lawder HJ, Pavlicek W (2010) Iterative reconstruction technique for reducing body radiation dose at CT: feasibility study. Am J Roentgenol 193(9):764 771
15. Herman GT, Lent A (1976) Iterative reconstruction algorithms. Comput Biol Med 6:273 294
16. Herman GT (1980) Image reconstruction from projections: the fundamentals of computerized tomography. Academic Press, New York
17. Jähne B (1991) Digital image processing: concepts, algorithms and scientific applications. Springer, Berlin
18. Jain AK (1989) Fundamentals of digitals image processing. Prentice Hall, Englewood Cliffs
19. Kak AC, Slanley M (1988) Principles of computerized tomographic imaging. IEEE Press, New York
20. Kaczmarz S (1937) Angenäherte Auflösung von Systemen linearer Gleichungen. Bull Acad Polon Sci Lett 35:355 357
21. Saquib SS, Bouman CA, Sauer K,(1998) ML parameter estimation for Markov random fields with application to Bayesian tomography. IEEE Trans Image Process 7(7):1029 1044
22. Sauer K, Bouman C (1992) Bayesian estimation of transmission tomograms using segmentation based otimization. IEEE Trans Nucl Sci 39(4):1144 1152
23. Sauer K, Bouman C (1993) A local update strategy for iterative reconstruction from projections. IEEE Trans Signal Process 41(2):534 548
24. Tanabe K (1971) Projection method for solving a singular system of linear equations and its applications. Numer Math 17:203 214
25. Thibault J B, Sauer K, Bouman C (2000) Newton style optimization for emission tomographic estimation. J Electron Imag 9(3):269 282
26. Thibault J B, Sauer KD, Bouman CA, Hsieh J (2006) A recursive filter for noise reduction in statistical iterative tomographic imaging. SPIE 6065
27. Thibault J B, Sauer KD, Bouman CA, Hsieh J (2007) A three dimensional statistical approach to improved image quality for multislice helical CT. Med Phys 34(11):4526 4544

Chapter 9
Evaluation of CT Devices

The production of tomographic images can be regarded as the transformation of the X-ray attenuation coefficient distribution in a patient's body into a reconstructed image. The final image is produced as a result of a whole chain of processes and is affected by a range of factors including the technical parameters of the scanner, the type of projection system, and finally the type of reconstruction algorithm applied.

Assessment of the physical and technical capabilities of CT scanners is made possible by the establishment of standardised, quantitative, comparative criteria.

9.1 Technical Parameters of CT Devices

As with any technical device, CT scanners can be described using standard parameters [1, 2, 4, 7, 8]. When planning the purchase of a scanner, a health service department should carefully analyse the models on the market using standardized parameters that describe both their properties and capabilities. In order to make the right decision concerning what is, after all, a considerable financial investment, they need to strike a balance between the price of the equipment and their expectations of the device. Parameters for the evaluation of the quality of a CT scanner include:

- *Cycle time* The total time taken to scan and reconstruct the image. Note that the smaller the cycle time, the greater the chance of avoiding the creation of artefacts caused by patient movement, including physiological movements such as the beating heart or chest movements while breathing;
- *Spatial resolution* [12] The minimum area in the image in which changes can be detected. This quantity is defined using the transfer function of the scanner $G(f_x, f_y)$ (called often the MTF, modulation transfer function [6]), an example of which is given in Fig. 9.1 (because the function is axially symmetrical about the

R. Cierniak, *X Ray Computed Tomography in Biomedical Engineering*,
DOI: 10.1007/978 0 85729 027 4 9, © Springer Verlag London Limited 2011

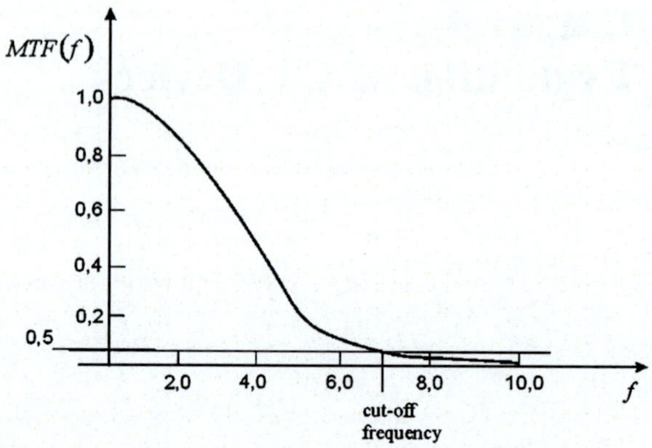

Fig. 9.1 An example transfer function

origin of the coordinate system, it can be represented by a single curve *MFT*(*f*)). The transfer function defines the frequency domain relationship between the original and the reconstructed image in the presence of noise, and determines the ability of the scanner to capture rapidly changing attenuation coefficients in the object. The spatial resolution is most often defined in terms of the cut-off frequency of the one dimensional transfer function, i.e. the value at which the function *MTF*(*f*) drops to the 50, 10 or 2% level. The value of this parameter depends solely on the properties of the detectors and X-ray source used in the scanner, on the method of sampling and on the method of reconstruction (the interpolation method and kernel filter used).

- *Low-contrast resolution* (contrast detail) [5] The ability to detect small differences of attenuation coefficient in tissues. It is defined as the ratio between the smallest detectable difference of attenuation coefficient (on the Hounsfield scale) and the average value within an object of a given size, for a specific radiation dose. This last factor is introduced because low-contrast resolution is proportional to the radiation dose. Current scanners have a resolution of between 0.3 and 0.4%. This can be increased by increasing the radiation dose or extending the scanning time.
- *Uniformity* [4] A measure of the homogeneity of the image (or rather the heterogeneity). This can be calculated from the average attenuation coefficients measured at selected areas of a uniform standard water phantom (Sect. 9.2), using the formula:

$$\text{heterogenity} = \frac{\mu^{\max}(x,y) - \mu^{\min}(x,y)}{\mu^{\max}(x,y) + \mu^{\min}(x,y)}, \tag{9.1}$$

where $\mu^{\max}(x, y)$ is the highest average attenuation coefficient from among all the selected areas of the phantom; $\mu^{\min}(x, y)$ is the smallest average attenuation coefficient from among all the selected areas of the phantom.

- *Linearity* (sensitometry) [4, 10] defines the relationship between the attenuation coefficients measured at the average energy of the scanner and the values assigned to them on the Hounsfield scale for all types of tissue, using the formula:

$$\text{linearity} = \sqrt{\frac{1}{I}\sum_{i=1} I(\mu_i - \mu_i^{\text{av}})^2}, \qquad (9.2)$$

where μ_i is the attenuation coefficient assigned to a given tissue, on the Hounsfield scale; μ_i^{av} is the attenuation coefficient measured at the average energy of the scanner; I is the number of the tissue under consideration.

A practical method for determining this parameter using a phantom is given in Sect. 9.2.

- *Slice thickness* The nominal thickness of the image cross-section. This is often determined using the value of the full width at half maximum (FWHM) of the scanner [3, 4], which is defined on the basis of the sensitivity function of the scanner. An example of a sensitivity function is presented in a simplified form in Fig. 9.2.

  To determine the sensitivity function, a phantom composed of metal strips or wires inclined at an angle is used (Sect. 9.2). The intensity of the X-rays is measured along the main axis of the patient with respect to a fixed point, and the results are then normalised relative to the maximum value. The slice thickness is the distance between the two points on the graph of the sensitivity function, which have values equal to half the maximum value. A typical value for this parameter would be in the range 0.4 10 mm.
- *Computed tomography dose index* (CTDI) This index is measured in milligrays (mGy). It defines what dose a patient absorbs when scanned by a particular CT apparatus, and is determined as follows:

$$\text{CTDI} = \frac{1}{|z_2 - z_1|}\int_{z_1}^{z_2} \text{Dose}(z)\,\mathrm{d}z, \qquad (9.3)$$

where Dose(z) is the distribution along the z-axis of the dose absorbed by a phantom during the test; z_1, z_2 are the start and endpoints on the z-axis of the measurements made by the dosimeter. The test measurements are made using an

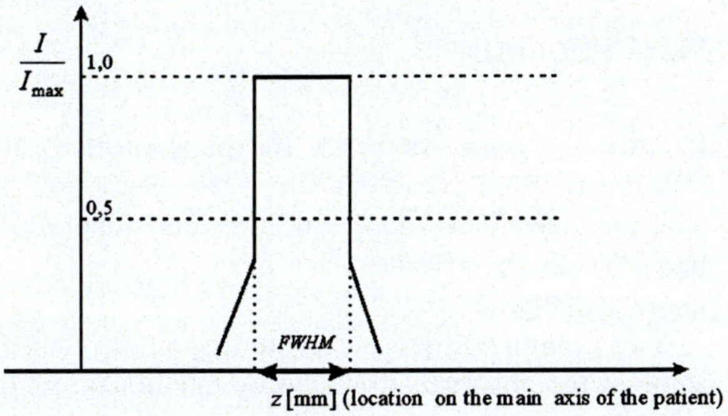

Fig. 9.2 A simplified example of the sensitivity function of a scanner

ionization chamber (diameter 10 mm, length 100 mm) placed inside a cylindrical phantom made from a substance similar to human tissue (e.g. polymethylmethacrylate). If we assume that the CTDI index varies linearly with the distance between points on the surface and the centre of the phantom, its average value for one scanned slice can be calculated using the formula:

$$ {}_{n}\mathrm{CTDI}_{w} = \frac{1}{Q}\left(\frac{1}{3}\mathrm{CTDI}_{100,c} + \frac{2}{3}\mathrm{CTDI}_{100,p}\right), \tag{9.4} $$

where Q is the current-time product during the test; the subscript 100 means that the measurement was made using an ionization chamber of length 100 mm; c means that the measurement was made at the centre of the phantom; p represents a value calculated on the basis of two to four measurements made at the periphery of the phantom. Note that the ${}_{n}\mathrm{CTDI}_{w}$ index can vary depending on the nominal thickness of the scanned slices. We can determine the value of the dose absorbed by the patient during a scan by using this parameter and taking into account other parameters such as: the high-tension voltage of the tube, the current-time product used during the scan, the thickness of the slices scanned and the number of those slices. Clearly, the total dose absorbed by the patient should not exceed permissible levels. Consequently, much of the efforts of manufacturers of tomographic equipment are currently directed towards minimising this dose. The most important approaches in this respect are presented in the paper [9].

- *Pitch* This factor is only relevant to spiral scan systems and is the ratio between the displacement of the table with the patient on it and the thickness of the scanned layer for one revolution of the scanner:

$$ \mathrm{pitch} = \frac{\lambda}{\mathrm{SW}}, \tag{9.5} $$

where λ is the relative travel of the spiral described by the tube as it moves around the test object in (mm/rad); SW is the nominal thickness of the layer in (mm) (see Eq. 7.5 and the appropriate comment below it).

9.2 Phantoms

In order to control or verify the parameters of a scanner, specially developed structures called phantoms are used. Some of these have become standards whereas, due to the widely differing functional requirements placed on CT scanners, the design of others has been specified by individual medical equipment manufacturers.

This section will present the most popular standard phantoms and examples of some of the phantoms provided by manufacturers of scanners.

Fig. 9.3 The ATS phantom

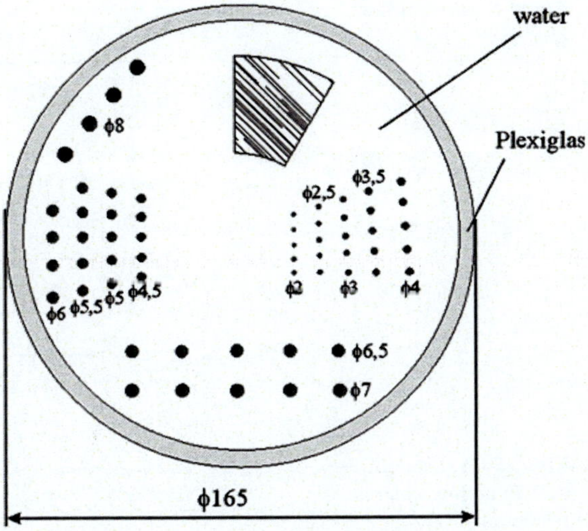

9.2.1 ATS Phantom

The ATS phantom was first proposed by the American Association of Physicists in Medicine and was designed to test low-contrast resolution, one of the key parameters that characterise tomographic devices. The design of this phantom, together with its dimensions, is shown in Fig. 9.3.

Situated inside the Plexiglas housing of this phantom are rows of circular inserts with diameters that change from row to row. These inserts have adjustable attenuation coefficient values, expressed on the Hounsfield scale. The whole of the inside of the phantom is filled with water.

During the measurement of low-contrast resolution, the phantom is subjected to radiation of constant, standard intensity.

9.2.2 Moström's Phantom

This phantom is used to measure the homogeneity of the image, as defined in the previous section of this chapter [4, 11]. In the example of the phantom illustrated in Fig. 9.4, the parameter $I = 5$.

9.2.3 Low-contrast Resolution Phantom

The earliest design of phantom used to measure low-contrast resolution is shown in Fig. 9.5.

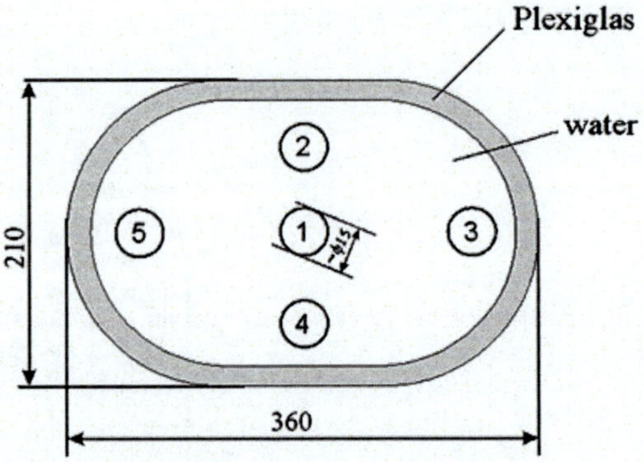

Fig. 9.4 Moström's phantom

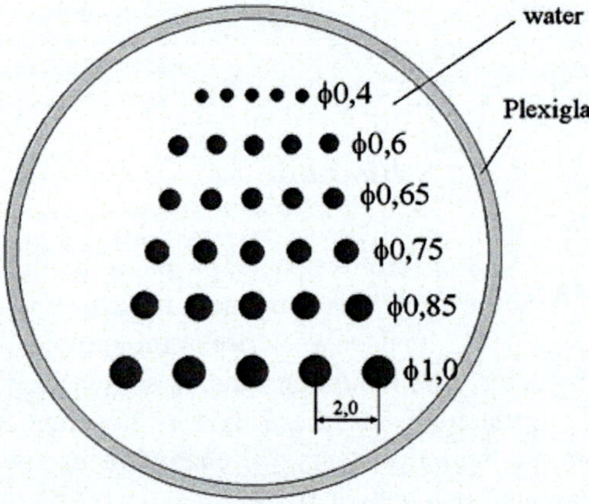

Fig. 9.5 A phantom used to determine low contrast resolution

The metal rods, shown immersed in water in the diagram, are arranged in rows, where both the diameter d_i and the distance between the rods $2d_i$ decrease as the index i of the row increases. The low-contrast resolution of the scanner is determined by the smallest diameter of rod, which is visible as a distinct element in the reconstructed image (see also [13]).

9.2.4 Spatial Resolution Phantom

Spatial resolution (units: lp/cm) is determined by the use of a phantom to measure the point spread function. In this phantom, a length of stainless steel wire is placed perpendicular to the test cross-section, as shown in Fig. 9.6 [4, 12].

The MTF, which directly determines the resolution of the scanner, can be calculated using the Fourier transform of the reconstructed image. Because the diameter of the wire is small in relation to the size of the pixels, it can be neglected in the calculation.

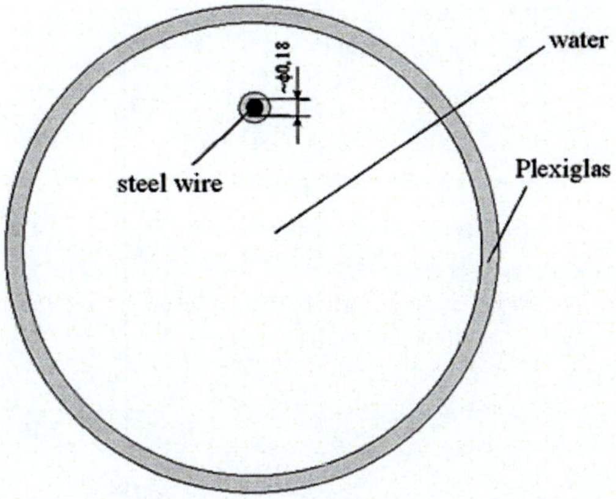

Fig. 9.6 A phantom to measure the point spread function

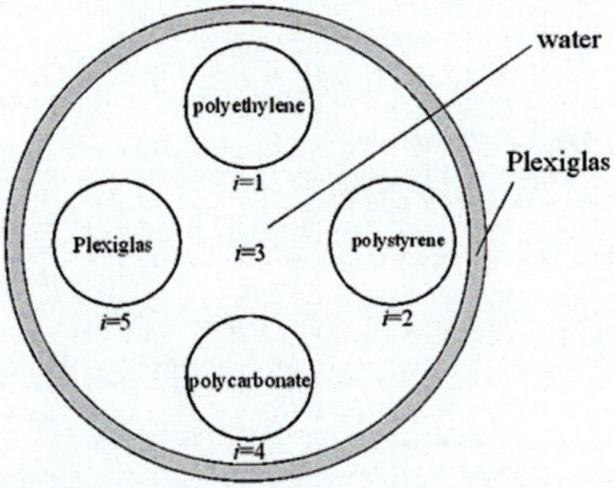

Fig. 9.7 An example of a CT linearity phantom

9.2.5 CT Linearity Phantom

The phantom described here is used to assess the linearity of the tomographic image as defined in Sect. 9.1. In the phantom illustrated in Fig. 9.7, the parameter $I = 5$ (Eq. 9.2).

The five materials used here are selected according to the Hounsfield number assigned to them. The Hounsfield numbers are chosen to cover the widest possible range of the scale.

By drawing a graph (see Fig. 9.8) of the relationship between the Hounsfield numbers assigned to these materials and their attenuation coefficients measured by the scanner (at the average radiation energy), we can establish the nonlinearity parameter based on Eq. 9.2.

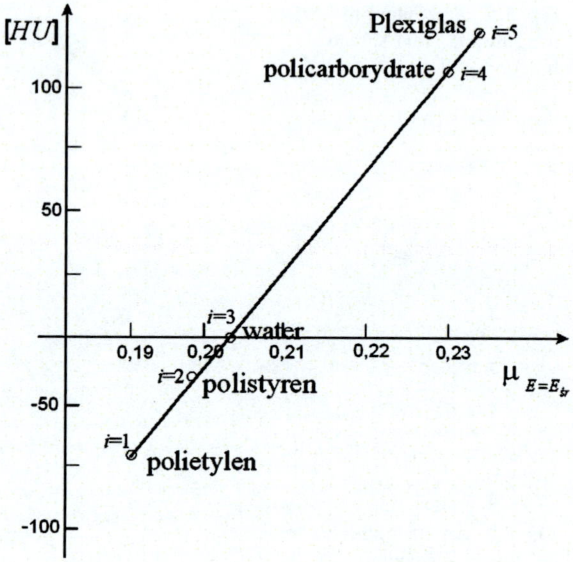

Fig. 9.8 Evaluation of the linearity of a CT scanner

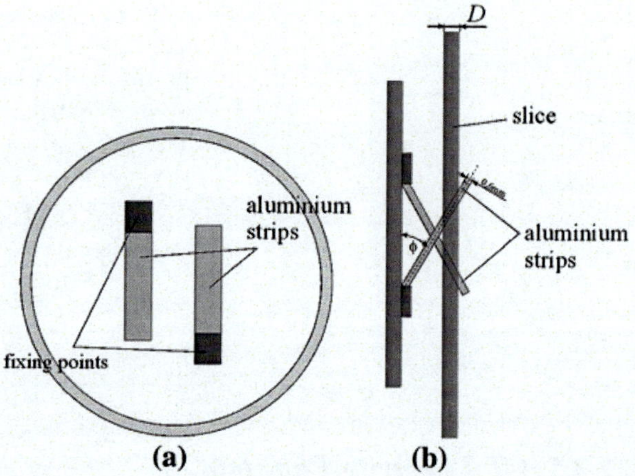

Fig. 9.9 Phantom to measure the slice thickness: **a** front view; **b** side view

9.2.6 Slice Thickness Phantom

The most popular solution to the problem of measuring the slice thickness is the method using the phantom shown in Fig. 9.9 [3, 4]. This phantom has two aluminium strips of thickness $b = 0.6$ mm inclined to the reconstruction plane at a fixed angle ϕ (this angle is usually either 30 or 45%).

Figure 9.10 shows how the length d of the shadow of one of the metal strips, which is visible in the tomographic image, is used to calculate the thickness of the cross-section D, using the formula:

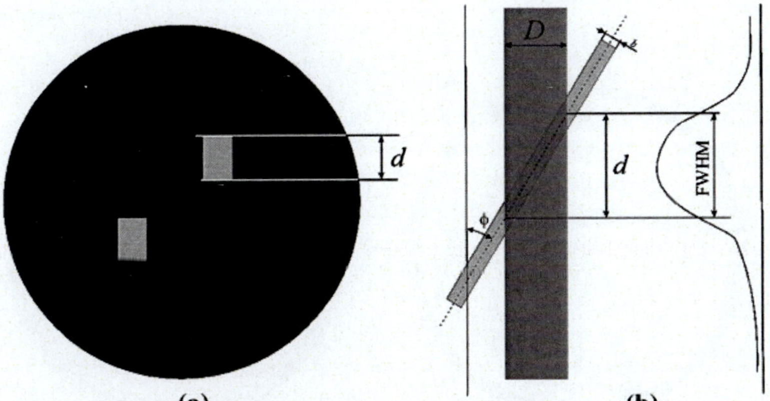

Fig. 9.10 Measurement of the slice thickness: **a** tomographic image of the phantom shown in Fig. 9.9; **b** the trigonometric relationships in the determination of the slice thickness

$$D = d \cdot \tan \phi. \tag{9.6}$$

The method of determining the slice thickness, described above, assumes a negligible thickness for the aluminium strips. The absolute minimum slice thickness that can be measured using this method is determined by the relationship:

$$D_{\min} = \frac{b}{\cos \phi}. \tag{9.7}$$

For the angle $\phi = 30°$ quoted earlier, the value $D_{\min}$ is approximately 0.7 mm. Since, in modern designs of scanner, slice thicknesses can be <0.4 mm, the method of calculating D outlined here had to be modified. The modifications included changes to the material used to make the metal strips in the phantom, the thickness of the strips and the angle at which they are set. The strips in modern designs of phantom are made from titanium, which gives better contrast; their thickness is 0.05 mm and the angle $\phi = 8°$. The minimum slice thickness, which can be determined with a phantom like this, is $D_{\min} \leq 0.1$ mm.

9.2.7 Phantom Simulating a Skull Bone

Filters are often used in reconstruction algorithms to compensate for the distortions to the image at the boundary between the skull and the brain. The use of the phantoms described above would cause these filters to have an adverse effect on the reconstructed image in the absence of a substitute for the skull bone. For that reason, a Teflon rim, as shown in Fig. 9.11, is usually fitted to one of the phantoms described above (for example Fig. 9.11b) to simulate the skull bone [4].

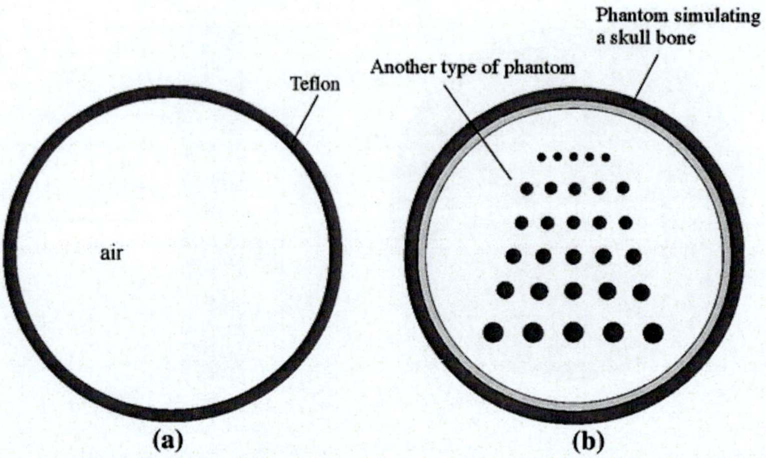

Fig. 9.11 A phantom simulating the skull bone: **a** the design of the phantom; **b** how the phantom is used to simulate the skull bone

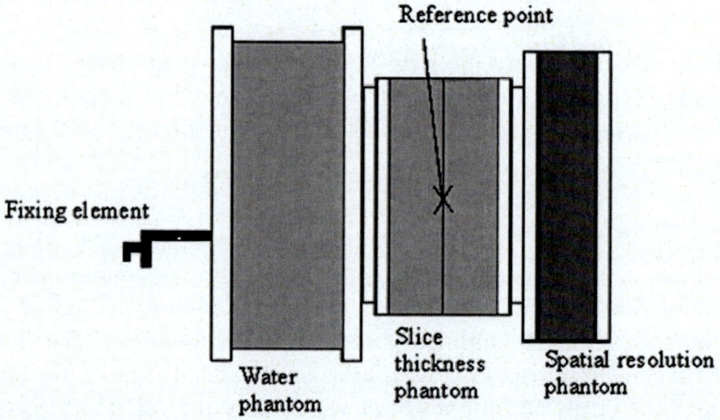

Fig. 9.12 A phantom set

9.2.8 Phantom Sets

In practice, phantom sets composed of several sections are often used; each section may contain several (usually two) of the basic phantoms described above. An example of a set of phantoms is shown in Fig. 9.12.

To facilitate accurate mounting of the phantom set, a reference point is marked on the second section. The position of this point can be adjusted using a special optical viewfinder in the gantry of the scanner.

A set like this enables quality control tests to be carried out on the whole measurement system of the CT scanner: the X-ray tube, the radiation detectors and the instrumentation.

9.3 Start-up and Test Procedures

To ensure reliable operation of the scanner throughout the whole of its working life, it is important that all the manufacturer's recommended procedures for start-up and testing are followed.

As soon as the scanner is turned on, the start-up window of the scanner's application software informs the operator of the progress of the start-up procedures. An example of a start-up window can be found in Fig. 9.13.

After sliding the table out of the scanner's gantry (*Feed Out*), the quality of the image is tested (*Test Image*), but without the emission of radiation. This is to confirm the correct operation of the imaging system. The next step is to prepare the tube for operation by heating it up (*Warm Up*). The next action (*Calibration*) takes place in the absence of any radiation-absorbing material in the gantry of the scanner. The measurements made at this time form the basis of the corrections that must be made to the projections obtained during the routine operation of the scanner. After calibration, procedures testing the operation of the scanner are carried out (*Quality*). The procedures performed at this stage can be divided into two types:

- qualitative tests, performed each day or weekly,
- stability tests, performed each month,
- annual tests.

A set of daily/weekly tests (performed by technicians) to check the quality of the reconstructed image might include:

- a test to measure the homogeneity of the image, using a phantom such as that shown in Fig. 9.6,
- a test of the point spread function, using a wire phantom as shown in Fig. 9.11,

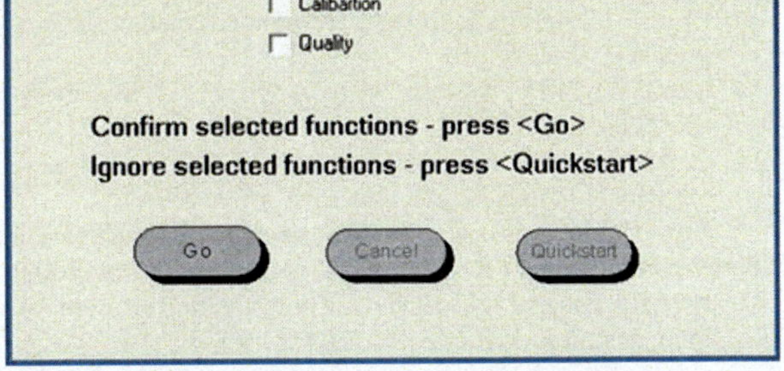

Fig. 9.13 An example of a start up window for a CT scanner

• a check of the X-ray tube voltage.

A battery of tests performed by service personel or technicians on a monthly basis might consist of the following items:

• spatial resolution,
• positioning accuracy,
• linearity,
• slice thickness.

Annual tests might be a combination of the following examinations (performed by physicists):

• daily/weekly tests,
• index accuracy and table positioning test,
• contrast scale test,
• distance accuracy test,
• patient dose.

In an emergency, if the time needed to perform the entire start-up procedure could affect the life or health of the patient, a fast start-up procedure (*Quickstart*) can be carried out, which excludes all the points selected in the start-up window shown in Fig. 9.13.

Appropriate tests should also be carried out on the scanner after the installation of the equipment and after any routine maintenance or servicing. Application software installed on the scanner's computer enables the results of the tests to be saved, so creating a history of the device for purposes of comparison.

References

1. AAPM (1977) Phantoms for performance, evaluation and quality assurance of CT scanners. Report No. 1 American Association of Physicists in Medicine
2. AAPM (1993) Specification and acceptance testing of computed tomography scanners. Report No. 39, American Association of Physicists in Medicine
3. Atkins FB, Goodenough DJ, Levy JR (1998) A new method to test CT scan plane angulation and rotation relative to a test phantom. Radiol 209(P):285
4. Catphan 500 and 600 Manual (2004) The Phantom Laboratory Inc., Greenwich
5. Cohen G, DiBianca FA (1979) The use of contrast detail dose evaluation of image quality in a computed tomographic scanner. J Comp Assist Tomogr 3(2):189 195
6. Droege RT, Morin RL (1982) A practical method to measure the MTF of CT scanners. Med Phys 9:758 760
7. Goodenough DJ, Weaver KE, Davis DO (1976) Development of a phantom for evaluation and assurance of image quality. Opt Eng 16:52 65
8. Goodenough DJ, Levy JR, Kasales C (1998) Development of phantom for spiral CT. Comp Med Imag Graph 22:247 255
9. Gunn MLD, Kohr JR (2009) State of the art: technologies for computed tomography dose reduction. Emerg Radiol published online 20 Nov 2009
10. Kriz RJ, Strauss KJ (1985) An investigation of computed tomography (CT) linearity. Med Imag Instrum SPIE 555:195 204

11. Möstrom U (1986) Evoluation of CT scanners for use in neuroradiology. Upsala University, Upsala
12. Rossman K (1969) Point spread function, line spread function and modu lation transfer function: tools for the study of imaging systems. Radiol 93:257 272
13. Suess C, Kalender WA, Coman JM (1999) New low contrast resolution phantoms for computed tomography. Med Phys 26(2):296 302

Chapter 10
Computer-Generated Projections for Simulations

Any new image reconstruction algorithm or indeed any modification of an existing method requires a computer simulation to verify its usefulness. In previous chapters, a number of reconstruction methods have been introduced and in order to facilitate their practical application, we took the opportunity to give their discrete versions. One of the biggest problems when it comes to testing reconstruction algorithms is the difficulty in obtaining a set of projection values measured physically by a CT scanner. Moreover, if we were to use measurements obtained from a scanner, we would really need a set of standard projections in order to compare the different image reconstruction algorithms, particularly as real, physical projections are affected by various types of distortion whose nature and degree are uncertain.

However, mathematical models of phantoms have been proposed [4, 7], which allow us to obtain virtual projection values. The main advantage of this approach is that it makes it possible to standardise the data for the reconstruction algorithms and therefore makes it much easier to compare results. It also becomes easier to compare the reconstructed image with the original cross-section. In addition, a number of studies have presented virtual models of organs and body parts such as the heart [3] and the thorax (http://www.imp.uni-erlangen.de/phantoms/).

The best way of obtaining the projection value data needed for a simulation is to use a mathematical model of a particular part of the body such as the model of a head phantom proposed in [7] and described, for example, in [1, 2, 5, 6]. A mathematical model of a phantom of this type should have the following characteristics:

- it should be possible to assemble the object from separate elements, each of which has a constant attenuation coefficient,
- it should be easy to calculate of the path of a ray that passes through an element of the phantom,
- the calculated projection values for the various elements of the phantom should be additive (a consequence of the linearity property of the Radon transform).

R. Cierniak, *X Ray Computed Tomography in Biomedical Engineering*,
DOI: 10.1007/978 0 85729 027 4 10, © Springer Verlag London Limited 2011

10.1 Mathematical Model for Parallel-beam Projections

When we consider the conditions set out in the preceding section, in particular, ease of calculation, the geometric shape most suitable for the construction of mathematical phantoms is the ellipse. A phantom made up of ellipses allows us to obtain the projection values for all points of interest on the screen, at any projection angle. An example of the structure of a mathematical head phantom is given in Fig. 10.1.

This model consists of elliptical elements each having a constant value of attenuation coefficient. Equations describing the individual ellipses and a table containing their parameters are given below (the symbols of the variables used in the model are illustrated in Fig. 10.2):

$$\frac{x^2}{a^2}+\frac{y^2}{b^2}\leq 1, \tag{10.1}$$

for an ellipse centred at the origin of the coordinate system,

$$\frac{(x-x_0)^2}{a^2}+\frac{(y-y_0)^2}{b^2}\leq 1, \tag{10.2}$$

for an ellipse with its centre displaced to the point (x_0,y_0),

$$\frac{((x-x_0)\cos\alpha_0+(y-y_0)\sin\alpha_0)^2}{a^2}+\frac{(-(x-x_0)\sin\alpha_0+(y-y_0)\cos\alpha_0)^2}{b^2}\leq 1, \tag{10.3}$$

for an ellipse displaced to the point (x_0,y_0) and rotated about its centre by an angle α_0 (Table 10.1).

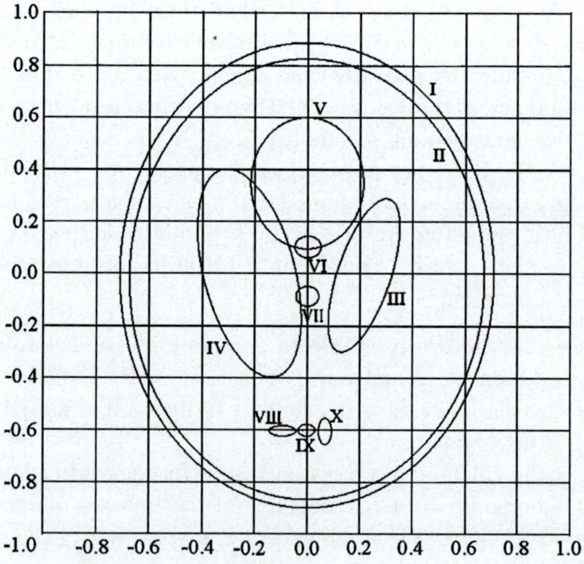

Fig. 10.1 The topology of a mathematical model of a head phantom

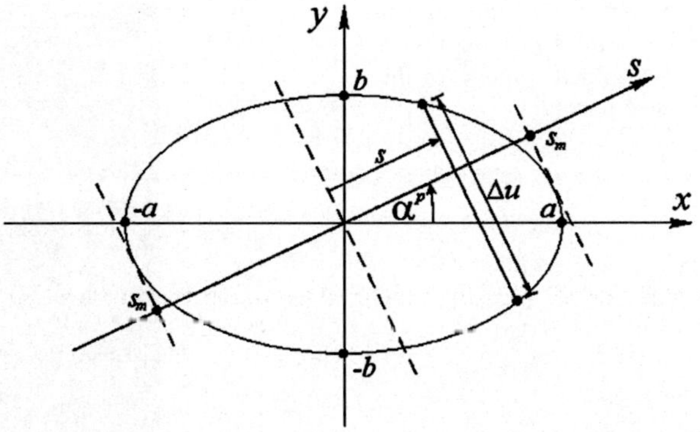

Fig. 10.2 Symbols used to describe the ellipses in the model of the head phantom

The image of the model head phantom is built up by superimposing successive elements of the phantom using ellipses defined by the following equations with appropriate parameters:

$$\mu_i(x,y) = \begin{cases} \mu_i^{\text{const}} & \text{for } \frac{x^2}{a^2} + \frac{y^2}{b^2} \leq 1 \\ 0 & \text{for } \frac{x^2}{a^2} + \frac{y^2}{b^2} > 1 \end{cases}, \tag{10.4}$$

for an ellipse centred at the origin,

$$\mu_i(x,y) = \begin{cases} \mu_i^{\text{const}} & \text{for } \frac{(x\quad x_0)^2}{a^2} + \frac{(y\quad y_0)^2}{b^2} \leq 1 \\ 0 & \text{for } \frac{(x\quad x_0)^2}{a^2} + \frac{(y\quad y_0)^2}{b^2} > 1 \end{cases}, \tag{10.5}$$

for an ellipse with its centre displaced to the point (x_0, y_0),

$$\mu_i(x,y) = \begin{cases} \mu_i^{\text{const}} & \text{for } \frac{((x\quad x_0)\cos\alpha_0 + (y\quad y_0)\sin\alpha_0)^2}{a^2} + \frac{(\;(x\quad x_0)\sin\alpha_0 + (y\quad y_0)\cos\alpha_0)^2}{b^2} \leq 1 \\ 0 & \text{for } \frac{((x\quad x_0)\cos\alpha_0 + (y\quad y_0)\sin\alpha_0)^2}{a^2} + \frac{(\;(x\quad x_0)\sin\alpha_0 + (y\quad y_0)\cos\alpha_0)^2}{b^2} > 1 \end{cases}, \tag{10.6}$$

Table 10.1 Parameters of the ellipses making up the mathematical model of the head phantom

Ellipse number	Coordinates of the centre		Semi major axis	Semi minor axis	Angle of rotation α_0 (deg)	μ^{const} (x, y)
	x_0	y_0	a	b		
I	0.0000	0.0000	0.6900	0.9200	0.0	2.00
II	0.0000	0.0184	0.6624	0.8740	0.0	0.98
III	0.2200	0.0000	0.1100	0.3100	18.00	0.02
IV	0.2200	0.0000	0.1600	0.4100	18.00	0.02
V	0.0000	0.3500	0.2100	0.2500	0.00	0.01
VI	0.0000	0.1000	0.0460	0.0460	0.00	0.01
VII	0.0000	0.1000	0.0460	0.0460	0.00	0.01
VIII	0.0800	0.6050	0.0460	0.0230	0.00	0.01
IX	0.0000	0.6050	0.0230	0.0230	0.00	0.01
X	0.0600	0.6050	0.0230	0.0460	0.00	0.01

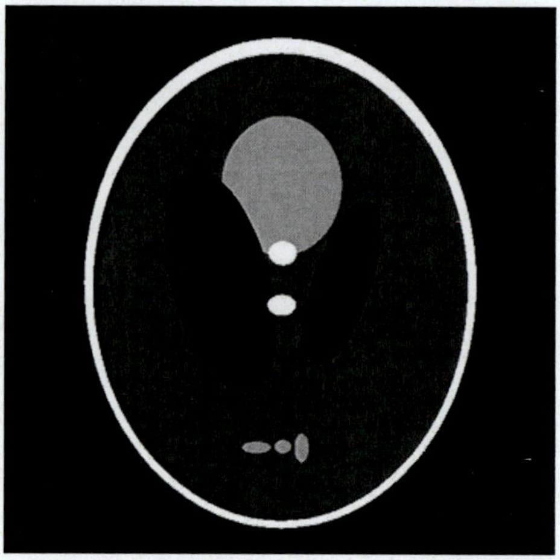

Fig. 10.3 The topology of the ellipses making up the mathematical model of the head phantom

for an ellipse displaced to the point (x_0, y_0) and rotated about its centre by an angle α_0. A phantom constructed in this way is shown in Fig. 10.3.

Assembling the mathematical model of the phantom from elliptical shapes as described above allows us to use the superposition property of the Radon transform. This means that for a given angle of incidence α^p, we can sum the separately evaluated projection values $p^p{}_i(s, \alpha^p)$ for the individual figures at each point s:

$$p^p(s, \alpha^p) = \sum_{i=1}^{10} p_i^p(s, \alpha^p). \tag{10.7}$$

For a single figure, the projection value at a given angle is expressed by:

$$p_i^p(s, \alpha^p) = \Delta u \cdot \mu_i^{\text{const}} = \begin{cases} \frac{2ab\sqrt{s_m^2 \quad s^2}}{s_m^2} \mu_i^{\text{const}} & \text{for} \quad |s| \le s_m \\ 0 & \text{for} \quad |s| > s_m \end{cases}, \tag{10.8}$$

where $s_m = \sqrt{a^2 \cos^2 \alpha^p + b^2 \sin^2 \alpha^p}$ is the distance of the ray (tangential to the ellipse) furthest from the centre of the ellipse.

Proof

$\frac{x^2}{a^2} + \frac{y^2}{b^2} \quad 1$	The equation of the ellipse
//Substituting $x \quad \frac{s - y \sin \alpha^p}{\cos \alpha^p}$	Using a relationship from Table 4.3
$\frac{(s - y \sin \alpha^p)^2}{a^2 \cos^2 \alpha^p} + \frac{y^2}{b^2} \quad 1$	
//Transforming the expression on the left hand side of the above equation	
$\frac{s^2 - 2sy \sin \alpha^p + y^2 \sin^2 \alpha^p}{a^2 \cos^2 \alpha^p} + \frac{y^2}{b^2} \quad 1$	
//Equivalently	

(continued)

(continued)

$b^2s^2 \quad b^2 2sy \sin \alpha^p + b^2y^2 \sin^2 \alpha^p + y^2a^2 \cos^2 \alpha^p \quad b^2a^2 \cos^2 \alpha^p$

//Rearranging all monomials to one side of the equation
//and rearranging the square trinomial

$y^2(b^2 \sin^2 \alpha^p + a^2 \cos^2 \alpha^p) + y(\ 2b^2 s \sin^2 \alpha^p) + b^2s^2 \quad a^2b^2 \cos^2 \alpha^p \quad 0$

//Calculating the discriminant Δ_0 of the square //trinomial — Substituting $s \quad s_m$

$\Delta_0 \quad (\ 2b^2 s_m \sin^2 \alpha^p)^2 + 4(b^2 \sin^2 \alpha^p + a^2 \cos^2 \alpha^p)(b^2 s_m^2 \quad a^2b^2 \cos^2 \alpha^p) \quad 0$

//Rearranging and simplifying the expression

$s_m^2 \quad a^2 \cos^2 \alpha^p + b^2 \sin^2 \alpha^p$

//Returning to the calculation of the discriminant of the square trinomial

$\Delta_{12} \quad (\ 2b^2 s \sin^2 \alpha^p)^2 \quad 4(b^2 \sin^2 \alpha^p + a^2 \cos^2 \alpha^p)(b^2s^2 \quad a^2b^2 \cos^2 \alpha^p)$

$4a^a b^4 \sin^2 \alpha^p \cos^2 \alpha^p \quad a^2b^2s^2 \cos^2 \alpha^p + a^4b^2 \cos^4 \alpha^p$

$4a^2b^2 \cos^2 \alpha^p (b^2 \sin^2 \alpha^p \quad s^s + a^2 \cos^2 \alpha^p)$

$4a^2b^2 \cos^2 \alpha^p (s_m^2 \quad s^s)$

//The first root of the quadratic equation in the y direction

$y_1 \quad \frac{2b^2 s \sin^2 \alpha^p - 2ab \cos^2 \alpha^p (s_m^2 - s^s)}{2s_m}$

//The second root of the quadratic equation in the y direction

$y_2 \quad \frac{2b^2 s \sin^2 \alpha^p + 2ab \cos^2 \alpha^p (s_m^2 - s^s)}{2s_m}$

//The square of the difference of the roots in the y direction

$(y_1 \quad y_2)^2 \quad \left(\frac{4ab \cos^2 \alpha^p (s_m^2 - s^s)}{2s_m}\right)^2$

//The first root of the quadratic equation in the x direction

$x_1 \quad \frac{2a^2 s \sin^2 \alpha^p - 2ab \cos^2 \alpha^p (s_m^2 - s^s)}{2s_m}$

//The second root of the quadratic equation in the x direction

$x_2 \quad \frac{2a^2 s \sin^2 \alpha^p + 2ab \cos^2 \alpha^p (s_m^2 - s^s)}{2s_m}$

//The square of the difference of the roots in the y direction

$(x_1 \quad x_2)^2 \quad \left(\frac{4ab \sin^2 \alpha^p (s_m^2 - s^s)}{2s_m}\right)^2$

//The Euclidean distance between the two points where the path
//of the ray s intersects the ellipse:

$Dist \quad \sqrt{(x_1 \quad x_2)^2 + (y_1 \quad y_2)^2}$

$\sqrt{\left(\frac{4a^2b^2 \sin^2 \alpha^p (s_m^2 - s^2)}{2s_m}\right)^2 + \left(\frac{4a^2b^2 \cos^2 \alpha^p (s_m^2 - s^2)}{2s_m}\right)^2}$

//Finally

$\frac{2ab\sqrt{(s_m^2 - s^2)}}{s_m} \sqrt{\sin^2 \alpha^p + \cos^2 \alpha^p} \quad \frac{2ab\sqrt{(s_m^2 - s^2)}}{s_m}$

□

For ellipses whose centres have been displaced by the vector (x_0, y_0) and/or rotated by the angle α_0, we can calculate the projection value using the following relationship:

$$p_i^p(s, \alpha^p, (x_0, y_0), \alpha_0) = p_i^p\left(s - s_0 \cos(\alpha^p - \alpha_0^{xy}), \alpha^p - \alpha_0\right), \tag{10.9}$$

where

$$s_0 = \sqrt{x_0^2 + y_0^2}, \tag{10.10}$$

$$\alpha_0^{xy} = \arctan\left(\frac{y_0}{x_0}\right). \tag{10.11}$$

The strategy in this case is to bring the centre of the displaced ellipse to the origin of the coordinate system, and then to simulate the projection values there, bearing in mind that the measurement was actually carried out on the screen at the appropriately displaced point. For an ellipse rotated by α_0 the simulation of the projection values is carried out at a projection angle α^p, adjusted by the angle α_0. The relevant trigonometric relationships and their interpretation are shown in Fig. 10.4.

To calculate the distance s_m^{xy}, between the ray passing through the centre of the ellipse and the furthest rays still just passing through it, we use the relationship:

$$s_m^{xy} = \sqrt{a^2 \cos^2(\alpha^p - \alpha_0) + b^2 \sin^2(\alpha^p - \alpha_0)}. \tag{10.12}$$

Note that in Eq. 10.12, there is no term related to the displacement of the centre of the ellipse. This means that ellipses whose centres have been displaced but not rotated do not require a correction during the calculation of s_m.

The determination of the parameters of the rays tangential to the ellipse is illustrated further in Fig. 10.5.

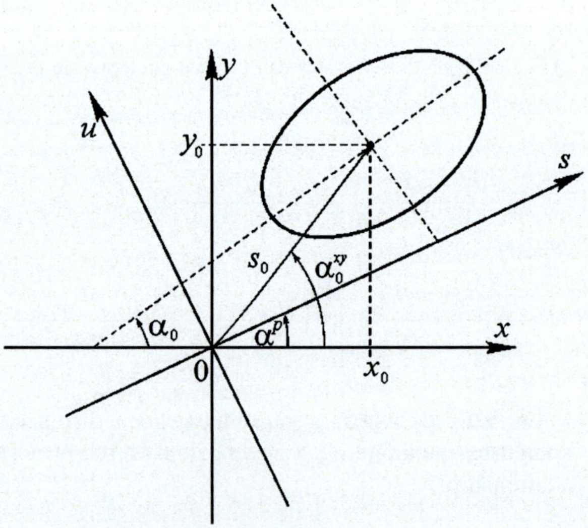

Fig. 10.4 Determining the projection value of an ellipse rotated through an angle α_0 and displaced by the vector (x_0, y_0)

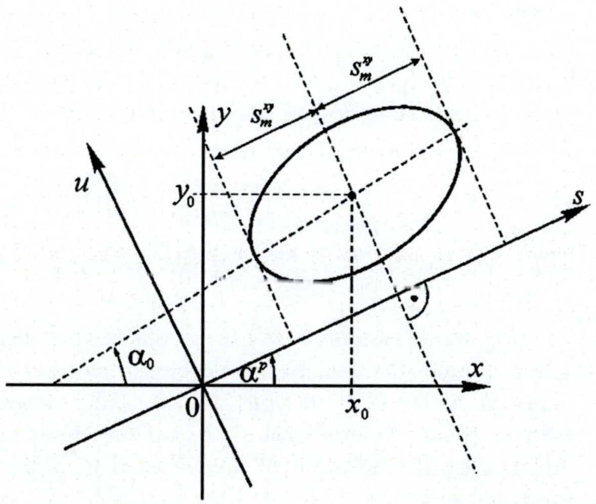

Fig. 10.5 Determining the tangents to an ellipse rotated through an angle α_0 and dis placed by the vector (x_0, y_0)

Now that we have constructed the phantom model we can move on to obtain the projections. To do this, we need to choose the resolution with which to calculate the projections and to choose the angle through which the system is rotated after each projection. The calculations are then performed using the procedure described above.

10.2 Mathematical Model for Fan-beam Projections

The problem of image reconstruction from fan-beam projections was introduced in Chap. 6. Here, we will apply the geometric relationships derived in that chapter to formulate a method of obtaining fan-beam projection values for the mathematical phantom just described in the previous section of this chapter. The most important conclusion we can draw from our earlier investigations is that for any ray in a fan-beam, we can find an equivalent ray in a hypothetical parallel-beam. Using equations (6.19) and (6.20), we can define relationships that allow us to express the parameters of a parallel-beam ray in terms of parameters specific to a ray in the fan-beam:

$$s = \mathrm{R}_f \sin \beta \tag{10.13}$$

and

$$\alpha^p = \alpha^f + \beta, \tag{10.14}$$

where β is the angle between the ray and the principal axis of the fan-beam, α^f the angle of rotation of the fan-beam projection system and R_f is the radius of the circle described by the tube.

The next step is to determine the parallel projection values $p_i^p(s, \alpha^p)$ for all the elements of the mathematical phantom, using the parameters established by Eqs. 10.13 and 10.14. This is carried out as described in Sect. 10.1. The sum of these projection values for all of the elements of the phantom gives us the projection value $p^f(\beta, \alpha^f)$.

10.3 Mathematical Model for Cone-beam Spiral Projections

For projection systems that use a cone shaped beam of radiation moving in a spiral around the patient, it becomes necessary to define the mathematical phantom in three dimensions [4, 5]. This means that Eq. 10.1, defining the ellipses (plane figures) that make up the mathematical phantom, needs to be replaced by the equation of an ellipsoid (a three-dimensional solid), as in the following equation:

$$\frac{x^2}{a^2} + \frac{y^2}{b^2} + \frac{z^2}{c^2} \leq 1, \tag{10.15}$$

for ellipsoids centred at the origin of the coordinate system. For ellipsoids displaced to the point (x_0, y_0, z_0), the equation takes the form:

$$\frac{(x - x_0)^2}{a^2} + \frac{(y - y_0)^2}{b^2} + \frac{(z - z_0)^2}{c^2} \leq 1. \tag{10.16}$$

If in addition, the ellipsoid is rotated in the (x, y) plane by an angle α_0 about the origin, then the above equation becomes:

$$\frac{((x - x_0)\cos\alpha_0 + (y - y_0)\sin\alpha_0)^2}{a^2} + \frac{(-(x - x_0)\sin\alpha_0 + (y - y_0)\cos\alpha_0)^2}{b^2} + \frac{(z - z_0)^2}{c^2} \leq 1. \tag{10.17}$$

The following table contains the set of parameters for the ellipsoids in a proposed mathematical model of a head phantom [5].

A perspective view of the complete mathematical phantom, whose parameters are given in Table 10.2, together with cross-sections in the (x, y) plane are shown in Fig. 10.6.

Any parallel projection in 3D space can be regarded as a projection made in the (x, y) plane by a beam of radiation parallel to the x-axis, after all the rays of the beam have been subjected to two transformations combined. The first of these transformations is rotation in the (x, y) plane by an angle α_1^p about the z-axis. This means that the coordinate system (x, y, z) can be replaced by the rotated system (s, u, z), where

Table 10.2 Parameters of the ellipsoids making up the mathematical model of the head phantom

Ellipse number	Coordinates of the centre			S. min. axis x	S. min. axis y	S. min. axis z	Angle of rotation	$\mu^{const}(x, y)$
	x_0	y_0	z_0	a	b	c	α_0 (deg)	
I	0.000	0.000	0.000	0.6900	0.9200	0.9000	0.0	2.00
II	0.000	0.000	0.000	0.6624	0.8740	0.8800	0.0	0.98
III	0.220	0.000	0.250	0.4100	0.1600	0.2100	108.0	0.02
IV	0.220	0.000	0.250	0.3100	0.1100	0.2200	72.0	0.02
V	0.000	0.350	0.250	0.2100	0.2500	0.5000	0.0	0.02
VI	0.000	0.100	0.250	0.0460	0.0460	0.0460	0.0	0.02
VII	0.080	0.650	0.250	0.0460	0.0230	0.0200	0.0	0.01
VIII	0.060	0.650	0.250	0.0230	0.0460	0.0200	90.0	0.01
IX	0.060	0.105	0.625	0.0400	0.0560	0.1000	90.0	0.02
X	0.000	0.100	0.625	0.0560	0.0400	0.1000	0.0	0.02

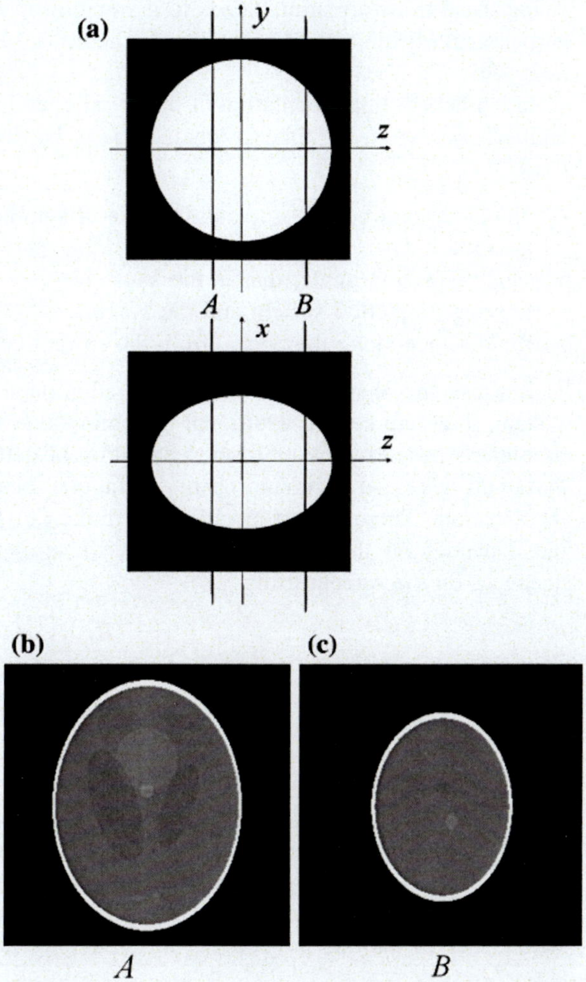

Fig. 10.6 Mathematical model of the head phantom from Table 10.2: **a** a perspective view, **b** a cross section in the plane A, **c** a cross section in the plane B

$$s = x \cos \alpha_1^p + y \sin \alpha_1^p \tag{10.18}$$

and

$$u = -x \sin \alpha_1^p + y \cos \alpha_1^p. \tag{10.19}$$

The second transformation is rotation of the (s, u, z) system by an angle α_2^p about the s axis. If we introduce a new, rotated coordinate system $(s, \dot{u}, t)$, the coordinates of any point in this space can be calculated using the following relationships:

$$t = z \cos \alpha_2^p + \left(-x \sin \alpha_1^p + y \cos \alpha_1^p\right) \sin \alpha_2^p \tag{10.20}$$

and

$$\dot{u} = -z \sin \alpha_2^p + \left(-x \sin \alpha_1^p + y \cos \alpha_1^p\right) \cos \alpha_2^p. \tag{10.21}$$

Using these transformations leads to a situation in which the parallel beam falls perpendicularly onto the screen to which the (t, s) coordinate system has been assigned.

In a practical implementation of the spiral cone-beam scanner, each of the rays emitted by the X-ray tube is characterised by the following parameters (see Chap. 7):

β the angle between the ray and the axis of symmetry of the moving projection system,
α^h the projection angle, that is the angle between the axis of symmetry of the moving projection system and the x axis,
$\dot{z}$ the distance along the z-axis, from the current centre of the projection system.

Because the shape of the screen of radiation detectors is cylindrical in this system, there are certain additional operations that we need to perform. A major problem is posed by the uniform distribution of detectors in the z-direction. Note that in this case there is no uniformity of angular distance between the rays striking the detectors. Therefore, to specify a ray in the (z, x) plane, it is better to consider the distances on the principal z-axis of the projection system rather than the distances on the screen, using:

$$\dot{z} = z \frac{\mathrm{R_f}}{\mathrm{R}_f + \mathrm{R}_d}, \tag{10.22}$$

where R_f is the radius of the circle described by the tube-screen system, R_d is the radius of the circle described by the screen.

In the y-direction, however, the cylindrical shape of the screen permits uniform spacing of the detectors both in terms of linear distance on the screen and in terms of angular distance between the rays striking the screen. In this situation, we can use the angle β to specify a given ray in the (x, y) plane.

We will now attempt to replace any projection value in the cone-beam system with a specific parallel projection value. The process of finding the parameters of the hypothetical parallel ray in the (x, y) plane is the same as in the case of the fan-beam (see Sect. 10.2). This occurs with the projection system rotated by the angle α^h about the z-axis, as indicated in Fig. 10.7.

Using this diagram, it is easy to find the trigonometric relationships between the parameters of the ray in question in the two projection systems:

$$s = \mathrm{R}_f \sin \beta \tag{10.23}$$

and

$$\alpha_1^p = \alpha^h + \beta. \tag{10.24}$$

Using Fig. 10.8, however, we can find the geometrical transformations allowing us to assign a ray in the (z, x) plane of the parallel-beam system to a ray in the

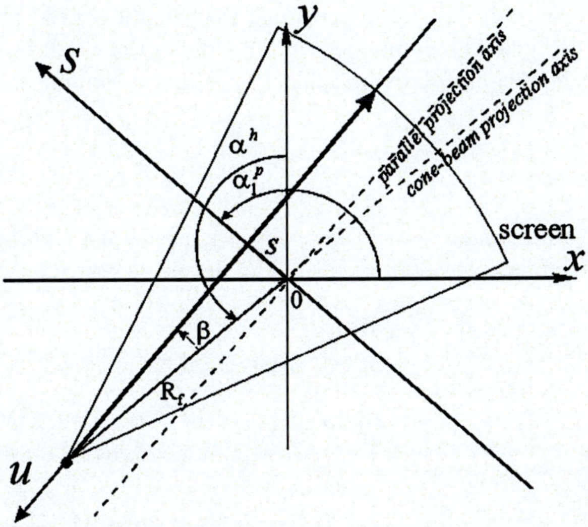

Fig. 10.7 Finding the ray in the (x, y) plane in the paral lel beam system equivalent to a ray in the cone beam

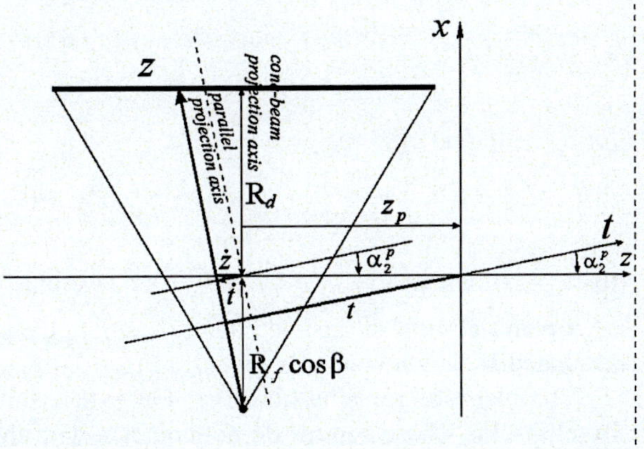

Fig. 10.8 Finding the ray in the (z, x) plane in the parallel beam system equivalent to a ray in the cone beam

cone-beam (in fact, to a segment of a fan-beam). The diagram also makes it easy to determine the following parameters for the parallel ray under consideration:

$$\dot{t} = \dot{z}\frac{\mathrm{R_f}\cos\beta}{\sqrt{(\mathrm{R}_f\cos\beta)^2 + \dot{z}^2}}, \tag{10.25}$$

where $\dot{z}$ is calculated using relationship (10.22) and:

$$\alpha_2^p = \arcsin\frac{\dot{z}}{\sqrt{(\mathrm{R}_f\cos\beta)^2 + \dot{z}^2}}. \tag{10.26}$$

It is easy now to determine the parameter t, using:

$$t = (\dot{z} + z_p)\cos\alpha_2^p. \tag{10.27}$$

As with the two-dimensional mathematical head phantom, the final result of the simulated measurement in three dimensions will be the sum of all the calculations for the ellipsoids in Table 10.2, using a formula similar to Eq. 10.7:

$$p^p(s, t, \alpha_1^p, \alpha_2^p) = \sum_{i=1}^{10} p_i^p(s, t, \alpha_1^p, \alpha_2^p). \tag{10.28}$$

In a similar way to Eq. 10.8, we can obtain a formula that allows us to find the projection value for a single ellipsoid in the 3D phantom:

$$\begin{aligned} p_i^p(s,t,\alpha_1^p,\alpha_2^p) &= \Delta u \cdot \mu_i^{\text{const}} \\ &= \frac{\mu_i^{\text{const}} \cdot 2abc}{d^2}[d_m]^{\frac{1}{2}} \\ &= \frac{\mu_i^{\text{const}} \cdot 2abc}{d^2}\Big[d^2 - s^2(c^2\cos^2\alpha_2^p + (b^2\cos^2\alpha_1^p + a^2\sin^2\alpha_1^p)\sin^2\alpha_2^p) \\ &\quad - t^2(a^2\cos^2\alpha_1^p + b^2\sin^2\alpha_1^p)\left(\frac{7+\cos(4\alpha_2^p)}{8}\right) \\ &\quad - 2st\sin\alpha_2^p\sin\alpha_1^p\cos\alpha_1^p(b^2 - a^2)\Big]^{\frac{1}{2}} \end{aligned} \tag{10.29}$$

for $d_m \geq 0$, and

$$p_i^p(s, t, \alpha_1^p, \alpha_2^p) = 0 \tag{10.30}$$

for $d_m < 0$, where $d = \sqrt{c^2(a^2\cos^2\alpha_1^p + b^2\sin^2\alpha_1^p)\cos^2\alpha_2^p + a^2b^2\sin^2\alpha_2^p}$.

A pictorial view of this method of obtaining the projection value of an ellipsoid irradiated by a cone-beam is given in Fig. 10.9.

A problem still remains, however: how to determine the parallel projection value for ellipsoids whose centres do not coincide with the point $(x, y, z) = (0, 0, 0)$ or

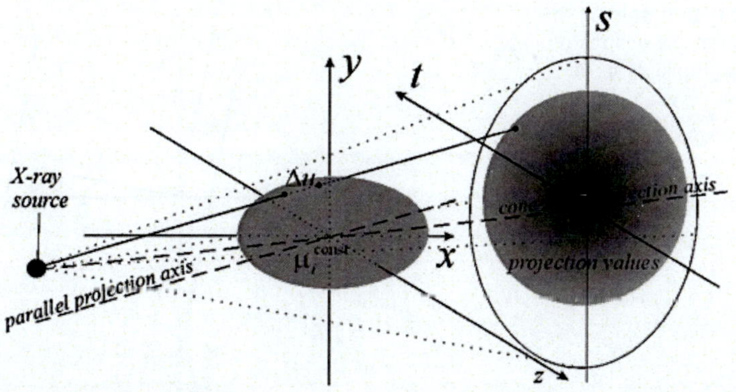

Fig. 10.9 Determining the projection value of an ellipsoid using a cone beam of radiation

are rotated with respect to one of the (x, y, z) axes. In the first case, the centre of the ellipsoid is translated by the vector (x_0, y_0, z_0), while in the second, it is rotated by the angle α_0 in the (x, y) plane only. To determine the projection value of a 3D ellipsoidal element of the model, which has been subjected to one of these transformations, we simply use the following relationship:

$$p_i^p\left(s,t,\alpha_1^p,\alpha_2^p,(x_0,y_0,z_0),\alpha_0\right) = p_i^p\left(s - s_0 \cdot \cos\left(\alpha_0^{xy} - \alpha_1^p\right), t - t_0 \cos \alpha_2^p, \alpha_1^p - \alpha_0, \alpha_2^p\right). \tag{10.31}$$

We will now attempt to determine correction parameters for the translated ellipsoids. The geometrical relationships shown in Fig. 10.10 are helpful in formulating expressions regarding correction in the s dimension.

Fig. 10.10 Determining the correction of the centres of displaced ellipsoids in the s dimension

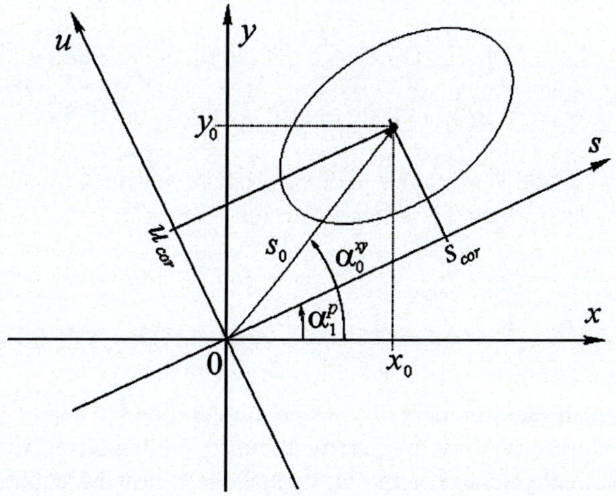

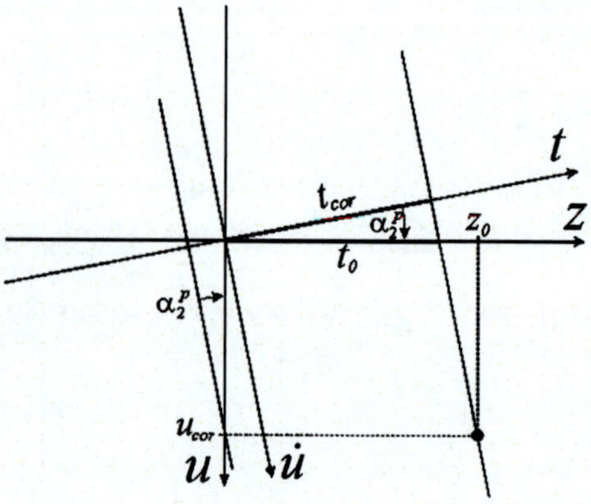

Fig. 10.11 Determining the correction of the centres of displaced ellipsoids in the t dimension

In a similar way to the 2D case, we can find the correction of the centres of displaced ellipsoids in the s dimension based on relations (10.10) and (10.11). Additionally, we can determine the following auxiliary parameter:

$$u_{\text{cor}} = s_0 \cdot \sin\left(\alpha_0^{xy} - \alpha_1^p\right). \tag{10.32}$$

In the case of the correction of the centres of displaced ellipsoids in the t dimension, Fig. 10.11 is very useful. It represents the geometrical relationships when the projection system is rotated by the angle α_2^p about the s-axis.

Based on Fig. 10.11 we can write:

$$t_0 = z_0 + u_{\text{cor}} \tan \alpha_2^p = z_0 + s_0 \sin\left(\alpha_0^{xy} - \alpha_1^p\right) \tan \alpha_2^p. \tag{10.33}$$

To calculate the value of d for ellipsoids rotated by α_0, we use the relationship:

$$d = \sqrt{c^2\left(a^2 \cos^2\left(\alpha_1^p - \alpha_0\right) + b^2 \sin^2\left(\alpha_1^p - \alpha_0\right)\right) \cos^2 \alpha_2^p + a^2 b^2 \sin^2 \alpha_2^p}. \tag{10.34}$$

Note that irrespective of the projection angle, translation of the centre of the ellipsoid does not affect the way we calculate this parameter. The trigonometric relationships and the basic symbols used in this problem are presented in Fig. 10.12.

The sum of the parallel projection values of all the elements of the phantom determines the projection value $p^h(\beta, \alpha^h, z)$.

10.4 Introduction of Noise to the Projections

All measurements of physical quantities are subject to noise. In order to simulate the effect of measurement noise on the projection values obtained using the mathematical phantom, we use the following equation:

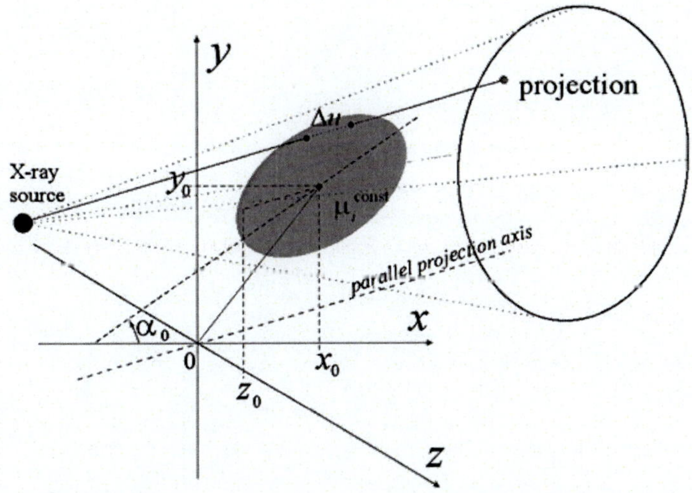

Fig. 10.12 Determining the projection value of an ellipsoid rotated through an angle α_0 and displaced by the vector (x_0, y_0, z_0)

$$p^p_{\text{normal}}(s, \alpha^p) = \left(1 + N\left(p_0, \sigma^2\right)\right) p^p(s, \alpha^p), \tag{10.35}$$

where $p^p{}_{\{\text{normal}}(s, \alpha^p)$ is the parallel projection value distorted by normal noise, $N(p_0, \sigma^2)$ is stochastic noise of normal distribution (p_0, mean value and σ^2, variance).

Suggested values [8] for the mean and the variance of the normal distribution are $p_0 = 0$ and $\sigma^2 = (0.05)^2$, respectively.

A method for the computer generation of noise with a normal distribution is given in Appendix B, for set values of p and σ^2.

References

1. Jähne B (1991) Digital image processing: concepts, algorithms and scientific applications. Springer, Berlin
2. Jain AK (1989) Fundamentals of digitals image processing. Prentice Hall, Englewood Cliffs
3. Kachelrieß M (2000) ECG correlated image reconstruction from subsecond multi slice CT scans of the heart. Med Phys 27:1881 1902
4. Kak AC, Roberts B (1986) Image reconstruction from projections. In: Young TY, Fu KS (eds) Handbook of pattern recognition and image processing. Academic Press, New York
5. Kak AC, Slanley M (1988) Principles of computerized tomographic imaging. IEEE Press, New York
6. Rosenfeld A, Kak AC (1982) Digital picture processing. Academic Press, New York
7. Shepp LA, Logan BF (1974) The Fourier reconstruction of a head section. IEEE Trans Nucl Sci NS 21:21 43
8. Wang Y, Wahl FM (1997) Vector entropy optimization based neural network approach to image reconstruction from projections. IEEE Trans Neural Netw 8:1008 1014

Appendix A
Functions and their Properties

A.1 The Dirac Delta Function

Definitions

The one-dimensional Dirac delta function:

$$\lim_{\varepsilon \to 0} \int_{\varepsilon}^{\varepsilon} \delta(x) = 1 \text{ where } \delta(x) = 0 \quad \text{for } x \neq 0 \tag{A.1}$$

Table A.1 Functions used in the book and their definitions

Section	Name of function	Definition
	rect	$rect(x) \quad \begin{cases} 1 & \text{for} \quad \lvert x\rvert \geq \frac{1}{2} \\ 0 & \text{for} \quad \lvert x\rvert < \frac{1}{2} \end{cases}$
	sign	$sign(x) \quad \begin{cases} 1 & \text{for} \quad x > 0 \\ 0 & \text{for} \quad x \quad 0 \\ \;\; 1 & \text{for} \quad x < 0 \end{cases}$
	sinc	$sinc(x) \quad \frac{\sin(\pi x)}{\pi x}$
	div	division with no remainder: $x \; div \; \Delta \quad c;\, c \in \mathbb{I}$; when $\lvert \Delta \cdot c \rvert \leq x \wedge \lvert \Delta \cdot (c+1) \rvert \geq x$
	mod	remainder after division: $x \; mod \; \Delta \quad c;\, c \in \mathbb{I}$; when $c + (x \; div \; \Delta) \quad x$
	Trunc	$Trunc(x, \Delta) \quad \begin{cases} \frac{(x-(x \, mod \, \Delta))}{\Delta} & \text{for} \quad x \geq 0 \\ \frac{(x-(x \, mod \, \Delta))}{\Delta} \quad 1 & \text{for} \quad x > 0 \end{cases}$
A.1	Dirac delta δ	$\lim_{x \to 0} \int_{-x}^{x} \delta(x) \quad 1$; where $\delta(x) \quad 0$ for $x \neq 0$
	comb	$comb(x) \quad \sum_{i \;\; -\infty}^{\infty} \delta(x \quad i)$
	Convolution	$fun_1(x) * fun_2(x) \quad \int_{-\infty}^{\infty} fun_1(x \quad \dot{x}) \cdot fun_2(\dot{x}) d\dot{x}$

(continued)

Table A.1 (continued)

Section	Name of function	Definition
A.2	Fourier transform	$FUN(f) \equiv F\{fun(x)\} \triangleq \int_{-\infty}^{\infty} fun(x)e^{-j2\pi fx}dx$
A.3	Radon transform	$p(s,\alpha) \equiv R\{fun(x,y)\} \triangleq \int_{-\infty}^{\infty} fun(x,y)\cdot\delta(x\cos\alpha + y\sin\alpha \quad s)dxdy$
	Hilbert transform	$Hfun(x) \equiv H\{fun(x)\} \triangleq fun(x) * \frac{1}{\pi x} \quad \frac{1}{\pi}\int_{-\infty}^{\infty}\frac{fun(\dot{x})}{x-\dot{x}}d\dot{x}$
	Cross correlation	$fun_1(x) \star fun_2(x) \quad \int_{-\infty}^{\infty} fun_1(\dot{x})\cdot fun_2(\dot{x} \quad x)d\dot{x}$

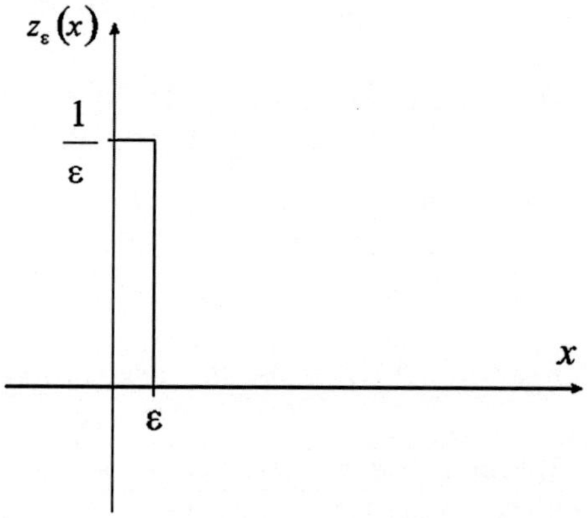

Fig. A.1 The form of function (3)

The two-dimensional Dirac delta function:

$$\lim_{\varepsilon\to 0}\int_{\varepsilon}^{\varepsilon}\int_{\varepsilon}^{\varepsilon}\delta(x,y) = 1 \text{ where } \delta(x,y) = 0 \quad \text{for } x \neq 0 \vee y \neq 0 \tag{A.2}$$

Proof of the scaling property of the Dirac delta function:

$$\delta(ax) = \frac{\delta(x)}{|a|} \tag{A.3}$$

An alternative definition of the Dirac delta function is:

$$\delta(x) = \lim_{\varepsilon\to 0} z_\varepsilon(x), \tag{A.4}$$

where $z_\varepsilon(x)$ is a function defined as:

$$z_\varepsilon(x) = \begin{cases} \frac{1}{\varepsilon} & \text{for } \; 0 \leq x \leq \varepsilon \\ 0 & \text{for } \; \text{the remaining } x \end{cases}, \tag{A.5}$$

the graph of which is shown in Fig. A.1.
Thus substituting:

$$\delta(ax) = \lim_{\varepsilon \to 0} z_\varepsilon(ax)$$

into equation (A.1) we obtain:

$$\lim_{\varepsilon \to 0} \int_{\infty}^{\infty} z_\varepsilon(ax)\mathrm{d}x = \frac{1}{|a|}.$$

Thus, if the mass

$$\int_{\infty}^{\infty} \delta(ax)\mathrm{d}x = \frac{1}{|a|} \int_{\infty}^{\infty} \delta(x)\mathrm{d}x,$$

we obtain:

$$\delta(ax) = \frac{\delta(x)}{|a|}.$$

□

Proof of the Dirac delta function of a function:

$$\delta(fun(x)) = \sum_l \frac{\delta(x - x_l)}{\left|\frac{dfun(x_l)}{d(x)}\right|} \tag{A.6}$$

If by definition we know that $\delta(x) = 0$ for every $x \neq 0$, then similarly:

$$\delta(fun(x)) = 0$$

Table A.2 Properties of the Dirac delta function

Property	Description
Scaling	$\delta(ax) \quad \frac{\delta(x)}{\|a\|}$
One dimensional shifting	$\int_{-\infty}^{\infty} fun(\dot{x}) \cdot \delta(x \quad \dot{x})d\dot{x} \quad fun(x)$
Two dimensional Dirac delta	$\delta(x, y) \quad \delta(x)\cdot\delta(y)$
Two dimensional shifting	$\int_{-\infty}^{\infty}\int_{-\infty}^{\infty} fun(\dot{x},\dot{y}) \cdot \delta(x \quad \dot{x}, y \quad \dot{y})d\dot{x}d\dot{y} \quad fun(x,y)$
Dirac delta function of a function	$\delta(fun(x)) \quad \sum_l \frac{\delta(x-x_l)}{\left\|\frac{dfun(x_l)}{d(x)}\right\|}$ where x_l are zero points of the function $fun(x)$
	$\int_0^{\pi} \delta((x \quad \dot{x})\cos\alpha + (y \quad \dot{y})\sin\alpha)d\alpha \quad \frac{1}{\sqrt{(x-\dot{x})^2+(y-\dot{y})^2}}$

for every value of *fun*(x) except where *fun*(x) $= 0$, i.e. the points at which $x = x_l$, where x_l are the zero points of the function *fun*(x). At these points, we can regard the derivative $\frac{dfun(x_l)}{dx}$ as the local gradient of *fun*(x), i.e. the linear coefficient appearing in *fun*(x) $= a_l x + c_l$, where:

$$a_l = \frac{dfun(x_l)}{dx}$$

and $c_l = x_l$ are the shifting constants.

Therefore, taking into consideration the scaling and shifting properties of the Dirac delta proved earlier and the presence of many places where *fun*(x) is zero, we can write the following:

$$\delta(fun(x)) = \sum_l \frac{1}{|a_l|}\delta(x - c_l) = \sum_l \frac{\delta(x - x_l)}{\left|\frac{dfun(x_l)}{d(x)}\right|}$$

□

Proof of the relationship:

$$\int_0^{\pi} \delta((x - \dot{x})\cos\alpha + (y - \dot{y})\sin\alpha)d\alpha = \frac{1}{\sqrt{(x - \dot{x})^2 + (y - \dot{y})^2}} \tag{A.7}$$

$$\int_0^{\pi} \delta((x - \dot{x})\cos\alpha + (y - \dot{y})\sin\alpha)d\alpha =$$

//$fun(\alpha) = (x - \dot{x})\cos\alpha + (y - \dot{y})\sin\alpha = \int_0^{\pi} \delta(fun(\alpha))d\alpha =$

//Considering property (A.6)

$$= \int_0^{\pi}\left(\sum_l \frac{\delta(\alpha - \alpha_l)}{\left|\frac{dfun(\alpha_l)}{d(\alpha)}\right|}\right)d\alpha =$$

//where: $fun(\alpha_l) = (x - \dot{x})\cos\alpha_l + (y - \dot{y})\sin\alpha_l$

$$= \int_0^{\pi}\left(\sum_l \frac{\delta(\alpha - \alpha_l)}{|-(x - \dot{x})\sin\alpha_l + (y - \dot{y})\cos\alpha_l|}\right)d\alpha$$

$$= \sum_l\left(\frac{1}{|-(x - \dot{x})\sin\alpha_l + (y - \dot{y})\cos\alpha_l|}\int_0^{\pi}\delta(\alpha - \alpha_l)d\alpha\right) =$$

//If $\alpha \in [0,\pi)$, then $l \in \{L\}$ and $\int_0^{\pi} \delta(\alpha - \alpha_l)d\alpha = 1$ in the function $\tan\alpha_l$

$$= \frac{1}{|-(x-\dot{x})\sin\alpha_L + (y-\dot{y})\cos\alpha_L|}$$

$$= \frac{1}{\sqrt{(-(x-\dot{x})\sin\alpha_L + (y-\dot{y})\cos\alpha_L)^2}} =$$

//Considering that: $-\frac{x\ \dot{x}}{y\ \dot{y}} = \tan\alpha_l = \frac{\sin\alpha_l}{\cos\alpha_l} \Rightarrow \frac{(x\ \dot{x})^2}{(y\ \dot{y})^2} = \frac{\sin^2\alpha_l}{\cos^2\alpha_l}$

$$= \frac{1}{\sqrt{(x-\dot{x})^2+(y-\dot{y})^2}}$$

□

A.2 The Fourier Transform

Definitions in one dimension:

The Fourier transform:

$$FUN(f) \equiv F_1\{fun(x)\} \triangleq \int_{\infty}^{\infty} fun(x) \cdot e^{\ j2\pi fx} dx \qquad (A.8)$$

The inverse Fourier transform:

$$fun(x) \equiv F_1^{\ 1}\{FUN(f)\} \triangleq \int_{\infty}^{\infty} FUN(f) \cdot e^{j2\pi fx} df \qquad (A.9)$$

Definitions in two dimensions:

The Fourier transform:

$$FUN(f_1, f_2) \equiv F_2\{fun(x,y)\} \triangleq \int_{\infty}^{\infty}\int_{\infty}^{\infty} fun(x,y) \cdot e^{\ j2\pi f(x\cos\alpha^p + y\sin\alpha^p)} dxdy \quad (A.10)$$

The inverse Fourier transform:

$$fun(x) \equiv F_2^{\ 1}\{FUN(f_1, f_2)\} \triangleq \int_{\infty}^{\infty}\int_{\infty}^{\infty} FUN(f_1, f_2) \cdot e^{j2\pi f(x\cos\alpha^p + y\sin\alpha^p)} df_1 df_2$$

(A.11)

Proof of the Fourier transform of the function:

$$-\frac{1}{(2\pi x)^2} \leftrightarrow |f| \qquad (A.12)$$

Table A.3 Fourier transforms of various functions

fun(*x*)/*fun*(*x*, *y*)	*FUN*(*f*)/*FUN*(f_1,f_2)
$\delta(x)$	1
$\delta(x \pm x_0)$	$e^{\pm j2\pi f x_0}$
$e^{\pm j2\pi a x}$	$\delta(f \pm a)$
rect(*x*)	*sinc*(*f*)
comb(*x*)	*comb*(*f*)
$\frac{1}{(2\pi x)^2}$	$\lvert f\rvert$
$\delta(x, y)$	1
$\delta(x \pm x_0, y \pm y_0)$	$e^{\pm j2\pi f_1 x_0} \cdot e^{\pm j2\pi f_2 y_0}$
$e^{\pm j2\pi a_1 x} \cdot e^{\pm j2\pi a_2 y}$	$\delta(f_1 \pm a_1, f_2 \pm a_2)$
rect(*x*, *y*)	*sinc*(f_1,f_2)
comb(*x*, *y*)	*comb*(f_1,f_2)

Table A.4 Properties of the Fourier transform

Transform property	Form of the function/equivalent after Fourier transformation
One dimension	$fun(x) \leftrightarrow FUN(f)$
Rotation	$fun(\pm x) \leftrightarrow FUN(\pm f)$
Linearity	$a_1 fun_1(x) + a_2 fun_2(x) \leftrightarrow a_1 FUN_1(f) + a_2 FUN_2(f)$
Scaling	$fun(ax) \leftrightarrow \frac{FUN\left(\frac{f}{a}\right)}{\lvert a\rvert}$
Shifting	$fun(x \pm x_0) \leftrightarrow e^{\pm j2\pi f x_0} \cdot FUN(f)$
Convolution	$fun(x) \quad fun_1(x) * fun_2(x) \leftrightarrow FUN(f) \quad FUN_1(f) \cdot FUN_2(f)$
Product	$fun(x) \quad fun_1(x) \cdot fun_2(x) \leftrightarrow FUN(f) \quad FUN_1(f) * FUN_2(f)$
Cross correlation	$fun(x) \quad fun_1(x) \star fun_2(x) \leftrightarrow FUN(f) \quad FUN_1(f) * FUN_2(f)$ where: $fun_2(x)$ is real
Two dimensions	$fun(x, y) \leftrightarrow FUN(f_1, f_2)$
Rotation	$fun(\pm x, \pm y) \leftrightarrow FUN(\pm f_1, \pm f_2)$
Linearity	$a_1 fun_1(x, y) + a_2 fun_2(x, y) \leftrightarrow a_1 FUN_1(f f_2) + a_2 FUN_2(f_1, f_2)$
Separability	$fun_1(x) \cdot fun_2(y) \leftrightarrow FUN_1(f_1) \cdot FUN_2(f_2)$
Scaling	$fun(ax, by) \leftrightarrow \frac{FUN\left(\frac{f_1}{a}, \frac{f_2}{b}\right)}{\lvert ab\rvert}$
Shifting	$fun(x \pm x_0, y \pm y_0,) \leftrightarrow e^{\pm j2\pi(f_1 x_0 + f_2 y_0)} \cdot FUN(f_1, f_2)$
Convolution	$fun(x, y) \quad fun_1(x, y) * fun_2(x, y) \leftrightarrow$ $\leftrightarrow FUN(f_1, f_2) \quad FUN_1(f_1, f_2) \cdot FUN_2(f_1, f_2)$
Product	$fun(x, y) \quad fun_1(x, y) \cdot fun_2(x, y) \leftrightarrow$ $\leftrightarrow FUN(f_1, f_2) \quad FUN_1(f_1, f_2) * FUN_2(f_1, f_2)$

$$fun(x) = \int_{\infty}^{\infty} \lvert f\rvert e^{j2\pi f x} df =$$

//Applying the approximation: $\lvert f\rvert \cong \lim_{\epsilon \to 0}\left(\lvert f\rvert e^{\epsilon \lvert f\rvert}\right)$

$$= \lim_{\epsilon\to 0} \int_{\infty}^{\infty} |f| \cdot e^{\ \epsilon|f|} \cdot e^{j2\pi fx} df =$$

//Applying: $|f| = f{\cdot}sign(f)$

$$= \lim_{\epsilon\to 0} \int_{\infty}^{\infty} f \cdot sign(f) \cdot \cdot e^{\ \epsilon f \cdot sign(f)} \cdot e^{j2\pi fx} df$$

$$= \lim_{\epsilon\to 0} \left(- \int_{\infty}^{0} f \cdot e^{\epsilon f} \cdot e^{j2\pi fx} + \int_{0}^{\infty} f \cdot e^{\ \epsilon f} \cdot e^{j2\pi fx} df \right)$$

$$= \lim_{\epsilon\to 0} \left(- \int_{\infty}^{0} f \cdot e^{(\epsilon + j2\pi x)f} + \int_{0}^{\infty} f \cdot e^{\ (\epsilon\ \ j2\pi x)f} df \right) =$$

//Applying the theorem of integration by parts

$$= \lim_{\epsilon\to 0} \left(\frac{\left[e^{(\epsilon + j2\pi x)f}\right]_{\infty}^{0}}{(\epsilon + j2\pi x)^2} - \frac{\left[e^{\ (\epsilon\ \ j2\pi x)f}\right]_{0}^{\infty}}{(\epsilon - j2\pi x)^2} \right)$$

$$= \lim_{\epsilon\to 0} \left(\frac{\epsilon^2 - (2\pi x)^2}{\left(\epsilon^2 - (2\pi x)^2\right)^2} \right) = \frac{-1}{(2\pi x)^2}$$

□

Proof of the inverse Fourier transform of the function:

$$FUN(f) = |f| \cdot \left(1 - \frac{\epsilon|f|}{f_0}\right) \cdot rect\left(\frac{f}{2f_0}\right) \qquad \text{(A.13)}$$

The derivation:

$$fun(x) = \int_{\infty}^{\infty} |f| \cdot \left(1 - \frac{\epsilon|f|}{f_0}\right) \cdot rect\left(\frac{f}{2f_0}\right) e^{j2\pi fx} df$$

$$= \int_{f_0}^{f_0} |f| \cdot \left(1 - \frac{\epsilon|f|}{f_0}\right) \cdot e^{j2\pi fx} df$$

$$= \int_{f_0}^{f_0} |f| \cdot e^{j2\pi fx} df - \frac{\epsilon}{f_0} \int_{f_0}^{f_0} f^2 \cdot e^{j2\pi fx} df$$

The first of these two components is calculated as follows:

$$\int_{f_0}^{f_0} |f| \cdot e^{j2\pi fx} df$$

$$= -\int_{f_0}^{0} f \cdot e^{j2\pi fx} df + \int_{0}^{f_0} f \cdot e^{j2\pi fx} df$$

$$= -\frac{f}{j2\pi x} e^{j2\pi fx}\Big|_{f_0}^{0} + \int_{f_0}^{0} \frac{1}{j2\pi x} \cdot e^{j2\pi fx} df + \frac{f}{j2\pi x} e^{j2\pi fx}\Big|_{0}^{f_0} - \int_{0}^{f_0} \frac{1}{j2\pi x} \cdot e^{j2\pi fx} df$$

$$= -\frac{f_0 \cdot e^{\ j2\pi f_0 x}}{j2\pi x} + \frac{e^{\ j2\pi f_0 x}}{(j2\pi x)^2} - \frac{1}{(j2\pi x)^2} + \frac{f_0 \cdot e^{j2\pi f_0 x}}{j2\pi x} + \frac{e^{j2\pi f_0 x}}{(j2\pi x)^2} - \frac{1}{(j2\pi x)^2}$$

$$= \frac{f_0\left(e^{j2\pi f_0 x} - e^{\ j2\pi f_0 x}\right)}{j2\pi x} + \frac{e^{j2\pi f_0 x} + e^{\ j2\pi f_0 x}}{(j2\pi x)^2} - \frac{2}{(j2\pi x)^2}$$

$$= \frac{f_0 \sin(2\pi f_0 x)}{\pi x} + \frac{2}{(j2\pi x)^2} - \frac{4\sin^2(\pi f_0 x)}{(2\pi f_0 x)^2} - \frac{2}{(j2\pi x)^2}$$

$$= 2f_0^2 \frac{\sin(2\pi f_0 x)}{2\pi x} - f_0^2 \left(\frac{\sin(\pi f_0 x)}{\pi f_0 x}\right)$$

As a rule, the second component is determined as shown in brief below:

$$-\frac{\epsilon}{f_0} \int_{f_0}^{f_0} f^2 \cdot e^{j2\pi fx} df$$

$$= -\frac{\epsilon}{f_0}\left(f^2 \frac{f^2}{j2\pi x} e^{j2\pi fx}\Big|_{f_0}^{f_0} - 2 \int_{f_0}^{f_0} \frac{f}{j2\pi x} \cdot e^{j2\pi fx} df \right)$$

$$= -\frac{\epsilon}{f_0}\left(f_0^2 \frac{e^{j2\pi f_0 x} - e^{\ j2\pi f_0 x}}{-j2\pi x} + \frac{2f}{(2\pi x)^2} e^{j2\pi fx}\Big|_{f_0}^{f_0} - \int_{f_0}^{f_0} \frac{2}{(2\pi x)^2} e^{j2\pi fx} df \right)$$

$$= -\epsilon\left(\frac{f_0 \sin(2\pi f_0 x)}{\pi x} + \frac{4\cos(2\pi f_0 x)}{(2\pi x)^2} - \frac{4\sin(2\pi f_0 x)}{f_0 (2\pi x)^3} \right)$$

Taking both these components and substituting $f_0 = \frac{1}{2\Delta_s^p}$, we obtain:

$$fun(x) = \frac{1}{2\left(\Delta_s^p\right)^2} \frac{\sin\left(\frac{\pi x}{\Delta_s^p}\right)}{\frac{\pi x}{\Delta_s^p}} - \frac{1}{4\left(\Delta_s^p\right)^2} \left(\frac{\sin\left(\frac{\pi x}{2\Delta_s^p}\right)}{\frac{\pi x}{2\Delta_s^p}} \right)^2 - \epsilon\left(\frac{\sin\frac{\pi x}{\Delta_s^p}}{2\pi x \Delta_s^p} + \frac{\cos\frac{\pi x}{\Delta_s^p}}{(\pi x)^2} - \frac{\Delta_s^p \sin\frac{\pi x}{\Delta_s^p}}{(\pi x)^3} \right)$$

□

A.3 The Radon Transform

Definition

$$p(s,\alpha) \equiv R\{fun(x,y)\} \triangleq \int_{\infty}^{\infty} fun(x,y) \cdot \delta(x\cos\alpha + y\sin\alpha - s)dxdy \qquad (A.14)$$

Table A.5 Properties of the Radon transform

Transform property	Form of the function	Equivalent after Radon transformation
	$fun(x, y) \quad fun(r, \phi)$	$p(s, \alpha)$
Linearity	$a_1 fun_1(x, y) + a_2 fun_2(x, y)$	$a_1 p_1(s, \alpha) + a_2 p_2(s, \alpha)$
Space limitedness	$fun(x,y) \quad 0$, for $\lvert x\rvert > R$ or $\lvert y\rvert > R$	$p(s, \alpha) \quad 0$ for $\lvert s\rvert > \sqrt{2}R$
Symmetry	$fun(x, y)$ is symmetrical	$p(s, \alpha) \quad p(\quad s, \alpha \pm \pi)$
Periodicity	$fun(x, y)$ is periodic	$p(s, \alpha) \quad p(s, \alpha \pm 2i\pi)$ where i is an integer value
Shifting	$fun(x \quad x_0, y \quad y_0)$	$p(s \quad x_0 \cos\alpha \quad y_0 \sin\alpha, \alpha)$
Rotation by α_0	$fun(r, \phi + \alpha_0)$	$p(s, \alpha + \alpha_0)$
Scaling	$fun(ax, ay)$	$\frac{1}{\lvert a\rvert} p(as, \alpha)$
Mass	$Mass \quad \int_{-\infty}^{\infty}\int_{-\infty}^{\infty} fun(x,y)dxdy$	$Mass \quad \int_{-\infty}^{\infty} p(s,\alpha)ds$

Appendix B
Sample Code for Selected Functions

B.1 Determination of the Fast Fourier Transform Using the Cooley Algorithm

We can use the implementation presented below of one of the FFT algorithms, namely the Cooley Algorithm, to obtain the Fourier or inverse Fourier transform. Firstly, we need to perform the following declarations using Java code:

```
Declarations public class Complex {

    public double re;
    public double im;

    public Complex() {
        this.re = 0.0;
        this.im = 0.0;
    }

    public Complex(double re, double im) {
        this.re = re; this.im = im;
    }
    public static Complex complex(Complex c) {
        return new Complex(c.re, c.im);
    }

    public void set(Complex c) {
        this.re = c.re;
        this.im = c.im;
    }
```

```
        public static Complex complex() {
            return new Complex();
        }
        public static Complex complex(double re, double im) {
            return new Complex(re, im);
        }
        public static void swap(Complex c1, Complex c2) {
            double i = c1.im;
            c1.im = c2.im;
            c2.im = i;
            i = c1.re;
            c1.re = c2.re;
            c2.re = i;
        }
    }
```

B.1.1 Determination of the FFT Transform

To determine the fast Fourier transform of a function represented by 512 samples, we can use the following program code written in Java:

```
class FFT {
    //the number of samples of the function to be transformed
    //(a multiple of 2)
    final public static int number_of_samples=512;
    //the number of bits needed to code the number of samples
    //in natural binary code
    final public static int bits = 9;
    //samples of the complex function
    private Complex [] s = new Complex[512];

    public FFT(Complex [] s) {
        this.number_of_samples = s.length;
        this.s = s;
    }

    public Complex [] calcFFT() {
        //samples in the frequency domain
        Complex [] f = new Complex[number_of_samples];
        for (int i=0; i<number_of_samples; i++) {
            f[i] = Complex.complex(s[i]);
        }
```

```
//changing the order of the samples
int jj=1;
for (int i=1; i<=number_of_samples-1; i++) {
  if (i<jj) {
   Complex.swap(f[i-1], f[jj-1]);
  }
  double k = number_of_samples/2;
  while (k<jj) {
   jj = (int)(jj-k);
   k = k/2;
  }
  jj = (int)(jj+k);
}
//the actual FFT algorithm
for (int l=1; l<=bits; l++) {
  int NE = 1;
  for (int i=1; i<=l; i++) NE = 2*NE;
  int NE_half = Math.round(NE/2);
  Complex U = Complex.complex(1.0, 0.0);
  Complex W = Complex.complex(Math.cos(Math.PI/NE_half),
   -Math.sin(Math.PI/NE_half));
  Complex var_complex = Complex.complex();
      for (int j=1; j<=NE_half; j++) {
       for (int i=1; i<=Math.round(number_of_samples/NE); i++) {
         int k1 = j+((i-1)*NE);
         int k2 = k1+NE_half;
         var_complex.re = f[k2-1].re * U.re - f[k2-1].im * U.im;
         var_complex.im = f[k2-1].im * U.re + f[k2-1].re * U.im;
         f[k2-1].re = f[k1-1].re - var_complex.re;
         f[k2-1].im = f[k1-1].im - var_complex.im;
         f[k1-1].re = f[k1-1].re + var_complex.re;
         f[k1-1].im = f[k1-1].im + var_complex.im;
       }
       var_complex.set(U);
       U.re = var_complex.re * W.re - var_complex.im * W.im;
       U.im = var_complex.re * W.im + var_complex.im * W.re;
      }
    }
    return f;
  }
}
```

B.1.2 Determination of the Inverse IFFT Fourier Transform

To determine the inverse fast Fourier transform of a function in the frequency domain represented by 512 samples, we can use the following program code written in Java:

```
class IFFT {
    //the number of samples of the function to be transformed
    //(a multiple of 2)
    final public static int number_of_samples=512;
    //the number of bits needed to code the number of samples
    //in natural binary code
    final public static int bits = 9;
    //samples of the complex function in the frequency domain
    private Complex [] f = new Complex[512];

    public IFFT(Complex [] f) {
      this.f = f;
      number_of_samples = f.length;
    }

    public Complex [] calcIFFT() {
      //samples of the complex function
      Complex [] sf = new Complex[number_of_samples];

       for (int i = 0; i < number_of_samples; i++) {
          sf[i] = Complex.complex(f[i]);
       }

       // changing the order of the samples
       int jj = 1;
       for (int i = 1; i <= number_of_samples - 1; i++) {
          if (i < jj) {
            Complex.swap(sf[i - 1], sf[jj - 1]);
          }
          double k = number_of_samples / 2;
          while (k < jj) {
            jj = (int) (jj - k);
            k = k / 2;
          }
          jj = (int) (jj + k);
       }
       // the actual FFT algorithm
       for (int l = 1; l <= bits; l++) {
          int NE = 1;
```

```
            for (int i = 1; i <= l; i++)
             NE = 2 * NE;
            int NE_half = Math.round(NE / 2);
            Complex U = Complex.complex(1.0, 0.0);
            Complex W = Complex.complex(Math.cos(Math.PI / NE_half),
             Math.sin(Math.PI / NE_half));
            Complex var_complex = Complex.complex();
            for (int j = 1; j <= NE_half; j++) {
             for (int i = 1; i <= Math.round(number_of_samples / NE); i++) {
                int k1 = j + ((i - 1) * NE);
                int k2 = k1 + NE_half;
                var_complex.re = sf[k2 - 1].re * U.re - sf[k2 - 1].im* U.im;
                var_complex.im = sf[k2 - 1].im * U.re + sf[k2 - 1].re* U.im;
                sf[k2 - 1].re = sf[k1 - 1].re - var_complex.re;
                sf[k2 - 1].im = sf[k1 - 1].im - var_complex.im;
                sf[k1 - 1].re = sf[k1 - 1].re + var_complex.re;
                sf[k1 - 1].im = sf[k1 - 1].im + var_complex.im;
             }
             var_complex.set(U);
             U.re = var_complex.re * W.re - var_complex.im * W.im;
             U.im = var_complex.re * W.re + var_complex.im * W.re;
            }
        }
        //obtaining the IFFT by scaling
        for (int i = 0; i < number_of_samples; i++) {
           sf[i].re = sf[i].re / number_of_samples;
           sf[i].im = sf[i].im / number_of_samples;
        }
        return sf;
    }
}
```

B.2 Generation of Normally Distributed Pseudo-random Numbers

For a normal distribution with parameters $(x_{av}, \sigma^2) = (3, 0.025)$, we can obtain a random variable x of type real using the following Java code:

```
public class Rand_normal {
    public static void main(String [] args) {
        final double sigma = 0.025;
        final double x_av = 3.0;

        double sum = 0.0;

        for (int i=0; i<12; i++)
            sum = sum + Math.random();
        sum = sum + x_av;

        double x = (sum-6)*sigma;
    }
}
```

Index